UNSHRINKING PSYCHOSIS

Understanding and Healing the Wounded Soul

John Watkins

MICHELLE ANDERSON PUBLISHING
MELBOURNE

First published in Australia 2010
by Michelle Anderson Publishing Pty Ltd
P O Box 6032 Chapel Street North
South Yarra 3141, Melbourne, Australia
Tel: 61 3 9826 9028
Fax: 61 3 9826 8552
Email: mapubl@bigpond.net.au
Website: www.michelleandersonpublishing.com

© Copyright: John Watkins 2010
Reprinted 2011
Cover design: Chameleon Print Design
Typeset by: Midland Typesetters, Australia
Printed by: Toppan Security Printing Pte. Ltd.

National Library of Australia cataloguing-in-publication entry

Author:	Watkins, John, 1951-
Title:	Unshrinking psychosis : understanding and healing the wounded soul / John Watkins.
ISBN:	9780855724009 (pbk.)
Notes:	Includes index.
Subjects:	Psychoses—Patients—Rehabilitation. Psychoses—Treatment.
Dewey Number:	616.89

To one degree or another this applies to all of us, for madness is everyone's concern: If you have a mind, it can go mad.

– Edward Podvoll

CONTENTS

Introduction

To many people psychosis means "madness" and "insanity", words which conjure primal images of deeply flawed human beings who, having lost touch with reality, are prone to incoherent raving and unpredictable swings from sullen withdrawal to irrational violence. While advent of contemporary medical conceptions of a treatable "psychotic illness" have muted these fearful impressions somewhat, the spectre of lunatic asylums, strait-jackets and padded cells lingers subconsciously. Even the most enlightened tend to see afflicted individuals as requiring long-term treatment with "anti-psychotic" medications to counter their enduring susceptibility to mental chaos and bizarre irrationality.

But consider this. While defining it as a state of "mental derangement" the Oxford Dictionary explains that psychosis is derived from an Ancient Greek term meaning "I give soul or life to". How could such seemingly irreconcilable meanings be linked to the same word? Interestingly, the word psychiatry itself literally means "healing of the soul". Could contemporary views of psychosis as a biologically-based mental disease have lost sight of notions once considered essential to a correct understanding of this most enigmatic human phenomenon? Consider the following vignettes from cases discussed in this book:

"I was suddenly confronted with an overwhelming conviction I had discovered the secrets of the universe, which were being rapidly made plain with incredible lucidity. The truths discovered seemed to be known immediately and directly, with absolute certainty. I had no sense of doubt or of the possibility of doubt."

"I became interested in a wide assortment of people, events, places, and ideas which normally would make no impression on me. Completely unrelated events became intricately connected in my mind. I had very little ability to sort the relevant from the irrelevant. I felt there was some overwhelming significance in all this, produced either by God or Satan, and I felt that I was duty-bound to ponder on each of these new interests. By the time I was admitted to hospital I had reached a stage of 'wakefulness' when the brilliance of light on a window sill or the colour of blue in the sky would be so important it could make me cry."

"Even worse than the demonic transformations of the outer world were the alterations that I perceived in my inner being. Every exertion of my will, every attempt to put an end to the disintegration of the outer world and the dissolution of my ego, seemed to be a wasted effort. A demon had invaded my body, mind, and soul. I jumped up and screamed, trying to free myself from him, but then sank down helpless on the sofa. I was taken to another world, another place, another time. My body seemed to be without sensation, lifeless, and strange."

"The trees took on a magnificent appearance. He recognised the work of the supernatural and thought the dawn of creation had come. He studied the formation of the clouds and the sky took on for him an appearance wonderful beyond expression. He heard an infinite voice say that six o'clock was the appointed time for the arrival of God's decrees. He visualised himself as passing from an earthly to a spiritual life. At one time he felt a light within him as though he had touched the Holy Grail."

"I was plunged into the horror of a world catastrophe. I was caught up in a cataclysm and totally dislocated. The earth had been devastated by atomic bombs and most of its inhabitants killed. Only a few people had escaped."

"The hallucinations just kept coming and coming. There were mostly big spider-webs, and sometimes spiders would fall off and crawl around on my body. Then there were grinning faces that would melt and turn into other faces, like demons in a horror movie. I felt I was being punished for the sins of humanity. When my friends tried to comfort me, I was sure they were all laughing at me because they gave me poison and planned to kill me, but only after they tortured me for a while first."

"He was convinced his next-door neighbour was using sophisticated electronic equipment linked to satellites to manipulate his thoughts and mood. He believed the voices he heard were those of renegade government spies plotting with his neighbour against him. He also felt his neighbour was making him sick by pumping toxic gas through a pipe he secretly constructed under the house."

"While writing my 'new Bible' I held internal conversations with the 'spirits' of eminent thinkers including Freud, Jung, Buddha and

Christ. I talked with them about the design of a new society that would herald a return to tribal living and I recorded the 'messages' I obtained from each of them. When I finally realised my friends and family members did not share my messianic vision I felt totally lost and confused and began to consider the possibility of committing suicide. The image of my skeleton spontaneously appeared to me on several sleepless nights. During the height of these difficulties I suddenly heard a voice say, 'Become a healer'. I was startled."

"Both the Devil and God were speaking in her ear constantly, in conflict, and especially God's voice was always hilariously funny, cracking jokes and laughing. She felt a cosmic struggle was going on. The Devil was hatching a plot to destroy the world by an explosion of radioactive substances that he was experimenting with. Opposing him was Christ, who was struggling against him to save the world. Each had followers, thus dividing the world into two camps."

According to protocols of conventional psychiatry these people would all be diagnosed as suffering from a psychotic disorder of one kind or another. Furthermore, it would likely be assumed their highly disparate experiences were consequence of a brain malfunction. In line with this interpretation these intriguing experiences and beliefs are merely the bizarre "symptoms" (all carefully catalogued in diagnostic manuals) of a biological illness devoid of personal meaning or significance.

But what is really happening to people undergoing remarkable experiences such as these? Are they all simply tragic victims of a reality-distorting mental illness – or is there more to it? Can the one-size-fits-all "chemical imbalance" hypothesis currently in vogue adequately account for the kaleidoscopic variability of psychotic phenomena, which can encompass terrifying, tormenting, and disabling experiences at one extreme, and joyous, enlightening, possibly healing or transformative ones at the other?

In their own way each of these people has entered a different reality, one which in many ways resembles a dream or psychedelic drug "trip". Could the highly individualised "symptoms" of psychosis reflect vital concerns of the person undergoing the episode, as happens in dreams? If so, could dream psychology shed light on the nature of psychotic experience? Can the findings of psychedelic research contribute to our understanding of psychosis? Could some of the profoundly moving experiences that occur during psychotic episodes involve genuine spiritual phenomena? Do emotional wounds sustained in early life contribute to people becoming prone to psychosis? Do inner and outer circumstances surrounding a psychotic episode reveal something about its specific nature and provide clues to what might aid its constructive resolution?

This book is the result of a lifetime of research and reflection on these and related questions. This enterprise has been bedevilled by the fact that we lack a suitable language for the phenomena under consideration. "Psychosis" is a clinical term invariably implying a diseased or pathological condition. Current thinking has been so thoroughly medicalised many now habitually speak of "psychotic illness", oblivious to the powerful subliminal effects of such terminology. (The same is true when "illness" is silent but implied.) Even among those with more humanistic views a crude biomedical model often lurks beneath the surface as a kind of default belief system. Many people, lay and professional, simply assume psychosis has been proven to be an essentially biological disorder or soon will be. Unthinking acceptance of this reductionist view provides a convenient rationale for those wishing to avoid the complex questions psychosis raises. It can also serve as justification for relying exclusively on physical methods of treatment (such as medication) rather than employing a holistic approach that acknowledges the importance of social, psychological, and spiritual influences in causation and treatment.

Although psychosis is often considered the epitome of severe mental disorder, this term actually encompasses a broad range of phenomena, only *some* of which conform to the common notion of "nervous breakdown". Few people today, including most mental health professionals, are aware of the long tradition in psychiatry in which psychosis has been seen not as an illness but as a profound mental/emotional crisis: a state of "dis-ease" rather than a medical disease. In this view an acute psychotic episode is considered to be a crisis that has *happened* in a person's life rather than a mental illness they have *got*. Such crises may hold the potential for positive as well as negative consequences.

Sensitive analysis reveals a "method in the madness" of many psychotic crises. To the extent that they are an attempt to solve pressing personal problems and meet urgent emotional needs some may function as a desperate psychological coping strategy. Acute psychotic upheavals sometimes reflect the occurrence of a profound developmental crisis or autonomous self-healing process. And, since some of the most tumultuous episodes are impelled by deep spiritual imperatives, they may appropriately be viewed as potentially transformative psychospiritual crises.

This book begins with a description of experiences and behaviours widely taken to be characteristic symptoms of psychosis and an overview of the psychotic disorders listed in standard diagnostic manuals. Some key assumptions of the conventional psychiatric approach to psychosis are challenged in *Chapter Two*. This is followed by an examination of early life experiences and psychosocial influences that can contribute to development of "psychosis proneness". A comparison of acute psychosis to the normal experience of dreaming is presented in *Chapter Four*, before the notion of psychosis as a psychological or psychospiritual crisis is introduced in *Chapters Five* and *Six*. The increasingly common phenomenon of drug-induced psychosis and intriguing realm of psychedelic experience are considered in detail in *Chapters Seven* and *Eight*.

People exhibiting "psychotic" behaviours could be having radically different inner experiences and undergoing very different personal crises. Many problems befalling such persons and their helpers are a result of widespread failure to distinguish the various kinds of psychotic crises and respond to them in appropriate ways. Guidelines for making such a distinction are outlined in *Chapter Nine*. Since spiritual or allegedly spiritual phenomena occur during many spontaneous or drug-induced psychotic episodes, practical guidelines for differentiating genuine and illusory experiences are provided in *Chapter Ten*.

Drawing on the accumulated wisdom of eminent mental health experts and people with first-hand experience of psychosis, the final two chapters outline ways of responding to psychotic crises that will foster healing and recovery. These practical strategies together constitute a *holistic approach* which treats body, mind, and soul as a unified whole. Some personal reflections on the mental health field are presented in the *Epilogue: Unshrinking Psychosis*. Included here is a discussion of various factors – such as the phenomenon of psychophobia – that impede general acceptance of the concepts and therapeutic strategies advocated in this book.

The mental health field is barely recognisable compared to what it was like a few decades ago. Happily, there have been many improvements in that time, among the most important of which has been the move to providing care in the community rather than in decrepit custodial institutions. Active involvement of service-users and carers in design and delivery of services is a mark of progress inconceivable not so long ago. Commonly prescribed medications have also changed considerably. Though the supposed benefits of so-called "atypical" neuroleptic ("anti-psychotic") drugs have been greatly exaggerated, debilitating side effects that once blighted the lives of numerous psychiatric patients have become less common.

Sadly, this is not a tale of unalloyed progress. Indeed, it is clear the changes that have occurred, important as they are, have not produced the results everyone hoped for. Healing and recovery remain as elusive as ever. Indeed, healing is still rarely mentioned in connection with psychosis. There is now much talk about recovery but little appreciation of what it really is or what is required to bring it about. This unfortunate state of affairs is unlikely to change until there is better understanding of what people are recovering from. This will entail tackling difficult questions: What is psychosis? Why does it occur? How does it affect people (before, during and after the crisis)? While making no claim to be the final word on these complex issues, this book will help anyone sincerely seeking answers to these vital questions.

In-depth study of psychotic experience has led many to conclude that the notion of discrete "mental illnesses", such as "schizophrenia" and "bipolar disorder", is outmoded. Psychosis is a complex phenomenon encompassing a broad spectrum of experiences and possibilities, positive and negative. Appreciating its constructive aspects, as well as those of a potentially detrimental nature, provides the soundest basis for supporting healing and recovery.

Chapter One

Psychosis Defined

Classification is one of the basic devices for bringing order out of chaos. It has been a method used by psychiatrists from the earliest times to attempt to understand the mystery of mental illness.

Karl Menninger[1]

In the minds of many people, lay and professional, psychosis is the embodiment of severe mental illness. In Western societies, at least, those exhibiting behaviours identifying them as victims of this enigmatic disorder have often been feared and reviled, with the result that prolonged incarceration in neglectful custodial institutions was their common fate for centuries. Although significant medical and social advances have occurred in recent times, fear, misunderstanding, and ignorance are still widespread and contribute to the rejection, stigmatisation, and inadequate treatment of those afflicted with "true madness".

Knowledge is the key to changing attitudes and beliefs. During the course of the past century a bewildering variety of different approaches have been employed as part of psychiatry's ongoing effort to understand and classify mental disorders. The most widely used and influential classificatory system currently in use is based on diagnostic criteria devised by the American Psychiatric Association and outlined in the fourth edition of its *Diagnostic and Statistical Manual of Mental Disorders*, commonly known as *DSM-IV*.[2] Most psychiatrists now follow the guidelines set out in this manual. Since it is regarded by many as the ultimate authority on diagnostic issues this ubiquitous handbook is sometimes known colloquially as "the psychiatrist's bible". Understanding some of the key technical terms and diagnostic labels routinely employed by mental health clinicians in the process of assessing, diagnosing, and treating psychotic disorders is a useful first step in reducing the apprehension and helplessness so often associated with these puzzling conditions.

1

Signs and Symptoms of Psychosis

The psychiatric term "psychosis" is applied to states of mental disturbance or disorder in which there is a profound alteration in ordinary patterns of thinking, feeling, perception, and behaviour such that, for a time at least, the affected individual is considered to be "out of touch with reality" to a greater or lesser degree. While psychotic disorders are classified into various types according to their specific characteristics, most will involve several or all of the following features at some stage:

- Delusions: fixed false beliefs, i.e. unshakable convictions not shared by others
- Hallucinations: unshared sensory experiences involving any of the five senses, most commonly auditory (e.g. hearing "voices") and visual ("seeing things")
- Thought disorder: markedly illogical or highly idiosyncratic patterns of thinking
- Emotional disturbances: e.g. excessive or inappropriate feelings, lack of emotions
- Behavioural disturbances: e.g. grossly disorganised behaviour, hyperactivity, social and/or emotional withdrawal, loss of motivation, bizarre or inappropriate behaviour
- Significantly reduced ability to perform usual daily activities such as self-care, work, school/study, domestic duties, household chores (e.g. shopping, cooking, cleaning)
- Difficulty communicating and initiating or sustaining inter-personal relations

As well as occurring in an almost limitless variety of combinations the various symptoms that characterise psychosis can vary significantly in intensity. Thus, false beliefs might be held relatively loosely in some instances (so-called "over-valued ideas"), or with absolute conviction in others ("delusions"). For example, a person is said to be experiencing "ideas of reference" if they suspect that random events in the external environment (e.g. radio or television commentary, newspaper headlines) could be referring specifically to them. On the other hand, a person who has become totally *convinced* that this is happening is likely to be diagnosed as having "delusions of reference".

2

In a similar way, some hallucinatory experiences are vague and unclear while others may be quite vivid and seem absolutely real (thus one person told his psychiatrist, "The voices I hear are as real to me as yours"). As with intensity, symptom duration can also vary greatly, ranging anywhere from a few hours or days to much longer periods in the order of weeks, months, or years.

People experiencing psychosis are often said to have impaired "reality testing". This refers to an individual's ability to differentiate experiences that are purely subjective (inner or unshared) such as hallucinations, from those that belong to objective (consensual or shared) reality.* Such impairment is often temporary and, except in very severe cases, is always only partial. Thus, even if they are experiencing florid psychotic symptoms, people rarely lose the ability to perform ordinary tasks, e.g. holding a conversation, going to the shops, catching a bus, all of which require a highly developed ability to correctly assess and interact with the outer world of everyday reality.

"Insight" is a complex concept with a number of possible meanings. In psychiatry this term generally refers to the extent to which a person realises he or she has a mental disorder. In this sense insight may be considered complete, partial, or absent. A psychotic individual is likely to be described as "lacking insight" if they do not realise the unusual experiences they are having are directly attributable to their disturbance and that others do not share them. While those in the throes of florid psychosis generally lack an awareness of its purely subjective nature, most will acquire at least some degree of insight as the intensity of the episode diminishes. It is worth noting, however, that symptoms may continue even if insight into their illusory nature is present. For example, a person may have sufficient insight to say "I know the voices I'm hearing are auditory hallucinations", but continue to hear them. Psychotherapy aims to foster a deeper level of insight,

---

* In order to determine whether a given individual is "out of touch with reality" it is, of course, necessary to define what a *correct* perception of reality would amount to. Strictly speaking, this task involves daunting philosophical questions and an appreciation of various often quite subtle cultural and religious influences. In practice, mental health clinicians often sidestep these complex issues and simply assume that "reality" is the shared, tacitly agreed-upon reality of everyday experience (also referred to as "consensual" reality). As will become clear later, the fact that human beings can experience various altered states of consciousness (ASCs) in which perceptions of self and the outer world are radically altered demonstrates the highly subjective nature of all conceptions of "reality".

e.g. into the psychological and emotional factors which may have contributed to the development of symptoms in the first place.

The terms "acute" and "chronic" are often used in reference to psychotic disorders. These terms provide clinicians with a convenient short-hand means of describing in a very general way the course of a disorder and its symptoms. Although no precise time frame is specified, "acute" generally indicates that the disorder and/or symptoms in question had a rapid onset and are expected to have a relatively short duration. Thus, an "acute psychotic episode" is one in which the symptoms began fairly abruptly, quickly reached a peak, and started to diminish in intensity relatively soon after onset. The term "chronic", by contrast, generally implies a disorder and/or symptoms which are long-standing. Some "chronic" conditions involve a very gradual or insidious onset of symptoms (over months or years), unlike the rapid onset (over hours, days, or weeks) which characterises acute conditions. It should be noted that neither term indicates anything about the *severity* of a disorder or its associated symptoms. Thus, while symptoms of a chronic disorder tend to persist over a prolonged period they may in fact be relatively mild. For example, some people diagnosed with "chronic" schizophrenia may hear "voices" (auditory hallucinations) for years on end but at such a low level of intensity they are easily ignored.

Mental health clinicians tend to suspect a psychotic disorder has a predominantly physical cause if the following symptoms are prominent: confusion, memory impairment, disorientation (affected individual is uncertain of the time, date, or where they are), and *non-auditory* hallucinations, e.g. seeing or smelling things, unusual physical sensations. (The *DSM-IV* states that "nine out of ten non-auditory hallucinations are the product of a Substance-Induced Psychotic Disorder or a Psychotic Disorder Due to a General Medical Condition".[3]) Psychoses in which physical factors have played a primary causal role are sometimes referred to as "organic" while those without a physical cause have traditionally been classed as "functional". For practical purposes "organic" and "functional" disorders might be thought of as occupying opposite ends of a continuum. Many cases are actually likely to involve a complex combination of physical and non-physical causal influences such that it is often difficult to determine the relative importance of each.

Types of Psychotic Disorder

The specific psychiatric diagnosis a person receives will be based to a large extent on their highly individual pattern of presenting symptoms. Information regarding the person's past experiences and behaviour, both recent and more distant, will also be taken into account, e.g. how long particular symptoms have been occurring, whether they began gradually or suddenly, whether similar symptoms have occurred previously, whether or not the person has been exposed to influences that may have "triggered" the episode (e.g. substance use, excessive stress, physical illness or injury affecting brain functioning).

In accordance with *DSM-IV* criteria, mainstream psychiatry currently recognises a range of different psychotic disorders, among the most commonly diagnosed of which are the following:

Brief Psychotic Disorder
A psychotic disturbance characterised by delusions, hallucinations, disorganised speech, or grossly abnormal behaviour that lasts at least one day but less than a month. In some instances the episode is very brief, e.g. a few days. The onset of symptoms may be quite sudden and often occurs in response to a highly stressful event or situation such as loss of a loved one or severe psychological trauma. Episodes of this kind were formerly referred to as a "Brief Reactive Psychosis" to emphasise the fact that they were understood to be a *reaction* to some psychologically overwhelming event or situation. The affected person typically experiences extreme emotional turmoil and confusion and may be prone to rapid, intense mood swings. While the ability to function may be severely compromised during the episode, psychoses of this type are invariably transient and such impairment is always temporary. Complete recovery with full return to the person's usual level of psychosocial functioning occurs within one month. For this diagnosis to apply it must be ascertained that the disturbance is *not* due to the effects of a substance (e.g. illicit drug, medication, toxin) or medical condition affecting the brain.

Substance-Induced Psychotic Disorder
In this disorder, often referred to simply as "drug-induced psychosis", symptoms occur as a direct consequence of exposure to a drug – whether illicit or prescribed – or some other toxic chemical substance.

Many drugs can induce psychotic symptoms during states of *intoxication*. These include common illicit drugs such as cannabis, amphetamines, cocaine and hallucinogens (psychedelics) as well as alcohol and inhalants (e.g. petrol, glue). Some prescription medications such as sedatives, anxiolytic (anxiety-reducing) and hypnotic (sleep-inducing) drugs could have this effect. Psychosis can occur during *withdrawal* from drugs like alcohol, sedatives, hypnotics, and anxiolytics. Chemicals known to be capable of inducing psychotic symptoms include carbon monoxide, carbon dioxide, heavy metals (e.g. mercury), and volatile organic solvents (e.g. in glues and paints). *Note: drug-induced psychoses are discussed in detail in Chapters Seven and Eight.*

Psychotic Disorder Due to a General Medical Condition
A mental disorder in which the psychotic symptoms are directly related to disturbances of brain functioning due to physical illness or injury. Sometimes referred to as an "organic" psychosis. A broad variety of medical conditions can give rise to psychotic symptoms. These include head trauma involving injuries that directly affect the brain, central nervous system infections (e.g. AIDS, neurosyphilis), brain tumours, epilepsy (especially temporal lobe), endocrine imbalances, metabolic disorders, and cerebrovascular disease. Severe and prolonged deficiencies of certain essential nutrients (e.g. vitamin B12) can result in a state of mental and emotional disturbance that may involve psychotic aspects.

Mood Disorder with Psychotic Features
In this disorder psychotic symptoms occur *exclusively* during periods of significant mood disturbance such as depression or elation. For example, a severely depressed person may experience auditory hallucinations in the form of accusatory "voices" or develop fixed erroneous beliefs (delusions) regarding their supposed guilt or worthlessness. Likewise, individuals in the throes of a manic or hypomanic episode (defined below) may develop highly unrealistic or grossly exaggerated beliefs regarding their identity or abilities, i.e. grandiose delusions.

Delusional Disorder
A psychotic disturbance in which a person experiences one or more *non-bizarre* delusions for at least one month in the absence of other

"positive" and "negative" schizophrenia symptoms (as described below). Non-bizarre delusions are defined as beliefs which, while not factually true, could conceivably be true, e.g. believing one is being followed, spied upon, taken advantage of, deceived, poisoned, etc. "Erotomania" involves a conviction that one is loved by another person even if the individual in question denies having such feelings. While auditory and visual hallucinations are not especially conspicuous, tactile (touch) and olfactory (smell) hallucinations may be prominent and occur in connection with the predominant delusional theme, e.g. a man who believes he is being poisoned may perceive unpleasant tastes in food which convince him of the correctness of his belief. The affected person's interpersonal and occupational functioning may be severely impaired, though this is not necessarily the case. Despite having delusional beliefs some people are able to function adequately and their everyday behaviour may not be particularly unusual. The term "circumscribed delusions" refers to erroneous beliefs confined to specific areas of a person's thinking while other areas remain relatively unaffected. For this diagnosis to apply the disturbance must *not* be due to the effects of a substance (e.g. illicit drug) or a medical condition affecting the brain.

Bipolar Disorder
Once known as manic depression, bipolar disorder is a severe mood disorder characterised by recurrent episodes of mania and depression. To receive this diagnosis the person must have had at least one manic episode or one "mixed episode" involving symptoms of both mania and depression. Bipolar disorder can begin with either mania or depression. Manic episodes involve a distinct period of abnormally and persistently elevated, expansive, or irritable mood lasting at least one week (or any duration if hospitalisation is necessary). During a full-blown manic episode the affected person experiences a "high" characterised by emotional euphoria, greatly increased physical and mental energy, grandiose ideas, and impulsiveness. To warrant a diagnosis of bipolar disorder, three or more of the following symptoms must have been present to a significant degree and persisted during the course of the manic episode:

• Hyperactivity (significantly increased goal-directed activity, e.g. work, socialising, sexual behaviour) or psychomotor agitation (restlessness, irritability)

7

- Inflated self-esteem or grandiosity
- Decreased need for sleep
- More talkative than usual or pressure to keep talking ("pressure of speech")
- Flight of ideas or subjective experience of racing thoughts
- Distractability (attention easily drawn to irrelevant external stimuli)
- Excessive involvement in activities with potentially negative consequences (e.g. unrestrained spending sprees, uncharacteristic risk-taking, ill-considered financial undertakings or business ventures, sexual indiscretion or promiscuity)

To qualify as a manic episode the disturbance must have been sufficiently severe to cause marked impairment in occupational, social, or interpersonal functioning. Furthermore, the episode must *not* be a direct result of the effects of substances (e.g. illicit drugs, certain prescription medications) or a general medical condition (e.g. hyperthyroidism).

If a manic episode is severe enough to warrant psychiatric hospitalisation (whether voluntary or involuntary), or it results in significant impairment of the affected person's usual functioning, the disorder is classed as bipolar I. Less severe episodes – referred to as "hypomania" – are classed as bipolar II. Individuals who have had four or more episodes of mania or depression during a twelve-month period are sometimes referred to as "rapid cyclers". People who experience recurrent mood swings less severe than those associated with bipolar II (i.e. mild depression or hypomania) may be diagnosed with *cyclothymia* rather than bipolar disorder.

Schizophrenia
Schizophrenia is classed as a psychotic disorder estimated to affect around 1%–2% of the entire human race. Most authorities now believe that, rather than being a single entity, "schizophrenia" is best understood as a diverse *group* of loosely related conditions sharing an overtly similar pattern of symptoms. By current convention clinical manifestations of schizophrenia are grouped into two broad clusters: so-called "positive" symptoms include those involving an excess or distortion of normal perceptual and thought processes, while so-called

8

"negative" symptoms entail a diminution or loss of normal responses, abilities, or functions.

"Positive" symptoms typically associated with schizophrenia include:

- *Hallucinations*: sensory experiences (seeing, hearing, touching, tasting, smelling) in the absence of an external stimulus. Most often take the form of hearing various kinds of "voices" which may be either pleasant, unpleasant, or a mixture of both
- *Delusions*: fixed false beliefs held with varying degrees of conviction. Commonly involve grandiose, persecutory ("paranoia"), sexual, somatic, or religious themes
- *Formal thought disorder*: irrational, non-linear, or highly circumlocutory thought processes which may be difficult or impossible for others to understand or follow
- *Grossly disorganised or catatonic behaviour*: catatonic behaviour may involve a marked reduction in responsiveness to the outer world – sometimes to an extreme degree (so-called "catatonic stupor"), i.e. complete absence of overt responses to the surrounding environment, mutism (not speaking), and physical immobility

"Negative" symptoms typically associated with schizophrenia include:

- *Blunted or flat affect*: significantly decreased range and intensity of emotional expressiveness manifesting as marked reduction in facial and vocal expression of feelings, e.g. mask-like face, monotonous voice, restricted body language
- *Poverty of thought ("alogia")*: involves an apparent impoverishment of thought processes as inferred from reduction in spontaneous speech, brief and concrete replies to questions, and speech which seems to convey very little information
- *Loss of motivation ("avolition")*: significantly reduced ability to initiate and/or persist in goal-directed tasks; lack of interest in occupational or social activities
- *Inability to experience pleasure ("anhedonia")*: reduced ability to enjoy work, relationships, sex, social and recreational activities (e.g. hobbies, sports)
- *Social isolation and withdrawal*: a tendency toward uncommunic-ativeness and a marked preference for being alone (may actively avoid social interactions)

A person is likely to be given a diagnosis of schizophrenia if their psychotic experiences are characterised by one or more of the following:

- Delusional beliefs which are *bizarre* in nature, i.e. ideas are clearly implausible, have no possible basis in fact, and are not derived from ordinary life experience
- Hallucinations, especially in the form of two or more imaginary "voices" which speak among themselves about the hearer or keep up a running commentary on his or her thoughts, feelings or behaviour ("third person voices")
- Markedly illogical and/or disorganised thought processes (as reflected in speech), e.g. the person's thinking seems to slip off the track ("loose associations"), answers may seem only vaguely related to questions asked ("tangential thinking"), or thought is so disorganised it is impossible for others to understand or follow ("incoherence")
- Severe emotional disturbances, especially inappropriate, blunted, or flattened affect

The duration of symptoms is extremely important as *DSM-IV* defines schizophrenia as a condition in which signs of the disorder have been occurring for a *continuous* period of at least six months. During this six-month period positive and negative symptoms must have been evident a significant amount of time during a one-month period (less if the person has been treated successfully). For a diagnosis of schizophrenia to apply it must also be established that the psychosis is *not* due to drug or alcohol use, physical illness or injury affecting the brain, or a severe mood disorder such as depression or mania.

DSM-IV divides schizophrenia into a number of subtypes according to the specific symptoms most prominent at the time of diagnosis. The distinguishing features of three of the main subtypes are as follows:

Paranoid Type: preoccupation with one or more delusional beliefs (typically persecutory, grandiose or both), or frequent auditory hallucinations (e.g. "voices") the content of which is often related to the predominant delusional themes.

Disorganised Type: markedly disorganised thought, speech and behaviour (e.g. lack of goal orientation); flat or inappropriate affect (e.g. silliness or laughter unrelated to overt speech content).

Delusions and hallucinations, if present, tend to be fragmentary and lack a coherent theme. (This subtype was once referred to as "hebephrenia".)

Catatonic Type: characterised by extremes of psychomotor behaviour, such as immobility or stupor at one extreme, or excessive and apparently purposeless activity at the other. The affected person typically demonstrates highly unusual responses to environmental stimuli, including mutism, negativism (resistance to verbal requests or instructions, maintaining a rigid posture against attempts to be moved), posturing (assuming inappropriate or bizarre postures), grimacing, echolalia (parrot-like repetition of words or phrases just spoken by another person), echopraxia (imitation of movements of another person), and stereotypical movements (repetitive, apparently purposeless, movements or gestures).

DSM-IV acknowledges that it is not uncommon for individuals to have symptoms of more than one schizophrenia subtype and that the assigned subtype could change over time.

Schizoaffective Disorder

This diagnosis is applied to psychotic disorders in which a mood disturbance (depression or mania) occurs at the same time as characteristic schizophrenia symptoms (as described above). For this diagnosis to apply the mood disturbance must be present for a substantial portion of the total duration of the disturbance. Delusions or hallucinations must also have occurred for at least two weeks in the *absence* of elation or depression.

Schizophreniform Disorder

A psychosis characterised by typical schizophrenia symptoms which continues more than one month but less than six months is referred to as a *Schizophreniform Disorder*. This diagnosis could eventually be changed to *Schizophrenia* or *Schizoaffective Disorder* if the symptoms persist for six months, though it is estimated that approximately one in three people experience full recovery within six months and therefore receive *Schizophreniform Disorder* as their final diagnosis.[4] Psychotic disturbances resembling schizophrenia in terms of symptoms but which resolve completely within a relatively short time were once referred to as "good prognosis" or "reactive" schizophrenia.

Researchers have noted that people who experience psychosis in developing countries often recover relatively quickly with the result that *Schizophreniform Disorder* tends to diagnosed more frequently in such societies. (Implications of this intriguing observation are discussed in *Chapter Two*.)

Psychotic Disorder Not Otherwise Specified
DSM-IV requires that this diagnosis be given when the specific criteria for one of the other disorders listed above are not meet. This diagnosis might also be applied when there is inadequate or contradictory information about an individual's symptoms such that it is not possible to confidently assign some other diagnosis. For example, *Psychotic Disorder Not Otherwise Specified* might be diagnosed if it is unclear whether the presenting symptoms are substance-induced or related to a medical condition affecting the brain.

Conclusion

Widespread adoption of the *DSM* system has had the desirable effect of increasing the likelihood that psychiatric clinicians will be able to agree among themselves as to which particular diagnosis a person ought to receive. While this undoubtedly reduces confusion, casual perusal of the preceding information could create the impression that psychiatry has largely succeeded in its effort to correctly identify, precisely define, and appropriately categorise the various psychotic disorders to which human beings are prone. It might be assumed, furthermore, that this achievement has been accompanied by a greatly enhanced understanding of these puzzling conditions and a significantly improved ability to treat them more effectively. Unfortunately, such assumptions would be premature. Indeed, the daily experience of clinicians and the people they treat provides abundant evidence of the fact that conventional approaches to understanding and treating psychosis have significant shortcomings. Some of these are discussed in the next chapter.

Chapter Two

The Myths Of Mental Illness

Much of what is now thought of as mental illness is a mist that will soon be cleared by winds sweeping round the mountain.

David Healy[1]

Recent research has revealed that, of the 170 senior mental health clinicians who helped devise the *DSM-IV* diagnostic criteria, more than half had undisclosed financial ties to the pharmaceutical industry.[2] Among those responsible for developing the criteria for Mood Disorders (which include depression and bipolar disorder) and Schizophrenia and Other Psychotic Disorders, 100% had such ties. The researchers investigating these links noted: "The connections are especially strong in those diagnostic areas where drugs are the first line of treatment". These facts raise concerns about potential conflicts of interest since it is now common policy for regulatory agencies not to approve use of a drug to treat a mental disorder unless the condition in question is listed in the *DSM*. Critics argue that sections of the pharmaceutical industry have deliberately set out to have various types of emotional distress formally recognised as mental disorders by campaigning to have them included in *DSM* in order to ensure a guaranteed world-wide market for their products.[3]

The undue influence of the pharmaceutical industry on contemporary psychiatry is a legitimate cause for concern. Important as this issue is, however, it is by no means the only reason to question practices now widely taken for granted in the mental health field. There are many who feel the entire "symptom and diagnosis" approach is fundamentally flawed. It is noteworthy that some of the strongest critics of the current paradigm (referred to disparagingly as "diagnosis by committee") are eminently qualified, highly-respected mental health experts.[*]

---

[*] While many of the quotations and supporting references in this and subsequent chapters refer specifically to schizophrenia, it is the author's belief that the ideas and concepts discussed are equally applicable to other psychotic disorders – and, in many respects, to human beings generally.

Why Do Diagnoses Change?

It is quite common for people receiving psychiatric treatment to be given a number of different diagnoses over a period of time. There are several possible explanations for this. First, the art of diagnosis remains far from foolproof, despite the advent of comprehensive lists of precisely defined clinical criteria. At its most basic level the diagnostic process is critically reliant on the quality and quantity of information available to the diagnosing clinician. Such information could be inadequate, inaccurate, or both. In some instances it might be inadequate simply because the person being assessed has not been asked for, or been given reasonable opportunity to provide, all the relevant facts. The information upon which a diagnosis is based could also be inaccurate for various reasons. For example, the person undergoing assessment may choose not to disclose certain crucial details, or they may respond to queries in ways that lead to them being misunderstood or misinterpreted. The appropriateness of a given psychiatric diagnosis is thrown into question if it is based on an incomplete or inaccurate account of a person's feelings, experiences, and behaviour and the specific circumstances in which their difficulties arose.

The duration of symptoms is another important consideration. As explained in the preceding chapter, the *DSM-IV* criteria require that certain symptoms must be present for specified periods of time before particular diagnoses can be made. For example, a person who has experienced psychotic symptoms for less than one month when they are assessed could be given a diagnosis of *Brief Psychotic Disorder*. However, if the same symptoms persist for six months the diagnosis might be changed to *Schizophrenia* (assuming various other *DSM-IV* criteria are also met). Since so much depends on how things unfold over an extended period it is relatively common for a person's initial psychiatric diagnosis to be a provisional one.

Subjective judgement plays a more significant role in the diagnostic process than many people realise. One reason for this is that it can be extremely difficult to determine whether or not certain key symptoms are present. For example, "bizarre" delusions are considered one of the hallmarks of schizophrenia, but bizarreness can be difficult to judge, especially if it occurs in relatively mild form. What strikes one examiner as bizarre might not seem especially odd to another.

So-called negative symptoms can also be difficult to assess. At what point does restricted emotional expressiveness become "blunt" or "flat" affect? When does sitting quietly for long periods become "avolition" or not talking much become "alogia" (poverty of thought)? There is no clear boundary between plausible and bizarre, nor is there a clear distinction between a mild degree of reduced motivation (such as might be associated with demoralisation) and a degree which could be considered a psychiatric symptom. Faced with dilemmas such as these the assessing clinician is forced to rely on clinical judgement, thus introducing a degree of subjectivity into the process. As a result, it is conceivable different clinicians could sometimes assign different diagnoses to the same patient.*

The subjective nature of clinical judgement becomes especially relevant in cases involving phenomena that may have spiritual, metaphysical, or supernatural significance – as often occurs in mental states labelled psychotic. Because there are no objective rules for assessing the validity of such experiences the clinician's attitudes and personal beliefs inevitably come into play. In such cases a psychiatrist with a vital interest in spirituality could make a very different assessment of a patient's experiences than would one who happens to be a committed atheist. Whereas the latter may have little inclination to listen to someone who claims to be hearing the "voice of God", the former could be open to the possibility of such experiences having genuine spiritual significance. At the very least, a spiritually aware clinician may be inclined to keep an open mind and hold off on making a formal diagnosis until the picture is clearer. In practice, the highly materialistic paradigm under which contemporary psychiatry operates leads many clinicians to quickly assign pathological labels, e.g. "religious delusions", to experiences that are inherently difficult to assess, let alone understand.

---

* Recent research carried out by forensic psychiatrist Dr Luke Birmingham suggests that even apparently irrelevant factors – such as a person's name – might sometimes influence the diagnosis they receive. The *What's In A Name Study* noted that patients named Wayne or Tracey were more likely to be diagnosed as having a Personality Disorder, while those called Matthew or Fiona were more likely to be diagnosed with Schizophrenia. (Source: "Psychiatrists Dispense a Dose of Prejudice", *The Age*, Melbourne, 6/7/00.)

Are Psychiatric Diagnoses Valid?

As important as the preceding issues are a bigger and in many ways far more significant question can be asked: Does a psychiatric diagnosis reflect the presence, within the person concerned, of a discrete mental illness such as schizophrenia or bipolar disorder? Many people now take this for granted and simply assume the several hundred disorders listed in *DSM-IV* – including various psychotic disorders described in *Chapter One* – are medical illnesses in the same sense as physical conditions like diabetes, cancer, and heart disease. These beliefs, together with the assumption that mental disorders have an essentially biological cause, form the basis of the so-called "medical model" in psychiatry.

Though they are accepted unquestioningly by many people, these notions continue to be the subject of vigorous debate among professionals and others in the mental health field. Open-minded readers may be interested to consider the following propositions since they raise crucial questions regarding the validity of concepts central to contemporary approaches to psychiatric diagnosis and treatment.

(1) *The precisely defined disorders in DSM-IV are artificial constructs. The experiences of real people – perhaps especially of those undergoing profound mental crises – are far too complex to fit into neat diagnostic categories, no matter how sophisticated.*

Experience soon teaches mental health clinicians that "classic" cases of the various mental disorders in *DSM-IV* are rarely encountered in everyday practice. As psychology professor Richard Bentall notes, "Patients do not fall into discrete types of psychiatric disorder as is commonly assumed".[4] In reality, most people will experience only *some* of the symptoms considered to be characteristic of a particular disorder. Furthermore, people often exhibit mixtures of symptoms that are supposedly associated with *different* mental disorders. (The category "Psychotic Disorder Not Otherwise Specified" was created partly in response to such dilemmas.) These clinical facts have been the subject of heated debate in psychiatry for well over a century. At issue is the question of whether distinct psychiatric disorders really exist and if there is a clear dividing line between psychosis and "normality".

16

Exhaustive analysis of historical efforts to classify mental disorders led Professor Bentall to assert that all current psychiatric diagnoses are to a large extent arbitrary and do not reflect the existence of separate illnesses.[5] Although mainstream psychiatry strongly resists their influence, a growing number of mental health experts now share this view.[6]

(2) *It is often assumed that a characteristic, fixed, and predictable pattern of symptoms is associated with a specific psychiatric diagnosis. In fact, the symptoms people experience very often change over time, sometimes to the extent that an entirely different diagnosis – or possibly none at all – might subsequently be warranted.*

Some mental health experts have come to believe that it would be more in keeping with the facts to view mental disorders as complex and dynamic *processes* rather than as fixed and discrete illnesses. In the opinion of psychiatrist Lawrence Kubie, for example, there is no justification for the deeply entrenched practice of assigning psychotic disturbances to separate diagnostic categories:

I affirm the existence of mental illnesses as processes, in spite of the fact that we do not yet know how to differentiate simply and clearly among them or to separate them into distinct clinical entities ... *in psychiatry much of that to which we have given names, which imply they are separate "illnesses", are in fact only transient cross-sections of long and constantly changing processes*, cross-sections which are marked by clusters of symptoms.[7]

These sentiments were echoed in an article in the *British Journal of Psychiatry* in which Professor Luc Ciompi argued it would be more appropriate to view the condition diagnosed as "schizophrenia" as an *open life process* rather than as a medical illness. In Ciompi's opinion, clinical evidence supports the notion that schizophrenia "more closely resembles a life process open to a great variety of influences of all kinds than an illness with a given course".[8] In this view, psychological and social influences play as important a role as biological factors in determining both the kinds of symptoms experienced and the long-term course and outcome of a psychotic disturbance. These suggestions emphasise the dynamic, multi-faceted nature of the states under consideration and are also consistent with the notion of there being no clear division between psychosis and normality.

(3) *There is no clear dividing line between "madness" and sanity.*

Psychiatry's influential pioneers maintained that the hallmark of psychotic disorders like schizophrenia is that the thinking and behaviour of affected individuals is so bizarre and far removed from the realms of ordinary human experience as to be "un-understandable". Though it is still widely accepted, this view has proven erroneous.

Professor John Strauss, an internationally-recognised authority on schizophrenia, was one of the first mainstream psychiatrists to show that, rather being a distinct medical entity, schizophrenia exists on a continuum with normality. Basing his conclusions partly on research he carried out as part of the World Health Organisation's (WHO) International Pilot Study of Schizophrenia, Professor Strauss believes it is more in keeping with what diagnosed individuals experience to view their symptoms – including the hallucinations and delusions considered hallmarks of this disorder – as understandable exaggerations of normal mental functions. Professor Strauss summarised his views in a paper published in the prestigious *Archives of General Psychiatry*:

> This conceptualisation of schizophrenia has often been made on the basis of theoretical principles, but the findings [of this research] give it added support based on the symptomatic experiences described by patients. *This view stresses the notion that schizophrenia and the symptoms that characterise it are understandable exaggerations of normal function and not exotic symptoms superimposed on the personality.* When the distortion and exaggeration of certain normal psychological functions reach a certain level of eccentricity or begin to impair social function they are called symptoms.[9]

Professor Manfred Bleuler's views on this subject are especially noteworthy. The son of Eugen Bleuler, the Swiss psychiatrist who introduced the term "schizophrenia" to psychiatry in 1911, Manfred Bleuler spent his entire professional life as a psychiatrist working alongside people with this diagnosis. Among his many important observations was the following:

> Schizophrenic thinking is a part of every human being's life. It occurs in our everyday functioning as daydreams, dreams, art, fantasy, and fanatic thinking, among other phenomena. In a normal person this type of thinking prevails in a small part of life and is under control;

in a schizophrenic it has become the predominant way of dealing with life and of communicating with oneself and with others.[10]

In Bleuler's view, psychosis simply exaggerates and reveals mental processes and tendencies which were already present:

> Schizophrenic life exists in normal people – sometimes dormant and concealed beneath the surface, but still a part of our personality and constantly helping to shape that personality ... *something is liberated in schizophrenia and in other psychoses as well, that had always been there.* It is released because organisation and the proper guidance have been weakened; nothing is newly created.[11]

The above ideas are consistent with recent research showing that large numbers of "normal", psychologically well-adjusted individuals have experiences which psychiatrists generally regard as symptoms of severe mental illness.[12] Such experiences include various psychotic-like phenomena like hearing voices and entertaining delusional beliefs. Though many people – including many mental health professionals – still consider voice-hearing to be a strictly pathological phenomenon, a considerable body of evidence has challenged this belief. Indeed, numerous surveys have established that large numbers of people in the general population have such experiences on a regular basis.[13] Furthermore, Professor Bentall has pointed out that "the apparently irrational beliefs of other cultures present a challenge to those who seek a clear dividing line between normal and abnormal beliefs".[14]

(4) *The DSM-IV conceptualisation of mental disorders reflects an extremely materialistic, Western view of reality. Phenomena psychiatrists routinely label psychotic are sometimes viewed quite differently in non-Western traditional cultures.*

It is instructive to realise that there are a vast range of different ways in which patterns of behaviour routinely attributed to "mental illness" have been viewed in other cultures, most particularly non-Western ones. Psychiatrist and anthropologist Richard Warner has noted, for example, that many people who would routinely be considered psychotic in modern Western societies are not necessarily viewed this way in the developing world. Indeed, he has demonstrated that throughout the non-industrialised world much typically "psychotic" behaviour is attributed to culturally-acknowledged psychosocial or spiritual causes. When these kinds of folk explanations are used, terms like "mentally ill", "psychotic" or "mad" may never be applied.[15] Professor Warner notes that this has the highly desirable effect of avoiding or at least minimising the stigmatisation and rejection that often accompanies a psychiatric diagnosis in Western society.

It has long been known that people in developing nations who are diagnosed with schizophrenia tend to have a significantly better prognosis and outcome than comparable individuals in modern industrialised societies.[16] Though this unexpected fact is yet to be adequately explained, some believe the relative absence of stigmatising psychiatric labels, together with a generally greater tolerance for aberrant behaviour, has a benign influence which facilitates recovery.

(5) *Social, psychological, and spiritual influences play an extremely important – though rarely acknowledged – role in determining the type of psychosis a person experiences. When such influences are taken into account it becomes clear some psychotic episodes are better understood as profound psychological or psychospiritual crises than as medical illnesses.*

A consequence of psychiatry's effort to adopt a more rigorously scientific approach is that many clinicians now tend to shy away from delving into subjective dimensions which are inherently difficult to define and understand. As a result, essential human phenomena such as feelings, hopes and fears, identity, relationships, spirituality and a host of others of a highly personal nature now tend to be excluded from consideration in favour of biological variables that are easier to quantify. Shift in interest away from inner aspects of psychotic experience has been accompanied by a tendency to over-emphasise the role of biological factors while that of social, psychological, and spiritual influences is systematically under-emphasised – if it is not ignored altogether.

This narrow focus differs markedly from the more holistic outlook of earlier times. Few people now realise there is a long tradition in psychiatry in which psychosis has been viewed not as an illness but as a mental/emotional crisis, i.e. a state of "dis-ease" rather than a medical disease.* In this view an acute psychotic episode is seen as a crisis that *happened* rather than an incurable illness a person has *got*. As Professor John Nemiah explained in the *British Journal of Psychiatry*, such crises are closely linked to the affected individual's total life situation and circumstances:

> When we listen to our patients tell us about their illnesses, they will often, if we allow them to, put their illnesses within the context of their personal lives. It then becomes apparent that the illness has occurred in association with an event in their lives – an event that involves changes in important human relationships. It further becomes evident that the patients undergo a reaction to that event with an internally *experienced* response that sets in motion psychological processes that are intimately related to the emergence and nature of the symptoms of their illness. The key words here are *reaction, response* and *process* … [these facts are] often overlooked and excluded in the practical aspects of our current approach to psychiatric illness.[17]

Carl Jung was one of the first psychiatrists to make an intensive study of psychotic disorders from a psychological perspective. In-depth analysis of numerous cases led him to conclude that many acute psychotic episodes could best be understood as reactions to extreme emotional circumstances:

> That is how mental illness looks from the psychological side. The series of apparently meaningless happenings, the so-called "absurdities", suddenly take on meaning. We understand the method in the madness, and the insane patient becomes more human to us. Here is a person like ourselves, beset by common human problems, no longer merely a cerebral machine thrown out of gear. Hitherto we thought that the insane patient revealed nothing to us by his symptoms except the senseless products of his disordered brain-cells, but that was academic wisdom reeking of the study. When we penetrate into the human secrets of our patients, the madness discloses the system upon which it is based, and we

---

* It is noteworthy that *DSM-I*, the first edition of the American Psychiatric Association's *Diagnostic and Statistical Manual of Mental Disorders* published in 1952, referred to psychotic disorders like schizophrenia and manic depression (bipolar disorder) as *reactions* rather than illnesses.

recognise insanity to be simply an unusual reaction to emotional problems which are in no wise foreign to ourselves.[18]

This view of psychosis (which is explored in detail later in this book) allows for the possibility that long-term dysfunction and disability, so often considered an intrinsic feature of severe "mental illness", might be largely – or entirely – avoidable if the initial crisis can be understood and successfully resolved.

(6) *There is no unequivocal scientific evidence demonstrating a causal link between brain abnormalities and specific psychotic symptoms.*

Though schizophrenia and other psychotic disorders are now routinely attributed to some kind of brain abnormality, e.g. a "chemical imbalance", there is in fact little unequivocal evidence to support this view. Indeed, despite well over a century of intensive research – in recent times involving extremely sophisticated brain imaging and other technologies – attempts to elucidate a purely biological causation of psychosis have proven unsuccessful. As one comprehensive review of current scientific knowledge noted: "Despite a hundred years' research, the neuropathology of schizophrenia remains obscure."[19]

Research aimed at establishing a definitive biological cause for schizophrenia and other psychotic disorders has been bedevilled by the realisation that all promising findings have invariably been shown to occur in only *some* diagnosed individuals but never in all. Furthermore, such findings often prove to be inconsistent (e.g. to be demonstrated in some studies but not others), to vary over time (studies sometimes yield different results when the *same* group of subjects are re-tested later), to only occur in relatively small sub-groups (e.g. severely disabled individuals), or to also be found in individuals who do *not* have a mental disorder – including some members of the "normal" population.[20] Professor Elliot Valenstein's four decades of neuroscientific research led to the following conclusions:

> Contrary to what is often claimed, no biochemical, anatomical, or functional signs have been found that reliably distinguish the brains of mental patients. While several investigators have reported that there is something different about the brains of schizophrenics, for example, other investigators have not been able to verify these

findings. Even in the studies reporting positive results, many schizophrenics do not have the reputed brain "abnormality", while some of the people in the normal "control" group do, even though they have no history of any psychiatric disorder. The evidence of brain abnormalities in other mental disorders is even more tenuous than it is with schizophrenia. Furthermore ... indirect evidence of a biochemical disorder based on the belief that the most effective drugs for each major class of mental disorder produce the same biochemical changes is much less convincing than is usually claimed.[21]

One type of research often said to have proven schizophrenia is a "brain disease" relies on evidence obtained from brain scans of various kinds. While these studies suggest some people with this diagnosis may have a mild degree of cerebral atrophy, the *majority* of diagnosed individuals have been shown to have normal scans.[22] Furthermore, when anomalies such as enlarged cerebral ventricles are studied in brain imaging research, it is found there is never one well-defined group with enlarged cerebral ventricles and another with normal-sized ventricles. Rather, the variations tend to be distributed along a smooth gradient from normal to large.[23] According to one authoritative estimate, only 20%–30% of people diagnosed with schizophrenia show evidence of neurological impairment.[24]

No unequivocal scientific evidence has shown that specific brain abnormalities are *causally* related to major psychotic symptoms like delusions, hallucinations, and thought disorder. In 2003 neuropsychologist Professor Christopher Frith and psychiatrist Professor Eve Johnstone, both world-renowned schizophrenia researchers, summarised this state of affairs as follows:

> Many studies have tried to find relationship between symptoms ... and the structural brain changes, but, on the whole, consistent findings have not been shown. The most robust results suggest that patients with enlarged ventricles are more likely to have general cognitive impairments and movement disorders.[25]

It is important to remember that even if scientific research *were* to show that the brains of people who experience psychosis differ from those of non-psychotic individuals, this would not necessarily mean such differences are the principal *cause* of psychosis. It is feasible that subtle differences in brain structure or function might constitute non-specific risk factors for psychosis rather than being its primary cause. For example, peculiarities in brain function (such as autonomic nervous system hypersensitivity) could render certain individuals more susceptible to the impact of stress and consequently more vulnerable to being overwhelmed by it.[26] It is known that high levels of stress can stimulate increased production of dopamine in brain areas such as the prefrontal cortex which are believed to be associated with schizophrenia and other psychotic disorders.[27] Interestingly, it is also known that the therapeutic action of neuroleptic ("anti-psychotic") medications is related to their ability to reduce activity of this key neurotransmitter in specific brain areas.

While efforts to elucidate the biological aspects continue apace it is important to consider the possibility that if brain changes of some kind were found to be inextricably linked to psychosis, they could be an *effect* of these extreme mental states rather than their primary cause. This notion raises a proverbial chicken-and-egg question which is yet to be satisfactorily answered.

The now well-accepted phenomenon of *neuroplasticity* is highly relevant to this issue. Neuroscientists now know that, far from being an inert mass of tissue, the structure and biochemical activity of the human brain can change substantially in response to inner and outer stimulation of various kinds.[28] Psychiatrist John Nelson summarises this notion as follows:

> Mind and brain operate as a *unitary system* in which changes in one go hand in hand with changes in the other. Within such a unity, cause-and-effect relationships blur beyond distinction, and the best we can say is that any force that changes either brain or mind also changes the other ... Although it is easier to demonstrate that physically altering the brain changes subjective experience, there is mounting evidence that mental events also leave their imprints within the brain. The old view that a computer-like brain's hardwiring is fixed at birth, or even at maturity, is now passé. Neuroscience has demonstrated again and again that life experience is at least as powerful as genetic programming in shaping both the cellular architecture and chemical activity of the brain. In other words, *plasticity* is a fact of brain functioning, even at the relatively coarse level of the cell and synapse.[29]

Researchers intent on unravelling the mysteries of psychosis will doubtless make many important discoveries in coming years. Any such discoveries must not be allowed to overshadow a fundamental but frequently forgotten fact: human beings live in the world of experiences, not in the world of their brain chemistry. Whatever the biological aspects may turn out to be, to the person undergoing it an acute psychotic episode is a profound psychological, social, and emotional *experience* which must be understood and responded to as such.

The Biomedical Status Quo: "Mindless Psychiatry"

In recent years phrases such as "genetic predisposition" and "chemical imbalance" have gradually found their way into common use and are now uttered with nonchalant ease by lay-person and professional alike. So familiar have such expressions become in the mental health field that they are now widely assumed to be statements of fact and only rarely seen for what they actually are: grossly oversimplified shorthand for complex and scientifically unproven hypotheses.

Despite a continuing lack of firm scientific evidence it is now widely accepted that the enormously diverse range of disorders referred to collectively as "mental illness" are diseases that specifically impair normal brain functioning. Partly because they entail such extreme and unusual patterns of behaviour, psychotic disorders in particular have come to be seen as "biologically driven craziness". Within the domain of mainstream psychiatry terms like "psychotic reaction" or even "psychotic disorder" have largely been replaced by "psychotic *illness*". The latter more medical terminology is unquestioningly accepted by mental health professionals of all disciplines – including many, such as social workers, who do not have a medical background – as well as by many psychiatric patients and their relatives. Although most psychiatrists know the psychotic disorders listed in diagnostic manuals cannot be sharply distinguished one from another and are separated by vague and imprecise boundaries, for a variety of complex reasons many remain firmly committed to the concept of discrete mental illnesses with a definite – if yet undiscovered – biological cause.

The firmly entrenched hegemony of biological psychiatry has resulted in a drastic narrowing of attention and attendant neglect of relevant psychosocial factors. Though the term "schizophrenia" is properly understood to encompass a diverse *group* of conditions which are certain to involve different causative factors, a remarkably uniform approach now prevails. Thus, in everyday clinical practice, some kind of brain abnormality is often simply *assumed* to be the underlying cause of every psychotic episode. This assumption justifies the standard routine, often beginning as soon as a diagnosis is made, of relying on "anti-psychotic" medications as the primary – if not the only – form of active treatment. Psychiatrist Colin Ross is not alone in lamenting this ubiquitous trend:

> Globally in psychiatry, I think, we have become sloppy clinicians in our study of schizophrenia because of the biological model of the illness. The tendency now is away from spending any amount of time talking with the schizophrenic patient in an attempt to understand his or her *mind*. Once we check off a few symptoms, make the diagnosis, and start medication, detailed study of the psychosis becomes clinically irrelevant, in much of daily practice. One monitors the patient only carefully enough to track treatment response, which is usually not very carefully. There is no reason to try to understand the patient's mind in detail, as there is in a long-term psychotherapy case, because the symptoms are just biologically driven craziness that needs to be suppressed with medication.[30]

Similar remarks could be made about the way the other psychotic disorders – and indeed most "mental illnesses" – now tend to be treated.

The Need for a New Paradigm

Some observers have gone even further than simply criticising mainstream psychiatry's narrow biological focus and suggested that the entire conceptualisation of psychosis as a medical "illness" ought to be abandoned and a more holistic approach adopted. One of the earliest proponents of this view was Anton Boisen, a psychologist and minister of religion who, after experiencing and recovering from several severe psychotic episodes, went on to found the clincial pastoral education movement in the USA. (Boisen's experiences and seminal ideas are discussed in detail later in this book.) Though the following remarks were made long before the advent of modern psychiatric classification of mental disorders, they are as relevant now as they were when Boisen made them:

The prevailing classification has been made on a descriptive basis and not on the basis of the significant dynamic factors. It is therefore subject to much confusion as one goes from one group of diagnosticians to another. The descriptive groupings are not without significance but we would probably be better off if our psychiatric staffs would stop giving so much attention to a meaningless classification and more attention to the attempt to understand the real meaning of the experiences with which they are dealing.[31]

Although most contemporary psychiatric practitioners accept the claim that major psychotic disorders are biologically-based "mental illnesses", a growing number of mental health experts have come to hold views similar to those of Boisen. Professor Luc Ciompi, an internationally-renowned authority on schizophrenia, questioned the biomedical status quo in an article published in the *British Journal of Psychiatry* under the provocative title "Is There Really a Schizophrenia?" After pointing out that "It is still doubtful whether the concept of a disease entity of schizophrenia is a correct one", Professor Ciompi urged that an "alternative formulation" should be tried.[32] Similar statements could be made regarding other psychoses – including bipolar, schizophreniform, and schizoaffective disorders – as evidence of their purely biological status is similarly unconvincing.

Psychologist Richard Bentall has long been one of the most articulate proponents of a radically new approach to understanding and treating psychosis. Instead of focussing narrowly on diagnostic categories, Professor Bentall believes it would be more beneficial to look beyond the symptoms in an effort to gain a better understanding of what diagnosed people actually experience. As well as getting closer to the lived experience of psychosis, Professor Bentall feels this approach would remove the need for stigmatising labels:

> The fundamental principle guiding this approach can be simply stated as follows: *We should abandon psychiatric diagnoses altogether and instead try to explain and understand the actual experiences and behaviours of psychotic people.* By such experiences and behaviours I mean the kinds of things that psychiatrists describe as *symptoms*, but which might be better labelled *complaints*, such as hallucinations, delusions, and disordered speech ... once these complaints have been explained, there is no ghostly disease remaining that also requires explanation. Complaints are all there is.[33]

In the following chapters an attempt is made to follow the recommendations of these luminaries. This challenging task commences with an examination of some of the constitutional and developmental influences which might contribute to a person becoming prone to psychosis at some time in their life. Studying these antecedent factors has the added benefit of providing invaluable insights into the nature of psychotic experience.

Chapter Three

The Roots of Psychosis

The older clinicians paid great attention to the psychological precursors of insanity, just as the lay public still does, following a true instinct.

Carl Jung[1]

A basic premise of this book is that psychosis is a singular variety of human experience originating in a complex interplay of social, psychological, spiritual and biological factors. The interaction of these, in varying combinations during the different ages and stages of a person's life, may result in the development of a high level of "psychosis proneness" in certain individuals. Furthermore, far from being a totally aberrant phenomenon that strikes "out of the blue", an acute psychotic episode often represents a dramatic crisis point in a course of events that has been gradually unfolding over a considerable period. Carl Jung's observations regarding the psychological precursors of schizophrenia are equally relevant to other psychoses:

> We took up this trail and carefully investigated the previous psychological history whenever possible. Our efforts were richly rewarded, for we found surprisingly often that the illness broke out at a moment of some great emotion which, in its turn, had arisen in a more or less normal manner. We also found that in the [psychosis] which ensued, there were a number of symptoms that could not be understood at all from the anatomical standpoint. These symptoms immediately became comprehensible when considered from the standpoint of the individual's previous history.[2]

As psychiatrist Edward Podvoll has suggested, "Rather than the comforting notion that psychosis is only a rare disease, psychosis may be the natural consequence of the way anyone has lived".[3] Since they are rooted in a host of emotionally significant formative experiences, crises of this kind are invariably rich in personal meaning.

The role of non-biological influences is heavily emphasised in this and subsequent chapters. This emphasis is *not* intended to imply that biological factors play no part in the complex sequences of events that culminate in the upheaval of acute psychosis.* However, biomedical theories of psychosis (and mental disorders generally) are now so predominant in mainstream psychiatry that psychosocial aspects are routinely neglected. The president of the American Psychiatric Association recently acknowledged that "as a profession, we have allowed the biopsychosocial model to become the bio-bio-bio model".[4] Focussing specifically on the relevant social, psychological, and spiritual issues may help redress this unfortunate cultural and professional myopia.

The matters discussed in this chapter are inherently complex and involve feelings, experiences, and concepts that are often subtle and difficult to describe. Since psychosis is such an individual experience it can only be discussed in a general way. Consequently, the situations and behaviours described below will not necessarily be relevant in every case. Furthermore, while rather extreme situations have been described to illustrate important concepts, readers should be aware that far milder scenarios are common.

Exquisite Sensitivity

It is now often claimed that certain people inherit a genetic "predisposition" to psychosis. However, scientific evidence regarding this is actually rather equivocal, as the research of Professors Frith and Johnstone reveals:

> Looking at large samples of schizophrenic patients it is very clear that by no means all have a family history of the condition. This was certainly the case in large studies we have conducted. In the study of all schizophrenic patients discharged from hospitals in Harrow between 1975 and 1985, all relevant case notes were scrutinised for information on family history. A family tree was drawn up for each

---

* Pioneering research by neuroscientist Professor David Horrobin has shown that deficiencies in omega-3 fatty acids (especially EPA and DHA) in brain cell membranes can contribute to poor cognitive functioning, impaired mood regulation, and heightened predisposition to certain types of psychosis. [Horrobin, D. et al (1994) The Membrane Hypothesis Of Schizophrenia. *Schizophrenia Research*, Vol. 13, 195–207.] Research cited in *Chapter Twelve* lends support to the proposition that nutrient deficiencies may play an important – though often neglected – role in the causation and treatment of some forms of psychosis.

patient in consultation with that patient and a relative. *In more than 70% of these cases no family history could be found, and this applied not just to schizophrenia but to psychotic illness generally.* Similarly, in his review Gottesman noted that 89% of patients have parents who are not schizophrenic, 81% have no affected first-degree relatives, and 63% show no family history of the disorder whatsoever.[5]

While researchers have not been able to identify specific genes for schizophrenia, bipolar disorder, or the other major psychoses, genetic factors could nevertheless be one thread woven into the constitutional fabric of some who experience psychosis. However, rather than "causing" the disorder, the principal effect of such genes may be to influence how an individual responds to his or her environment. Professor Joseph Zubin describes this vital – though frequently misunderstood – role of human genes as follows:

> It is well known that genetic endowment does not determine an individual's traits (including the disorders he may develop); rather, the genes determine the responses of body and mind to environmental forces.[6]

While there are no specific "psychosis genes" as such, it is nevertheless possible that genetic factors – in combination with a wide range of non-genetic influences – might contribute to the acquisition of characteristics which profoundly influence an individual's psychological, social, and emotional development. There are a number of ways this could occur.* For example, it has long been noted that individuals diagnosed with schizophrenia are often extremely sensitive. Indeed, a distinguishing characteristic of many such persons is that they seem to be endowed with an *exquisitely sensitive nervous system.* From a very early age many possess what could be described as a kind of "hypersensitivity" to sensory and emotional stimulation. This might be partially genetically determined, as suggested in the

---

* Professor Manfred Bleuler has suggested that rather than involving specific genes, hereditary aspects of schizophrenia might involve genetic factors that are not in themselves harmful, but which happen to occur in disharmonious combinations: "The hereditary predisposition might rather consist of a lack of harmony among different inborn dispositions, an incompatibility of certain constellations of genes." Bleuler, M. (1970) Some Results of Research In Schizophrenia. *Behavioural Science*, Vol.15, 211–219. p. 216.

following statement from the highly regarded psychiatric reference, *Comprehensive Textbook of Psychiatry*:

> All schizophrenics are, at least originally, more sensitive than the average person. It is likely that increased sensitivity and heightened responsiveness to sensory and emotional stimulation is present in schizophrenics from an early age, possibly from birth. Schizophrenia may be characterised by a genetic hypersensitivity that leaves the patient vulnerable to an overwhelming onslaught of stimuli from without and within.[7]

It is important to stress that genes are not the only factors which determine innate sensitivity. Indeed, the very fact that a large proportion of diagnosed individuals have no family history of psychosis underscores the importance of *non-genetic* influences.

Growing Up Different

Physical and emotional hypersensitivity may represent one of the major building-blocks in the development of a predisposition ("vulnerability") to schizophrenia and other psychotic disorders. In order to understand how this might occur it is instructive to consider the wide range of ways in which an individual's emotional and social development may be affected by long-standing sensitivity to inner and outer stimuli. As well as influencing the kinds of life experiences a person has, extreme sensitivity can also increase the likelihood they will develop certain psychological characteristics, some of which might contribute to further increasing their sensitivity and subsequent vulnerability to psychosis.

Whatever may have contributed to a person being hypersensitive, the end result is that they will tend to experience many aspects of life with greater intensity than those who are inherently less sensitive. Esso Leete has described what this might be like with respect to both sensory (physical) and interpersonal (social) stimuli:

> For many individuals with a mental illness, we must learn to go through life experiencing our surroundings with a greater intensity than others do. Sounds are louder, lights brighter, colours more vibrant. These stimuli are distracting and confusing for us, and we are unable to filter their impact to lessen their effect. In addition, I believe we are more sensitive in an interpersonal sense as well. I have

noticed that others like myself are easily able to pick up emotional non-verbal cues and feelings that may be "hidden".[8]

Hypersensitivity itself is not necessarily a negative or undesirable characteristic. Studies of young children considered at risk of developing schizophrenia have found that many exhibit a marked degree of "openness" to their environment. These children often engage in highly constructive and imaginative play and appear rather more creative than others of comparable age.[9] This observation helps explain a consistent finding of genetic research – that siblings of diagnosed individuals who do *not* develop a mental disorder frequently display a range of creative abilities and artistic talents.[10] It seems reasonable to conclude that, while innate hypersensitivity might increase a person's risk of eventually developing psychological problems, it may also contribute to their acquisition of *desirable* attributes and abilities.

In an ideal world all hypersensitive children would grow up in environments that nurtured their development by responding appropriately to their distinctive temperamental characteristics. In particular, they would be exposed to appropriate kinds of stimulation at an optimal level of intensity, thus ensuring they were neither over- nor under-stimulated. Most importantly, their social environment would emphasise safe, nurturing relationships which allowed their attributes and abilities to develop in a natural way. Unfortunately, the real world is far from ideal and is not an easy place for highly sensitive individuals of *any* age, let alone young, dependent children. Even with the support and protection of a loving family many are bound to face numerous difficulties in life. Ordinary play with peers or the everyday rough and tumble of the schoolyard or playground could leave exceptionally sensitive children feeling as if they were in a veritable jungle in which "survival of the fittest" is a rule that seems to distinctly favour the thick-skinned and bold.

Experiencing callous or insensitive treatment at the hands of others is sometimes simply a matter of bad luck. It is impossible, after all, to predict or control the behaviour of the numerous people one encounters on an everyday basis such as neighbours, strangers in public places, school teachers, fellow students, and many others. Furthermore, people sometimes act in a negative, perhaps even hostile, manner as a result of their own reaction to subtle qualities they perceive (possibly unconsciously) in a hypersensitive child. One woman has described her experience of such a situation:

> I believe that several incidents during my lifetime occurred because of something "different" about me; perhaps I was physically and emotionally abused because my abusers sensed some vulnerability in my nature. I have learned that some of the basic elements of my illness may have been present since early childhood, in which case the way I related to my family and early acquaintances must have been affected and probably influenced the way other people related to me, even on an unconscious level. If this is true, the confusion I felt about myself was compounded by what seemed irrational or conflicting actions directed toward me. A child destined to become schizophrenic must deal not only with the seeds of illness within himself but also with the attitudes of others toward his "idiosyncrasies", whether these feelings are voiced openly or subtly manifested in everyday life ... the scars of emotional confusion remain, felt perhaps more deeply by a greater sensitivity and vulnerability.[11]

Relationships within the family ordinarily involve greater intimacy and emotional intensity than are generally experienced elsewhere. These conditions may have unforseen effects on young, hypersensitive children.

Early Childhood Experiences

There is no evidence to support the proposition that families are somehow responsible for causing their children to develop mental illness. However, the relationships and emotional atmosphere within any family have a deep and lasting effect on every one of its members and undoubtedly play a crucial role in laying the foundations of the children's subsequent psychological development. In the case of those later diagnosed with psychosis, certain early experiences may have a range of effects no one could have predicted – or even been aware of – at the time.

A child is not born into the world a completely blank slate. Rather, as a result of a combination of genetic and other factors each is born with a unique emotional disposition and repertoire of temperamental characteristics. This fact has important ramifications. In particular, while it is obvious a newborn baby will be profoundly affected by the way it is nurtured by its parents, its *own* behaviours – including subtle characteristics such as how it responds to being touched or picked up and its fluctuating pattern of feeding and sleep habits – will also have a significant effect on its parents. The parents of children who later experience psychosis sometimes say they felt there was something "different" about that particular child from the moment he or she was born. The baby in question may have been unusually quiet and undemanding, e.g. hardly ever crying even when hungry. On the other hand, such babies are sometimes extremely difficult to care for due to their irregular and unpredictable feeding and sleeping patterns, extreme touchiness, or bouts of inconsolable crying or screaming.

It is very difficult for parents and other care-givers to always respond to an infant in adequate and appropriate ways. For a child endowed with a hypersensitive nature even the most well-intentioned actions of others could be magnified or exaggerated until they assume a significance they may not otherwise have had. How can anyone possibly know what is going on within such a child? How can they know what is the "right" thing to do in every situation? In such difficult circumstances some parents find themselves becoming frustrated or exasperated at times. Such feelings, though understandable, could contribute to an emotional climate that has a lasting impact. In particular, a hypersensitive baby may grow into a young child experiencing an intensity of feelings he or she is not emotionally or psychologically equipped to handle.

The occasional periods of disharmony and discord which are a *normal* aspect of family life may provoke emotional responses out of all proportion to the events occurring. In such cases the crucial issue is not how people such as parents or siblings behaved, but what the hypersensitive young child felt and experienced. As Professor Silvano Arieti explains, innate sensitivity could cause children to experience family or other emotionally intense situations in an exaggerated or distorted way:

> The early environment of the child is certainly important and affects the rest of his whole life, including his proclivity to develop schizophrenia. However, this is only part of the picture. Among

the psychological causes of schizophrenia we must include the way the child experienced his environment. An undue sensitivity or a special biological predisposition probably made him react too strongly to some stimuli, especially to unpleasant ones. In addition, we must see how the child's experiences of the environment were assimilated, that is, became parts of his psyche. If the experiences were unduly strong, it is possible that they remained as disturbing components of his psyche and promoters of trouble and unrest ... early childhood is lived intensely by the patient, within family situations that he experiences too strongly and incorrectly.[12]

During the first few years of life a child's innocence and emotional bond with its parents provide effective protection from many potential threats and dangers. However, as a child grows older it can no longer be completely shielded from the harsh realities and demands of everyday life. Ironically, hypersensitivity may cause some children to awaken *prematurely* from the state of innocence that previously protected them. And, for reasons outlined above, a hypersensitive child may have already been emotionally "wounded" as a result of early experiences within the family and elsewhere, even if others always acted with the best intentions.

Highly sensitive children may experience particular difficulty in situations such as the classroom where sitting still and paying attention for extended periods is emphasised. Since they habitually experience both outer and inner stimuli as vivid and intense, such children may find it hard to resist distraction, leading to the accusation of "daydreaming" in class. Ordinary social interactions may be particularly fraught as they require an ability to rapidly process complex verbal and non-verbal information to decipher the meaning of spoken words, facial expressions, bodily gestures, and a host of other signals. Since these wide-open souls are often extremely alert to the subtle nuances and covert meanings in interpersonal behaviour, they may quickly pick up on *hidden* feelings or motives. The fact that people do not always "say what they mean and mean what they say" may become a source of constant confusion and distress which make the demands of the playground and classroom increasingly difficult to cope with. Sadly, those who hesitate, become confused, or fail to act decisively, may be picked on or ridiculed by others – victimisation that only serves to compound their problems.

A growing sense of being "different" may begin to undermine a child's emotional security. Some in this situation may find temporary relief in solitary pursuits – but there is the constant demand from others to mix, make friends, and fit in. Such expectations could exacerbate growing feelings of insecurity and inferiority which in turn provoke even more withdrawal. Lack of friends and playmates may lead a child to feel increasingly lonely, insecure, and odd. Destructive vicious circles of withdrawal and avoidance may develop as the acutely sensitive child becomes only too aware of how he or she is looked upon by others – even if their true feelings are politely disguised by superficial friendliness. *He or she is different and knows it.* Marcia Lovejoy describes the painful ordeal she endured at school:

> My classmates quickly noticed that I was "different" and reacted to me "differently" … my physical abilities lagged far behind those of other children. Simple skills such as balancing in hopscotch, catching a ball, or running into a twirling jump-rope were extremely difficult for me. The more I tried and practiced at home, the more difficulty I experienced. My classmates ridiculed my efforts and I reacted to their rejection by isolating myself from them, knowing that I did not belong. I learned at an early age that I was not like other children, and that I must conceal my difference.[13]

Some highly sensitive children are traumatised by experiences their more resilient peers are able to take in their stride. If this is true of experiences which for most are part of the normal trials and tribulations of growing up, it is not difficult to imagine how deep could be the emotional impact, in early childhood, of such exceptionally distressing events as loss of a parent or other loved one, parental separation, or family breakdown. Beyond such "normal" life events, some children are subjected to various kinds of physical and emotional neglect that has lasting effects. Tragically, some may be victims of deliberate physical, emotional, or sexual abuse.[14] (There is a growing view that trauma and/or abuse in early childhood play a role in predisposing people to psychosis later in life.[15] While there is no doubt this does occur, leading researchers stress that it is not true of every case: "It is clearly important to consider the possible role of trauma in the development and maintenance of distressing psychotic experiences and to ask about it. However, there are multiple paths to psychosis, and while trauma is clearly involved for some people ... there are many others with no history of trauma."[16])*

Even apparently "trivial" incidents could have a significant effect. The cumulative impact of a series of such incidents could profoundly affect critical aspects of a child's emotional and psychological development. A self-perpetuating cycle may be set in train as each traumatising incident further sensitises an already extremely sensitive child. In time some children, having come to *expect* hurt and rejection at every turn, seem to develop a kind of "psychological radar", a hyper-vigilant alertness with which they constantly scan their surroundings for signs of danger.

Personality Development

Early experience plays a major role in shaping the development of the human personality. Professor Arieti believes that, partly as a result of difficulties they experience in early life, hypersensitive children tend to develop one or other of two characteristic personality types (both of which involve traits many people possess in milder form). The so-called *schizoid* personality is marked by emotional aloofness and detachment, attributes which reflect a deeply-ingrained strategy of self-protective social withdrawal and "emotional shut-down". Such defensive strategies may sometimes reach an extreme degree, as psychiatrist Ainslie Meares explains:

> The child is aware of his own sensitivity, and he reacts to it. He uses both outward and inner defences to protect himself. His outward defence is the avoidance of the stimuli which hurt him on account of his sensitivity. He achieves this by withdrawal. He isolates himself, and so avoids the company of others, where he is exposed to psychological hurt. He also develops a complicated inner defence against his sensitivity. This really amounts to an inhibition of his feelings. A state of mind comes about in which things are

---

* Because mental health personnel are often reluctant to inquire about childhood trauma and/or abuse such occurrences tend to be systematically under-recognised, especially among individuals who have experienced psychosis. Failure to acknowledge these tragic facts amounts to denial and serves to perpetuate the culture of silence that has long surrounded this delicate subject. Such denial only does further disservice to those who have already been abused and victimised.

neither good nor bad, things neither please nor hurt. In order to save himself from his sensitivity, a kind of obliteration of all feelings is induced. He cannot be hurt now. It simply does not matter whether they tease him or not. He does not feel it any more ... Both these methods of defence, by isolating himself and by blotting out his feelings, protect him from the hurts of the world.[17]

Social withdrawal and emotional shut-down may provide necessary protection to those whose sensitivity renders them vulnerable to a multitude of hurts. Individuals who develop a schizoid personality may appear to become less sensitive to the world around them but, like a tortoise that retreats into the safety of its shell, deep within their original sensitivity remains, now hidden behind an "armour of detachment". While their emotional shut-down shields them from pain it also curtails their ability to experience *pleasurable* feelings. Indeed, many such individuals report a long-standing inability to derive much enjoyment from life.[18]

An altogether different personality structure may develop which Professor Arieti calls the *stormy* type. Such individuals find other people distressing and tend to respond to them in inconsistent and unpredictable ways, e.g. being compliant and accommodating at certain times, demanding or aggressive at others. A nagging inability to "find" themselves leads some into a series of crises as they search for a role in the world and a stable sense of identity. Some resort to alcohol or drug abuse or indulge in bouts of reckless sensation seeking. Though their inner unrest may be concealed behind a shallow attitude of humour and good spirits, even relatively minor incidents often have the power to precipitate such individuals into intense emotional turmoil. As Arieti asserts, "The life of these persons in general is a series of crises."[19]

As they grow older some hypersensitive children become markedly introverted. The extreme shyness and sensitivity of highly introverted children may make interacting with people outside their immediate family difficult and anxiety-provoking, with the result that some tend to become increasingly emotionally isolated from the world at large. While some of their personality traits make relating with others difficult, the peculiar sensitivity of such individuals often allows them to remain closely attuned to the rich inner world of imagination and fantasy in which they may find great comfort at times.

A "False Self" and "Façade of Normality"

Those who rely on social and emotional withdrawal for self-protection may be noticeably aloof and disengaged from others. Some may even seem almost entirely devoid of human feelings (though this outward appearance often masks a vibrant inner life). Interestingly, schizoid individuals do not always appear cold or distant. This seeming contradiction is a result of the way some people protect themselves from perceived dangers by concealing their real feelings and thoughts behind a "façade of normality" which, whether strong or fragile, thick or thin, may in time become a habitual coping strategy. Some people may even become skilled actors with a sophisticated ability to create and project a socially-acceptable personality, a strategy that allows their inner or "true" self to remain safely hidden from scrutiny while what is displayed to others is merely an outer "false" self that is, by its very nature, less vulnerable to harm.

It is a fact of human life that *everybody* develops a social "mask" which serves to mediate interactions with others while enabling private thoughts and feelings to be safely concealed. (The word "personality" is derived from the Latin *persona*, "an actor's mask".) This natural state of affairs reaches an extreme degree in certain individuals. Psychiatrist John Nelson believes it is especially evident among those whose early lives were blighted by a painful sense of being fundamentally different to others:

> This difference was not celebrated as a tribute to the uniqueness of the individual human spirit, but as a humiliating stigma best concealed from view. In the childhood of such a predisposed person, there often develops an exaggerated need to dissemble, to assume roles that are socially appropriate but do not reflect what he truly feels. Concealed behind this papier-mâché armour is soft flesh of a child for whom the consensual world is untrustworthy, of an adolescent whose raw sensitivity confers an exquisitely felt vulnerability to rejection, of a young adult who sees through the superficiality of others, whom he despises and envies for their social grace.[20]

The erroneous idea that individuals diagnosed with schizophrenia have a "split" personality may originate in an intuitive recognition of the true self/false self dichotomy.* Many with this diagnosis do, indeed, describe having endured a long and painful struggle to find an authentic identity. Mary McGrath said of her situation before being diagnosed: "Sometimes, though, I wonder if I ever knew myself, or merely played the parts that were acceptable, just so I could fit in somewhere ... hoping to find a comfortable position in which to be just me."[21] Another person was described as follows: "The patient has grown up with an intense sense of inferiority ... In her efforts to be found pleasing to her parents, she created a shell identity which others would find acceptable and which shielded her inner world and its insecurities."[22]

While the split into "true" and "false" selves may provide vital protection it could pave the way for a series of events that culminate in a self-perpetuating downward spiral. Since highly schizoid individuals never allow their true self to be touched or even seen, they do not engage at a *feeling* level with other people and the world of everyday reality. In time those whose schizoid withdrawal is extreme may come to experience themselves more and more as purely "mental" beings devoid of physical limits or attachments. With an increasingly tenuous connection to their body some may eventually feel they are not actually "in" it, or even that it is not really their own.

A disembodied onlooker who is always playing a part, always impersonating, may one day realise their secure fortress has turned into a suffocating prison. Even when they are with other people they remain cut off at an emotional level. Their peers may begin to perceive them as awkward or strange – and some may not bother to hide their discomfort and disapproval. Hypersensitivity magnifies the impact of their rejection. Since emotional isolation prevents them from being nourished and enriched by life, schizoid individuals may become increasingly prone to losing themselves in wishful fantasy and make-believe. Some may eventually live more and more in an inner world that continues without being confronted by the demands of reality. Sensing they do not belong and cannot fit in, some attempt to

---

* In the early 1960s renegade British psychiatrist Ronald Laing wrote an exquisitely insightful account of this phenomenon in the first of a series of books in which he summarised the results of his life-long effort "to make madness and the process of going mad comprehensible". See: R.D. Laing (1965) *The Divided Self*, Harmondsworth: Penguin.

create a realm in which they can find a home. A nobody in reality may become anybody in fantasy.

The "No Exit" Situation

Since positive experiences play a crucial role in fostering emotional and social growth, early isolation and aloofness tend to hamper development in these areas. In some cases a young person's confidence and self-esteem are so poor they may simply give up any effort to change or improve the situation. As a result, their social, academic, and occupational achievements may all be seriously compromised, further contributing to what may already be a long-standing pattern of gradual personal decline. Some hypersensitive individuals enter adolescence haunted by unrelenting feelings of emptiness, aloneness and uncertainty about who and what they are. Since social interactions provide the natural setting in which a sense of identity develops, prolonged isolation may result in evolution of a self-image that is both fragile and unstable.

It is no surprise psychosis often first occurs in late adolescence or early adulthood since unresolved personal problems and emotional difficulties are often greatly intensified during these critical periods. High levels of stress and emotional turmoil occur naturally when a young person is faced – often for the first time – with growing pressure to cope with new roles, responsibilities, and challenges. While these demands are difficult enough for any young person, those burdened with a fragile identity and deep feelings of personal inadequacy may feel they are surrounded by insurmountable obstacles.

To add to their difficulties some discover that behaviours they once relied upon are no longer effective or acceptable. The aloofness and detachment of those who coped by developing a "schizoid" personality may start to attract increasing criticism and rejection, while a "stormy" person's emotional intensity and unpredictability may finally exceed the tolerance of peers, employers, and family. In their different ways both personality types may come to feel increasingly like "strangers in a strange land".

Prior to the onset of their first psychotic episode many young people have endured a prolonged period of feeling different, alienated from others, and socially isolated. When they later reflect on this time many say things like, "I never really felt I knew who I was" and "I didn't know what to do with my life". The emotional distress accompanying these dilemmas may not be evident to others since maintaining a façade of "normality" may have long been a full-time occupation. Despite outward appearances, a gnawing sense of anguish may have been steadily growing beneath the surface. While it sometimes seems a psychotic episode has occurred "out of the blue", in fact it is often preceded by a looming psychological crisis centred on a range of vital personal concerns. As psychiatrist Edward Podvoll has put it, "There is almost always a *psychotic predicament*. No one goes crazy without first having arrived at a predicament".[23] Conflicts related to the following issues are often especially relevant to the onset of acute psychosis:

- *Individuation*: A young person endeavouring to establish a stable sense of identity must grapple with a host of complex questions: Who am I? What is life all about? What am I capable of? How should I live? and many more. Developing an acceptable identity inevitably entails much experimentation and periods of great uncertainty. Alcohol and illicit drugs are increasingly likely to play a part in this process (see *Chapter Seven*).
- *Independence*: The task of establishing an identity separate from one's family of origin can be extremely stressful, as can leaving home or school for the first time, entering the workforce, and endeavouring to gain financial and emotional independence. The desire for independence is often accompanied by a great deal of fear and uncertainty. Many are plagued by the question, "Am I strong enough to cope on my own?"
- *Relationships*: Developing intimate emotional and sexual relationships imposes many new demands which can be difficult to deal with, even more so for those burdened with low self-confidence and unresolved conflicts regarding identity and independence. The responsibilities and commitments associated with marriage and parenthood (planned or otherwise) also involve considerable stress.

Acute psychosis often seems to occur at a time when a person has become "stuck" in an intense emotional dilemma they are unable to cope with or escape from.[24] Those trapped in such an impasse experience escalating anxiety and an ever-deepening sense of despair. The straw that finally "breaks the camel's back" and triggers the onset of a psychotic episode often comes in the form of an event or situation which delivers a severe blow to a person's already fragile self-esteem. Common triggers include break-up of an important relationship, feeling rejected by a significant person such as a friend, teacher or employer, or feeling like a total failure as a human being. In the wake of such emotionally traumatic events a person may finally reach a point of feeling completely trapped. Expressions like "There was no way out" or "I had nowhere to turn" describe the claustrophobic feeling of being caught in a "no exit" situation which is impossible to fight or flee. If this sense of entrapment grows and no escape is possible, an intense emotional panic may be evoked that heralds the beginning of a psychotic crisis.

Professor Arieti believes that for many people a critical point is reached when they come to believe not only that their life is bad, but that it will *always* be bad no matter what they might do to improve the situation. Such people may conclude, furthermore, that the reason they are in such a terrible state is that they, themselves, are irredeemably bad and worthless:

> Sooner or later the person ... reaches the conclusion that the future will not redeem the present or the past ... he comes to believe that the future has no hope, that the promise of life will not be fulfilled, and that the future may be even more desolate than the present ... He is excluded from the busy, relentless ways of the world. He does not fit; he is alone. He experiences ultimate loneliness; he becomes unacceptable even to himself ... It is at this point that a state of panic occurs.[25]

It is not difficult to imagine how innate hypersensitivity would greatly increase the intensity of such crises, making all ordinary solutions impossible. A century ago pioneer psychiatrist Carl Jung made these observations about schizophrenia:

> Many cases originate in a psychologically critical period or following a shock or a violent moral conflict ... the psychological predisposition leads to a conflict, and thus by way of a vicious circle to psychosis ... most cases of [schizophrenia] are driven by their congenital predisposition into psychological conflicts, but these conflicts are not essentially pathological, they are common human experiences. *Since the predisposition consists in an abnormal*

sensitiveness, the conflicts differ from normal conflicts only in emotional intensity. Because of their intensity they are out of all proportion to the other mental faculties of the individual. They cannot, therefore, be dealt with in the ordinary way, by means of distraction, reason, and self-control. *It is only the impossibility of getting rid of an overpowering conflict that leads to [psychosis].* Only when the individual realises that he cannot help himself in his difficulties, and that nobody else will help him, is he seized by panic, which arouses in him a chaos of emotions and strange thoughts.[26]

Though Jung was here referring specifically to schizophrenia, similar observations could be made about other types of acute psychosis.

A Strange New World

Intense as they may be, crises such as described above do *not* inevitably lead to psychosis. Sometimes the person in crisis is fortunate enough to receive support of a kind that allows an impending psychotic episode to be averted. Meeting someone on a similar "emotional wavelength" may allow a distressed person to feel they are not totally alone, sparing them what Jung called "the disastrous shock of complete isolation".[27] By ameliorating anxiety and morbid self-concern this kind of timely encounter might arrest a spiralling emotional chain-reaction before it is too late.[*]

Sometimes, however, a point may finally be reached when it is no longer possible to fight a rising tide of churning emotions. Mental and emotional exhaustion may prevent further struggle and an overwrought person may then simply surrender, giving free rein to whatever feelings, ideas, or images happen to appear. Letting go in this way might even provide blessed relief from the long battle to remain in control of an increasingly turbulent inner world. At this crucial juncture some may make a conscious decision to surrender to experiences that beckon them toward a different world and new

---

[*] Averting psychosis in this manner probably happens more often than is generally realised. Jung estimated that, for every person who experiences overt psychosis, there are at least ten latent or potential cases. Many people probably experience "mini" psychotic episodes – brief periods during which symptoms flare up, but which they are able to pull themselves out of before the experiences become too intense and overwhelming to control.

state of being. For some, the feeling that a long-awaited personal transformation is about to occur may evoke great excitement and exhilaration:

> In the psychotic predicament one takes the opportunity of the explosion to "switch" into another dimension of concern and another plane of activity. This new domain is vaster and endlessly more fascinating than ordinary circumstances. It is filled with a sense of insight and power, electric with the play of energy, perception, and messages, a compelling drive toward completion that offers promises of bliss and happiness of all kinds. One's attention is thoroughly absorbed away from the pettiness of the mundane world from which one has switched-out.[28]

Individuals on the edge of psychosis feel themselves moving ever further from the solid and familiar world of everyday reality as they are drawn inexorably into a realm in which everything seems to be taking on new meaning and significance. Thoughts, feelings and sensations might become muted or extraordinarily intense and change unpredictably. Attention is captured by novel ideas and images that suddenly appear as if from nowhere. A magical dimension seems to be opening up:

> The individual experiences an escalating inner arousal ... His awareness becomes suffused with sensations from subconscious realms, archetypal images that assume terrifying visages as they filter through his fear and confusion, or repressed primal urges that seem alien and foreboding as they return from years of exile ... he feels precariously differentiated from his environment, more insubstantial than solid, in danger of engulfment by powers that would blot out his personal identity ... There follows a death struggle against this insistent chaos, a struggle to impose order and meaning at any cost ... the collective standards of society no longer apply, and only a solitary insight prevails: *all is not what it seems.* But soon a transformed self arises from the ashes of the old ... The earlier terrifying sense of inner disorder is replaced by a profound sense of relatedness that fills both inner and outer worlds. The individual feels that no event occurs anywhere that does not immediately affect him. And all that he thinks and feels directly influences not only other people, but even the inanimate world ... An avalanche of

discovery of hidden relationships between previously disconnected events exposes what had been concealed ... all the strange things happening must be clues of some sort ... Events of vast proportions are unfolding – dangerous events! – and it is clear that he has an important role in what is being played out.[29]

For a time the one entering psychosis may feel lost, tossed about in a living sea, rudderless, alone. In the midst of this turmoil there may be brief periods when everything seems to become clear again, when the person *knows* – perhaps with utter certainty – what is going on and why. Many event-filled moments may pass that each seems an eternity. Since conventional time means nothing to one who is no longer part of the ordinary world, the duration of these experiences is inestimable.

Chapter Four

Dreaming While Awake

A dream is a short-lasting psychosis,
and a psychosis is a long-lasting dream.

Arthur Schopenhauer[1]

Though widely believed to be bizarre and totally imcomprehensible, many facets of psychotic experience are more intelligible – and more familiar – than most people realise. Indeed, there are striking similarities between psychosis and mental states that *all* human beings experience on a regular basis. These facts have important implications. As well as reducing fear and stigmatisation, they suggest it may be possible for helpers to develop far greater empathic understanding of psychotic experience than is usually thought possible. Furthermore, throwing light on the meaningfulness of the ideas, feelings, and images that attend psychosis might enable those directly affected to better understand themselves and their experiences.

To gain insight into the nature of psychosis it is helpful to compare it to another mental state in which thinking, feeling, and perception are profoundly altered. Though this state also involves temporary "loss of contact with reality", it is nevertheless a common and undoubtedly quite *normal* variety of human experience.

A Dream is a Psychosis

A friend told me she had once found herself mowing the lawn at the bottom of the sea and went on to describe in detail how it had felt to push a lawn-mower under water. It would be understandable if our immediate response to such a tale involved wondering about this woman's sanity because we know what she reported is not only bizarre but impossible. But what if we knew she was describing something that occurred in a *dream*? Knowing this we would undoubtedly view her story very differently since everyone knows that such unusual happenings – and indeed far stranger ones – are a common feature of dreams.

The fact that experiences in psychosis are similar to those that occur in dreams has long been known to the most eminent authorities on the workings of the human mind. For example, Sigmund Freud, who developed techniques for unlocking the hidden meaning of his patients' dreams, formed the opinion that:

> A dream, then, is a psychosis, with all the absurdities, delusions and illusions of a psychosis. A psychosis of short duration, no doubt, harmless, even entrusted with a useful function ... None the less it is a psychosis.[2]

Significantly, Freud devoted a section of his seminal book, *The Interpretation of Dreams*, to discussing the relationship between dreams and mental disorder and was in no doubt that "we are working towards an explanation of the psychoses when we endeavour to elucidate the mystery of dreams."[3] Freud's erstwhile protégé, Carl Jung, recognised the existence of an intriguing relationship between these states: "It is no exaggeration to say that the dreamer is normally insane, or that insanity is a dream which has replaced normal consciousness."[4]

The similarities these and other eminent investigators noted between dreaming and psychosis more than justifies closer scrutiny of these enigmatic mental states. Hughlings Jackson, the father of British neurology, was convinced studying dreams would enrich our understanding of psychosis: "Find out all about dreams, and you will have found out all about insanity."[5]

The Nature of Dreams

Dreams generally occur during short periods (around 20–30 minutes) of so-called rapid eye movement (REM) sleep. On average, human beings dream for about two hours every night (though since dreams are often quickly forgotten, on waking many people mistakenly assume they did not have any). While nobody knows exactly why we dream it is certain dreaming must serve some important psychological purpose. If this were not so it is hard to explain why we spend around *one twelfth* of our entire lives dreaming!

The human mind functions very differently in the dream state. Ordinary waking patterns of thinking, feeling, and perceiving change profoundly and our sense of personal identity is often dramatically altered:

> While dreaming we appear to enter a world of our own. In it we appear to be doing all kinds of exciting, frightening, horrifying, delightful or absurd and impossible things. We can return to the selves we once were and to the places we once knew. Or we can become what we hope or once hoped to become – or what we fear or once feared we might become.[6]

In dreams we routinely experience all of the following:

• Altered sense of reality
Nothing is impossible in a dream! We can have extraordinary experiences and feel we possess remarkable, even magical, powers, e.g. the ability to fly, be in two places at once, read people's minds. The places we find ourselves in may seem strange or mysterious and ordinary objects or familiar people may take on new meaning or significance. We might experience a sense of *directly knowing* things even though the evidence does not support, and might even contradict, what we "know", e.g. I meet a woman whom I *know* is my mother even though she looks nothing like my "real" mother.

• Altered sense of self
In dreams the person we perceive ourselves to be is often very different from usual. We may be older or younger, have different physical characteristics, or look like a different person. We might feel we have actually *become* somebody different, or taken on the guise of an animal or unfamiliar creature. We might even temporarily lose our sense of having a recognisable "self".

• Altered sense of time
Time might speed up, slow down, or even stop. We may feel we have gone backwards in time and are living in the past, or have moved forward in time to some future era.

• Altered sense of place
We may feel we are somewhere else, perhaps a familiar place from the past or somewhere we do not recognise, or even somewhere we could

not possibly be when awake, e.g. under the sea, floating through the sky, on the moon or some other planet.

• **Altered sense of control**
Our usual waking sense of having control of our thoughts and actions may be partially or completely suspended. Dreams seem to "come" to us from somewhere else and involve events that occur "all by themselves". Though we routinely use expressions like "I had a dream", it would be more appropriate to say "A dream had me". Our attention is totally absorbed by whatever images happen to present themselves to us. Dreams are not bound by the rules of ordinary logic and the flow of a dream can change unpredictably following some enigmatic inner law.

We enter another world when we dream, one we do not consciously choose or create. In a sense we are "off the planet" temporarily! In this "other" world we tend to accept without question the apparent reality of our experiences and just go along with what is happening. Since our ability to test reality is temporarily suspended we do not say to ourselves, "Hold on, this is impossible!" If what is happening is pleasant we enjoy it; if it is frightening or painful we experience it as unpleasant but have to go through it anyway. Only when we awaken do we realise we were "only" dreaming.* Then, if the dream we were having was enjoyable, we may feel a little disappointed to be back in everyday reality – which is often not nearly as interesting as the dream world. On the other hand, if a dream is unpleasant (e.g. if we were having a nightmare) we may be relieved when it comes to an end and we realise it was all "just a bad dream".

---

* So-called *lucid dreaming* – in which a person becomes aware they are dreaming while still in a dream – is an exception to this general rule. A somewhat similar state of dual consciousness occurs when people are able to recognise the illusory nature of psychotic experiences while they are occurring. Such a person might say, for example, "I know the voices I am hearing are auditory hallucinations". This kind of awareness is often evident when a psychotic episode is ending, at which time the recovering person may question the truthfulness of beliefs and perceptions they previously accepted implicitly.

The Nature of Psychotic Experience

The dream-like quality of psychotic experience is evident in many first-hand descriptions. Such accounts tell how an episode often begins with quite subtle changes, such as colours seeming more intense or sounds becoming louder and more vibrant. These sensations may be accompanied by a growing conviction that some new meaning or deeper significance is being revealed:

> Most of the patients who experienced this change reported that for a time everything around them looked fascinating, objects standing out vividly in contrast to the background. These initial changes in mental function were experienced as pleasant, and a number of patients at this stage went through a transient period of mild elation. Coincident with this alteration in perception, these patients appeared to regard everything with new significance, and there was a general tendency for their interest to be turned to ruminating about the world and life in general, and to religion, psychology, philosophy, art and literature.[7]

Norma MacDonald's psychotic experiences began with the gradual development of a heightened state of awareness that made her feel as though some previously dormant part of her mind had suddenly awoken:

> I became interested in a wide assortment of people, events, places, and ideas which normally would make no impression on me ... I made no attempt to understand what was happening, but felt that there was some overwhelming significance in all this, produced either by God or Satan, and I felt that I was duty-bound to ponder on each of these new interests ... a hodge-podge of unrelated stimuli were distracting me from things which should have had my undivided attention ... By the time I was admitted to hospital I had reached a stage of "wakefulness" when the brilliance of light on a window sill or the colour of blue in the sky would be so important it could make me cry. I had very little ability to sort the relevant from the irrelevant ... Completely unrelated events became intricately connected in my mind.[8]

The experience of heightened awareness sometimes involves the return of vivid memories of events that occurred long ago. As the sense of being able to see beneath the surface of things grows some people feel they are drifting away from the everyday world into a different reality, perhaps one rich in mystery and meaning. Some people feel there is a spiritual dimension to what is occurring:

> I was in a higher and higher state of exhilaration and awareness. Things people said had hidden meaning. They said things that applied to life. Everything that was real seemed to make sense. I had a great awareness of life, truth, and God. I went to church and suddenly all parts of the service made sense. My senses were sharpened and I became fascinated by the little insignificant things around me. There was an additional awareness of the world that would do artists, architects, and painters good. I ended up being too emotional, but I felt very much at home with myself, very much at ease. It gave me a feeling of power. It was not a case of seeing more broadly, but deeper. I was losing touch with the outside world and lost my sense of time.[9]

Some psychotic episodes resemble "good" dreams in which the dreamer becomes engrossed in a realm of fascinating and pleasurable experiences. By contrast, some are more like "bad" dreams or even nightmares. Esso Leete's experience provides a graphic illustration of the latter:

> It was evening and I was walking along the beach near my college ... Suddenly my perceptions shifted. The intensifying wind became an omen of something terrible. I could feel it becoming stronger and stronger; I was sure it was going to capture me and sweep me away with it. Nearby trees bent threateningly toward me and tumbleweeds chased me. I became very frightened and began to run. However, though I knew I was running, I was making no progress. I seemed suspended in space and time. I panicked but with effort pointed myself in the direction of my dormitory and continued on. Finally, after what seemed like hours, I arrived back at my dormitory. By this time I was hearing voices and responding to them. I was confused, disoriented, and frightened, and remained in a different reality ... Over the next few weeks I continued to have auditory hallucinations, still not comprehending that I was out of touch with reality as others knew it. That reality had given way to the multiple realities I would now live.[10]

As they become increasingly absorbed in dream-like inner experiences people may find it difficult to interpret their surroundings correctly. This task is especially problematic when ordinarily insignificant objects, events, and people have assumed larger-than-life meanings. A dreamer often feels he or she is at the very centre of everything that is going on and something similar can occur in psychosis. Some people become convinced aspects of their environment refer to them in a directly personal way (a phenomenon known as "ideas of reference"). The words or actions of other people may seem to convey special "messages" or have hidden meaning. In the psychotic "dream world" it often seems that everything "means" something, a feeling which could lead a person to suspect some kind of elaborate conspiracy is going on:

> Wherever he turns his glance, he sees something that seems to stand in some relation to himself. His world has been transformed into one large "testing ground" where everything has been "arranged", "set up", and prepared to test him, like the stage set of a peculiar sort of theatre. They want to see if he will "tumble to it", if it will "register on him", even though they have "taken pains" to make things "as subtle as possible". They have also used "tricks" and "deceptions"; they are trying to "trap" him. They pretend to be "surprised"; they "conceal" things from him; they do not want him to notice that everyone else has "instructions", has "agreed" on things, has an assignment to carry out. Even the people passing in the street are part of the act. At the height of the episode he himself gives off a kind of aura, so that everything that meets his eye acquires a strangely distorted expression and is laden with tension.[11]

Though the above examples only refer to specific aspects of psychotic experience, their resemblance to what occurs quite normally in dreams is clear. If the words, "I had a dream in which ..." preceded any of these vignettes, their close similarity to the sorts of experiences *anyone* could have while dreaming would become obvious.

Dreams and Schizophrenia

In the classic monograph in which he first proposed the term "schizophrenia", Professor Eugen Bleuler stressed the similarity of psychotic symptoms to dreams: "We encounter hallucinations and delusions in the dreams of healthy people."[12] In a section of his seminal text entitled "The Relation of Schizophrenia to Dreams" he said: "In the healthy psyche, only the dream forms a sufficient analogy to what goes on in schizophrenia."[13] Professor Manfred Bleuler has made similar observations:

> Just as the schizophrenic does not permanently lose his normal inner life, so the normal person is also no total stranger to a schizophrenic inner life. *The dream experiences of normal people do perhaps differ in some details and nuances from the symbolic thinking and imagination of schizophrenics, but certainly only in details and nuances* ... The similarity between the dream life of normal people and schizophrenic existence ... is so close that Jung was fully justified in formulating his famous sentence: "If the dreamer could speak and act, he could not be distinguished from the schizophrenic." ... Even Freud was impressed with this similarity [though] he paid less attention to how similar the emotional life in dreams can be to that of many schizophrenic states.[14]

The peculiar non-rational thought processes associated with psychosis so resemble those in dreams that in both states a novel "language" rich in symbols and images often comes to the fore. Ordinarily this kind of non-rational thinking only occurs in a relatively small range of circumstances, e.g. dreams, creative reverie, drug-induced states. However, in psychosis such thinking may become a person's *predominant* way of interpreting the world and communicating with others. Because this dream-like thinking is so different to the rational thought of the waking state it may appear utter nonsense to others, with the result that those exhibiting it might be considered to suffer severe "thought disorder" of a type characteristic of schizophrenia.

Contemporary research on sleep and dreams throws further light on these matters. Thus, people who are prevented from dreaming by being woken during periods of REM sleep usually dream more the next night, as if trying to catch up on missed dream activity (a phenomenon called "REM rebound"). Interestingly, acutely psychotic individuals tend *not* to dream more the day after a period of experimental dream-deprivation.[15] In fact, they seem to need *less* REM sleep than usual.[16] These facts suggest that dream-like delusions and hallucinations of psychosis might temporarily take the place of sleeping dreams.

Psychosis: Dreaming While Awake

Arguably the most striking characteristic of psychosis is the fact that this dream-like state occurs while a person is wide awake. A century ago Jung's pioneering research on the psychology of schizophrenia led him to liken this condition to a "waking dream":

> To say that insanity is a dream that has become real is no metaphor. The phenomenology of the dream and of schizophrenia are almost identical, with a certain difference, of course; for one occurs normally under the condition of sleep, while the other upsets the waking or conscious state."[17]

Jung pointed out that it is difficult to distinguish the dreams of people diagnosed with schizophrenia from those of persons without this diagnosis. Indeed, it is known that their dreams tend to be rather *less* bizarre than those of "normal" people![18]

States can occur which resemble *partial* "waking dreams" that only affect a person in a limited way, e.g. they may have odd perceptual experiences or unusual thoughts or feelings for brief periods from time to time. In some experiences involving hearing voices (auditory hallucinations) it seems as if "fragments" of a dream have intruded into waking consciousness. By contrast, there may be times when virtually *every* aspect of a person's thinking and behaviour is so strongly influenced by compelling inner images and feelings that they completely over-shadow the outer world. The resulting mental state is referred to as an "acute psychotic episode". The fact that subsequent psychotic episodes often involve similar themes suggests a comparison with a *recurring dream* in which certain images and feelings are repeated over a prolonged period.

Similarities Between Dreams and Psychosis

Table One summarises some of the remarkable similarities between dreams and psychotic experience:

TABLE ONE: Similarities between Dreams and Psychosis

PSYCHOSIS	DREAMS
A psychosis is a *spontaneously occurring mental state* in which people think, feel, and perceive themselves and the world in ways which are *radically different to usual.*	A dream is a *spontaneously occurring mental state* in which people think, feel, and perceive themselves and the world in ways which are *radically different to usual.*
A person in psychosis is *"out of touch with reality"*, experiencing an *imaginal world not shared by others.*	The dreamer is *"out of touch with reality"*, experiencing an imaginal world not shared by others.
A person in psychosis may *see, hear, and experience things others do not* (hallucinations).	The dreamer may *see, hear, and experience things others do not.*
A person in psychosis may *hold unusual beliefs which are not shared by others* (delusions).	The dreamer may *hold unusual beliefs which are not shared by others.*

Differences Between Dreams And Psychosis

While dreams and psychosis are similar in a number of ways there are highly significant *differences* between them. For example, dreams are quite brief, often lasting no more than a few minutes, while psychotic episodes last far longer. Furthermore, a person asleep and dreaming is usually unaware of their physical surroundings whereas those in psychosis are often convinced that their experiences relate to the world around them and that others are also aware of them.

A crucial difference is the fact that a person who is asleep and dreaming is, for the duration, in a state of "suspended animation" so that everything in their dream occurs only in their mind while their body remains passive.* By contrast, people in psychosis often act on their delusional ideas or hallucinatory experiences. Indeed, those absorbed in the drama of an intense psychotic episode many feel *compelled* to do so.

---

* Dreams are often accompanied by a state of temporary physical paralysis. Some believe this may occur to safeguard the dreamer from possible negative consequences of "acting out" their forbidden dream impulses (e.g. sexual fantasies, violent or aggressive feelings).

Table Two summarises some of the important differences between the dream state and psychosis:

TABLE TWO: *Differences between Dreams and Psychosis*

PSYCHOSIS	DREAMS
A psychotic person *may act upon delusional beliefs or hallucinatory experiences.*	A dreaming person *does not act upon dream experiences* (state of "suspended animation").
A psychotic person *retains awareness of the physical environment* during the psychosis (though this awareness may be somewhat distorted at times).	A dreamer is usually *unaware of the physical environment* while absorbed in the "other world" of their dream.
A psychosis *may last days, weeks, or even longer.*	Dreams are *relatively brief* and end spontaneously.

An Inevitable Clash of Realities

Since a person who is asleep and dreaming is effectively in a state of suspended animation they are protected from any adverse consequences that might result should they attempt to act on their inner experiences. Most importantly, they do not have to interact with other people or cope with situations in the "real" world since it is temporarily non-existent for them. *Those experiencing psychosis are in a very different situation.* A person dreaming while awake is fully aware of the world around them and interacts with it. Consequently, it is almost inevitable a host of problematic situations will develop during the course of an acute psychotic episode.

Since a "waking dream" *seems* real to the one experiencing it – just as a sleeping dream does – it is only natural to want to act on it. However, a person who attempts to live it out is certain to encounter numerous difficulties. It is as if they were living in their inner (dream) world and the outer (physical) world *at the same time*, often without realising this is what they are doing (i.e. they "lack insight"). Because the "dream world" and the "real world" are fundamentally incompatible, it is only a matter of time before conflicts occur. Waking dreamers often find themselves on a collision course with consensual reality until a potentially tumultuous "clash of realities" becomes inevitable.

As a person's life fills with contradiction and disagreement they may begin to feel increasingly uncertain about what is going on. Growing confusion about what is real and what is not may cause their anxiety to rise dramatically. Dr Podvoll describes one aspect of their dilemma:

> Inside or outside? Where is all of this happening? Inside or outside? That is always the question. Perception teeters on the brink of doubt as to whether what is happening is inside one's mind or in the environment. Or whether it is happening at all! One appears to have fits of inattention when all one's concern becomes fixed on a dangerous interior.[19]

People in this situation often try desperately to explain their unusual experiences in an attempt to regain control. Angry that nobody seems to understand or agree with them, some may begin entertaining highly idiosyncratic ideas about themselves and the world which impose a reassuring sense of order and predictability. Because they seem strange or implausible to others, such beliefs may be called "delusions" – even if they make perfect sense from the waking dreamer's own point of view. (Such beliefs are called *secondary* delusions to distinguish them from *primary* delusions which arise spontaneously within a waking dream carrying an unshakable sense of conviction.) Elizabeth Farr explains how easily delusional ideas take root during periods of great uncertainty:

> In high school I became engrossed in religion, the occult, and the arts as a possible way to help explain what was going on. The central driving feature in my behaviour was to understand my experiences. The delusions started insidiously. I do not know where religion, the occult, and the arts left off and the crazy ideas started. All I know was that I thought there had to be an explanation for my experiences and I had to be active in my pursuit of an Enlightenment to resolve the conflict between my reality and the reality that everybody else seemed to be experiencing. Everything had to be connected up somehow, I thought. I had to make sense out of it all and connect it up with what I was trying to do in my life ... The reason for my becoming so interested in religion, ESP, and the occult was that these were the closest things I could find that seemed to have any relation to the things I was experiencing. I was susceptible to

kooky ideas ... I did the best I could to make order of the confusing state of my existence and all the conflicting evidence in front of me.[20]

A vicious circle may be set in train as an acutely psychotic individual's extreme or unusual behaviour is often highly disturbing to others. Anxiety and emotional turmoil can escalate dramatically if other people – who do not share the waking dream – insist it is not real and accuse the individual concerned of behaving irrationally. Because the "dream" is very real to the one having it a gulf may soon develop between them and others, including well-meaning family and friends. Fear and anger may feed the psychosis until a "good" waking dream rapidly becomes a "bad" one – or even a nightmare. It is easy to imagine how fear and suspicion occurring as part of a waking dream can be reinforced if the well-meant actions of others are interpreted by psychotic individuals as attempts to harm or control them. If "everything means something" the words and actions of those trying to help must also mean something ... but what?

The fear produced in a waking dreamer by the feeling of being increasingly cut-off from other human beings may cause them to withdraw even further into a private reality. Rachel Corday provides a glimpse into how perplexing the situation can become. Feeling increasingly alone and isolated from others, she was unable to decide whether she or other people were perceiving reality incorrectly:

The woman asked if I was hearing things. She spoke as if from a great distance, and I could not fathom her words. I could not interpret their meaning ... She said something but I could not decipher it. Other voices came into my head. Was there a crowd nearby? ... I looked at the woman next to me. Her eyes were large with fright. How could I tell her that I was seeing the same things she was seeing, but she wasn't seeing the same things I was seeing? She didn't know this scene was here just for now, that it had been inserted into reality like an extra frame being spliced into the reel. How could I tell her this was an alien world and I did not know if it was I or she who was strange?[21]

In the early stages of acute psychosis it is as if the person concerned must either "wake up" or go further into the separate reality of their inner world. As one young man explained, "There were two realities:

60

the world in which I lived and my day dreams, and the latter were more real."[22]

Themes and Images in Waking Dreams

Because the thinking and behaviour of psychotic individuals generally appears bizarre and unintelligible to others it is often judged to be psychologically meaningless. Indeed, it is common for psychotic symptoms to be dismissed as aberrations of a dysfunctional brain, or likened to the nonsensical output of a malfunctioning computer. A consequence of such limiting conceptions is that scant attention is paid to their possible symbolic meaning and metaphorical significance.

Contemporary attempts to account for psychosis in purely biological terms leave unanswered the question of why psychotic experiences vary so much from one individual to another. For example, if everyone experiencing psychosis has a "chemical imbalance" that is the cause of their symptoms, why do some hear harshly critical voices while others hear voices that are friendly and supportive? Why do some hear a mixture of "good" and "bad" voices while others hear no voices at all? What causes one person to believe he is a hugely popular celebrity, even a new Messiah, while another is convinced he is worthless and has been singled out for destruction? Though there are no simple answers to these questions, looking beyond brain chemistry to the way in which the "waking dream" of psychosis resembles a sleeping dream throws light on how hallucinations and delusions become individualised.

We would not expect different people to have exactly the same dream even though very similar patterns of biochemical and electrical activity occur in their brains while they are dreaming. This is because the content of dreams is not determined by brain physiology but by an array of variables which include the dreamer's biographical history, personality, social circumstances, and current psychological state. Despite the tremendous variability of dreams, several generic themes are common. Examples include flying, falling, running but getting nowhere, being naked or absurdly dressed in a public place, finding oneself in an unfamiliar house, being pursued by dangerous animals or hostile people, hurrying and getting lost in a crowd, and fighting with useless weapons.[23]*

Dreams can be highly creative and inspiring, and are potentially a valuable source of insights or glimpses of truths not available during the waking hours. Some may reflect aspects of the dreamer's personality or life situation which they are unaware of or have not fully accepted. The following are frequently expressed in dreams:

• **Wishes, hopes, and desires**
These could be wishes the dreamer is aware of (e.g. dreaming of winning the lottery may reflect a desire to have more money) or others of which they were unaware (e.g. someone with a secret longing to feel accepted dreams they are a famous movie star). As Jung has noted, "All strong wishes furnish themes for dreams, and the dreams represent them as fulfilled, expressing them not in concepts taken from reality but in vague dream-like metaphors."[24]

• **Fears and concerns**
Personal fears and concerns (past or present) are often expressed symbolically in dreams, e.g. a person who fears being misunderstood has a dream in which everybody they meet speaks in a strange, unintelligible language.

• **Current life situation**
Dreams often reflect some psychologically significant aspect of the dreamer's life which they need to become more aware of or do something about, e.g. a woman who has been neglecting her health dreams of having a life-saving operation.

The themes and imagery of dreams are determined by a complex combination of inner and outer influences. The form and content of hallucinations, delusions, and other aspects of a "waking dream" are

---

* Anyone interested in dream interpretation is advised to remember Jung's sage advice: "Here I ought to add a word of warning about unintelligent or incompetent dream analysis … it is plain foolishness to believe in ready-made systematic guides to dream interpretation, as if one could simply buy a reference book and look up a particular symbol. No dream symbol can be separated from the individual who dreams it, and there is no definite or straightforward interpretation of any dream." Jung,C.G (1994) *Man and His Symbols*. New York: Anchor Press. p.53.

also related to the psychotic individual's psychological conflicts and unresolved emotional issues, a view Professor Eugen Bleuler formed long ago. Voices, he said, "express ever the same wishes, hopes and fears", while persecutory delusions often reflect unresolved inner conflicts: "In many instances the persecutor is nothing else than the personification of the patient's conscience". The wish-fulfilling nature of delusional ideas led Bleuler to declare: "I have never seen a delusion in schizophrenics which did not also contain elements of disappointed aspirations."[25]

Sigmund Freud stated that "ideas in dreams and in psychoses have in common the characteristic of being *fulfilments of wishes*."[26] Jung's attempts to understand the cryptic communications of one of his female psychotic patients led him to conclude: "The patient describes for us, in her symptoms, the hopes and disappointments of her life, just as a poet might who is moved by an inner, creative impulse."[27] Many others who have studied the psychology of psychotic experience in depth share the views of these pioneers. Professor Silvano Arieti summarised their findings thus:

> Delusions and hallucinations should not be interpreted as nonsensical beliefs or false perceptions that are to be disregarded ... they have a purpose and therefore a meaning ... Freud demonstrated that the apparent nonsensical content of a dream has a meaning that it is important to know. Carl Jung applied to the symptoms of schizophrenia the same technique that Freud applied to dreams and became the first psychiatrist to give a full psychological interpretation to schizophrenic delusions ... Most delusions and hallucinations can be considered as metaphorical (especially the delusions of persecutions) or compensatory (especially the delusions of grandeur).[28]

Certain themes occur regularly in waking dreams. During his life-long research on schizophrenia Professor Manfred Bleuler observed that the hallucinations and delusions of women with this diagnosis often centred on their relationships with family members and other close persons, while those of men frequently concern competition with other males, homosexual issues, and ambivalent attitudes toward authority.[29]

A common theme in waking dreams involves feeling one is being unjustly treated or even persecuted by others. This can take the form of a simple conviction involving few people (e.g. "My neighbour is spying on me"), but could develop into a vast conspiratorial web involving many. The dream-like mood that pervades a psychosis makes it extremely difficult for the person concerned to recognise that these feelings and beliefs – which they experience as totally convincing – have been constructed in the theatre of their own mind. Furthermore, since the non-rational thought processes of a waking dream are not bound by rules of logic or evidence, a person's determined efforts to "figure it all out" may have the contrary effect of deepening their confusion.

If a waking dreamer assumes his or her experiences and beliefs are correct and acts on them as if they were literally true, an escalating cycle of accusations and recriminations may soon develop. This might eventually result in a person being called *paranoid* because of the mistaken beliefs they hold (*"persecutory delusions"*). Often it is only when a person emerges from their psychotic "dream" that they are able to see that what they thought was going on around them, and the things they accused others of doing to them, were actually an elaborate fantasy.

In waking dreams some people become convinced they possess special powers or abilities, are uniquely talented, or have been selected to perform some important mission. Such beliefs (*"grandiose delusions"*) take a wide variety of forms. Spiritual and religious themes are often prominent. If a person assumes such beliefs are literally true and acts on them as if they were incontestable facts, they may find themselves becoming increasingly isolated and cut-off from human contact. Growing loneliness and frustration might feed their anxiety and suspicion, driving them further into an unshared inner world.

As in ordinary dreams, the themes of acute psychotic experiences are expressed in a highly idiosyncratic symbolic form. This could be so obscure at times that it is difficult even for experienced therapists to correctly interpret psychotic imagery.* If others are hard pressed to discern the concealed meaning of delusions and hallucinations it is not hard to imagine the difficulty the person experiencing psychosis is likely to have distinguishing fantasy from reality! As their emotional

---

* While Jung emphasised the many similarities between the symbolic content of dreams and psychosis, he felt that in schizophrenia *collective* and *archetypal* imagery tend to predominate over those of a personal, biographical nature. (See *Appendix: Archetypal Imagery in Acute Schizophrenia*.)

turmoil deepens such a person's thinking may become increasingly idiosyncratic until the outer world is submerged by dream, wish, and fantasy.

Waking From the Dream of Psychosis

Individuals in the throes of acute psychosis must find a way of negotiating two extremely different "realities" (the inner and outer worlds) simultaneously. Daunting as this task is it is not the only one – nor even the most difficult – that must be faced. As a waking dream finally comes to an end, a host of new challenges present themselves.

Everyone waking from an ordinary sleeping dream passes through a brief period in which they feel disoriented, no longer in the "other world" of dreams, but not yet fully "here" in everyday reality. For a short time after waking we often feel uncertain: did that really happen or was I only dreaming? The Chinese sage Chuang-Tzu has given a poetic account of this in-between state in describing the confusion he experienced upon waking from an enchanting dream:

> Once upon a time I dreamt that I was a butterfly, fluttering hither and thither, to all intents and purposes a butterfly. I was conscious only of following my fancies as a butterfly, and was unconscious of my individuality as a man. Suddenly I awoke, and there I lay, myself again. Now I do not know whether I was then a man dreaming I was a butterfly, or whether I am now a butterfly dreaming I am a man.[30]

The *feelings* associated with an experience or situation are often remembered long after other details have been forgotten. So, too, may feelings invoked by a dream remain with the dreamer long after they awaken. A powerful "waking dream" may leave lingering emotions too deep for words to express. Certain aspects of an intense psychotic episode may be so disconcerting the recovering person refuses to speak about them. The emotional impact of such experiences could be deep and prolonged and might even be sufficient to provoke a post-traumatic stress disorder (PTSD).[31]

Some psychotic episodes involve extremely *positive* experiences such as feelings of emotional or sensory intensity, heightened creativity, awe, wonder and, in certain cases, a greatly enhanced sense of personal importance, power, and purpose. Such exhilarating experiences, once so tantalisingly real, may be reduced to quickly fading memories as the psychosis ends. While abatement of a "waking dream" is usually a relief to all concerned, in some cases feelings of loss and emptiness, even an echoing sense of regret, may remain long afterward. Such feelings sometimes contribute to the development of so-called "post-psychotic depression", a state not uncommon in the wake of acute psychosis.[32]

Since "waking dreams" often involve profound (though usually transient) changes in how people see themselves and the world around them, troubling questions regarding identity and the true nature of reality may remain when the episode ends. For example, a person once certain he was the new Messiah may now be unsure: "Was it just a dream or could I really be the unrecognised Messiah?" A person sure he was being spied upon may wonder whether people really were watching him or if that once-certain belief was just a convincing fantasy.* Nagging doubts may persist long after delusions and hallucinations fade (with or without treatment) and recovering individuals often have great difficulty finding satisfactory answers to their heart-felt questions. In such cases it is possible an emotional crisis or excessive stress could stir deep-seated doubts and uncertainties which, in the absence of adequate support, could intensify until they once again threaten mental equilibrium.

Conclusion

While likening psychosis to dreaming is not meant to imply the two states are identical, they are nevertheless sufficiently similar to justify comparing them. Doing so helps make psychosis more understandable in human terms, for instance by showing how the specific themes of delusions and hallucinations are determined. And even if it proves impossible to discover the symbolic meaning of a particular symptom, it is reassuring to know that even the most seemingly bizarre ideas and experiences contain at least a few "grains of truth", as Jung and others

---

* Certain experiences may be inherently more difficult for the recovering person to "reality test" than others. If someone dreams their house is burning down they will soon realise they were "only dreaming" when they wake and find their house intact. Such tangible evidence is not always available. For example, if during a psychotic episode a person feels talked about or spied upon, how can they ever be sure this was only part of a "waking dream"? After all, if people really *were* conspiring against you, would they admit as much?

insisted. This serves as a reminder that in the apparent disorder of acute psychosis are to be found reflections of a unique life story with its rich tapestry of hopes, wishes, and fears.

Appreciating the many points of similarity between psychosis and normal dream activity challenges the idea that this enigmatic state is a direct result of some type of brain malfunction. Such views, now so prevalent and influential, see the psychotic individual as the tragic victim of the meaningless chaos of his or her symptoms. If we are able to look *beyond* this apparent chaos, we may discover the truth of what Carl Jung pointed out long ago regarding schizophrenia:

> Though we are still far from being able to explain all the relationships in that obscure world, we can maintain with complete assurance that ... there is no symptom which could be described as psychologically groundless and meaningless. Even the most absurd things are nothing other than symbols for thoughts which are not only understandable in human terms but dwell in every human breast. In [psychosis] we do not discover anything knew and unknown; we are looking at the foundations of our own being, the matrix of those vital problems on which we are all engaged.[33]

Because of the complexity of the issues involved it may take considerable time for a person who has been floridly psychotic to re-establish a secure grounding in consensual reality. The task of rebuilding a stable and personally acceptable identity may necessitate a commitment to some form of counselling or therapy. Those undertaking this challenging work may find it helpful to know that, just as ordinary dreams can provide glimpses of otherwise hidden psychological truths, so too may some of the images and experiences that arise in the course of psychosis. As such, they may hold the potential to contribute to personal growth and emotional healing.

As well as highlighting the meaningfulness of psychotic experience, likening it to a waking dream has yet another value. Thus, rather than seeing psychosis as a rare and strange anomaly totally alien to "normal" people, we may begin to see that, while a person undergoing it truly has entered "another world", it is one which in many ways resembles the mysterious realm *all* human beings visit every time they dream.

Chapter Five

Varieties Of Psychotic Experience I: Psychological Crises

Many of the more serious psychoses are essentially problem-solving experiences.
Anton Boisen[1]

Though psychosis is often considered the epitome of psychological chaos and disorder – a "breakdown in the machinery of the mind" – this diagnosis actually encompasses a broad range of phenomena, only *some* of which conform to conventional images of irredeemable mental collapse. Sensitive analysis reveals that, far from being the nonsensical result of a reality-distorting brain malfunction, there is, in fact, a "method in the madness" of many psychotic crises. While this claim is supported by an abundance of clinical and anecdotal evidence, the meaningfulness of such experiences is often obscured by the peculiar, and at times frightening, behaviours that attend them.

Psychotic crises can take a variety of distinct forms. To the extent that they are an attempt to solve overwhelming personal problems and satisfy pressing emotional needs some may function as a desperate psychological coping strategy. In certain instances the upheaval of acute psychosis may reflect the occurrence of a profound developmental crisis or autonomous self-healing process. Spiritual issues and concerns lie at the heart of some psychoses. Indeed, since some of the most florid and tumultuous episodes are impelled by deep spiritual imperatives, they may appropriately be viewed as potentially transformative psychospiritual crises.

Every Psychotic Experience Is Unique

The preceding statements contrast sharply with the prevailing view that the various kinds of psychosis are fundamentally similar "illnesses" triggered by the impact of excessive stress on genetically-predisposed ("vulnerable") individuals. While biological theories are enticingly simple they cannot account for some of the most distinctive

68

characteristics of this highly diverse group of conditions. A truly comprehensive approach must address the following issues:

1. Timing of Episodes

Why does an initial experience of psychosis occur at the particular time it does – often late adolescence or early adulthood? If there are further episodes (so-called "relapses"), why do these occur when they do? It is known that acute psychosis is often preceded by severe threats to self-esteem. The fact that people often feel trapped in an intolerable emotional dilemma immediately beforehand suggests some episodes may be attempts to escape such a "no exit" situation. Others may reflect a massive breach of psychological defences or the collapse of an unstable personality structure in the face of unremitting inner conflict.

2. Individualisation of Symptoms

The highly idiosyncratic nature of psychotic symptoms cannot be explained by simplistic biochemical theories. As with dreams, the form and content of delusions, hallucinations, and other symptoms is meaningfully related to an affected individual's psychological state and predominant social, emotional, and spiritual concerns. As explained below, the kind of experiences a person has will be strongly influenced by the particular type of psychotic crisis they are undergoing.

3. Variability of Outcome

A broad range of outcomes are possible for individuals who experience psychosis. While some may emerge with a stronger identity and clearer sense of purpose, others not only fail to recover but go on to develop severe, possibly lasting disability. Treatment that does not adequately address crucial psychosocial issues could compound a person's difficulties. An innate self-healing tendency plays a key role, both in the genesis of certain episodes, and in subsequent recovery. Failure to recognise and co-operate with this benevolent inner resource increases the risk healing will be compromised.

4. Spiritual and Metaphysical Dimensions

People sometimes have experiences in psychosis which they feel are profoundly spiritual, e.g. "There was a cosmic battle of good and evil", "I had a sacred mission and was to play a crucial role in the salvation of the human race". Though such ideas are often summarily dismissed as "religious delusions" they may reflect genuine spiritual experiences, such as occur in an awe-inspiring encounter with numinous images from the depths of the psyche. Dr Podvoll's study of psychosis and mysticism led him to conclude: "The psychotic inner world often explodes with states of ecstasy, feelings of profound truth, contact with an ultimate reality, and excruciating insights into the nature of self that have always been the characteristic and life-changing qualities of the mystic experience."[2] These facts raise vital questions about the nature of psychosis and the best way to help those who have, willingly or otherwise, come face to face with the deepest mysteries of life.

Psychosis is Not a Unitary Phenomenon

A great deal of confusion has resulted from the fact that the label "psychosis" is routinely applied to mental states sometimes only superficially similar. Although they share certain features, this diverse group may be related to a variety of causes and have distinctively different subjective qualities and personal significance. Mainstream psychiatry's failure to acknowledge this diversity, and its practice of lumping together all such experiences and assuming they have a common biological cause, has only exacerbated what is already an extremely complex and challenging situation.

Acute psychosis can, in fact, assume a wide variety of forms and occur for many different reasons. In this chapter psychoses reflecting an intense *psychological crisis* are discussed under the following headings:

• Psychosis as a Psychological Breakdown
• Psychosis as a Psychological Coping Strategy
• Psychosis as a Psychological Irruption

In the next chapter psychoses reflecting occurrence of a profound *psychospiritual crisis* are divided into two types:

• Psychosis as a Self-Healing Process
• Psychosis and Spiritual Emergency

In *Chapters Seven* and *Eight* the increasingly common phenomenon of psychoses which occur in the context of illicit drug use are discussed under two headings:

- Drug-induced Psychosis
- Psychedelic Experience

Note: There are no sharp boundaries between any of the above categories and a mixture of elements from the various types could be present in any particular case.

Psychosis as a Psychological Breakdown

It was suggested in *Chapter Three* that some people reach adolescence or early adulthood not having developed a strong, stable, and secure identity (a liability sometimes referred to as "ego weakness"). Partly as a result of the way innate hypersensitivity shaped their social and emotional development, such individuals may have grown into psychologically fragile young adults with little confidence in their ability to cope with the ever-increasing demands placed upon them. Lack of a clearly-bounded identity together with an unstable, poorly-integrated personality renders such persons exquisitely vulnerable to the impact of stress. The pressures associated with increasingly complex social roles, expectations, and responsibilities could eventually trap them in an emotional impasse ("no exit" situation) with potentially drastic consequences.

A self-perpetuating cycle of escalating anxiety and uncertainty may develop as a person's strategies for coping with mounting emotional stress are increasingly challenged. Individuals in this situation may initially utilise simple self-protective manoeuvres such as withdrawal and avoidance in an effort to limit stimulation. If these prove ineffective, more extreme defences may be mobilised, e.g. emotional shut-down. If the pressure continues, a progressive retreat from the outer world into a private inner realm may result in an already tenuous adjustment being further compromised until the person's coping mechanisms are overwhelmed. As Professor Ciompi notes: "Every crisis must be understood as the acute over-taxing of a coping system …We can thus regard acute psychotic manifestations in large measure as reactions of sensitive, vulnerable individuals to stress that has become too great for them."[3]

The prevailing psychiatric view is that the mental and emotional turmoil of acute psychosis reflects the occurrence of a far-reaching psychological collapse. The expression "nervous breakdown" is sometimes used (albeit incorrectly) to refer to such a dire state of affairs. In this conceptualisation the personality of the affected individual is likened to a faulty or unstable structure such as a bridge or house which, having been over-stressed, finally collapses under the pressure of an unbearable load. As Jung recognised, this may be an appropriate metaphor for some psychotic episodes:

> The possibility of a future psychosis ... has everything to do with whether the individual can stand a certain panic, or the chronic strain of a psyche at war with itself. Very often it is simply a matter of a little bit too much, of the drop that falls into a vessel already full, or the spark that accidentally lands on a heap of gunpowder ... It is quite consistent with such a state of mind if some particularly unruly parts of the patient's psyche then acquire a certain degree of autonomy ... It is as if the very foundations of the psyche were giving way, as if an explosion or an earthquake were tearing asunder the structure of a normally built house. I use this analogy on purpose, because it is suggested by the symptomatology of the initial stages.[4]

The stressors that provoke this type of collapse are often highly idiosyncratic. For example, while everyone naturally experiences a blow to their self-esteem as distressing and hurtful, those harbouring deep uncertainty about their identity and worth may take it as incontestable proof that they are a total failure as a human being and will always be so. A psychotic breakdown may be provoked by a single emotionally distressing event which has an overwhelming impact ("big bang"), or by the cumulative effect of a series of minor events occurring over time ("Chinese water torture"). The emotional consequences of the latter might not be obvious if a person's growing despair and sense of impending calamity are hidden behind a "façade of normality".

As devastating as "breakdowns" of this type may be they do not necessarily result in *permanent* psychological or social disability. While extremely traumatic, such an event might only occur once in a person's lifetime. With sincere effort and adequate support, in time many people are able to fully recover.

Individuals who have experienced breakdown are often encouraged to "pick up the pieces" of their shattered lives in the hope of salvaging enough to recreate what existed before things fell apart. In this endeavour it is worth reflecting on why such a collapse occurred. If the pre-psychotic personality was fragile or inauthentic, simply replicating it is likely to leave the individual concerned susceptible to further breakdowns. Undergoing a total collapse may create an opportunity for a person to reconstruct their life in a new way. This could be likened to *renovating* a structurally unsound house or bridge rather than simply rebuilding it, so it will be more resilient in future.

As dire as it seems at the time, if a "breakdown" can be successfully negotiated it may open a way toward constructive change and personal growth. Such a drastic crisis could provoke a radical reassessment of outmoded beliefs, attitudes, goals, and identity. Many who have undergone such crises speak of the opportunity they provided to abandon self-limiting habits and behaviours and replace them with healthier, life-affirming ones. Should this occur, what may have begun as a breakdown could eventually open the way to a breakthrough of sorts.

Psychosis as a Psychological Coping Strategy

Some psychotic episodes occurring in the context of an insoluble emotional impasse may be manifestations of a desperate attempt to reduce mounting anxiety and escape emotional distress. This idea has many eminent advocates. For instance, in his classic monograph on schizophrenia, Professor Eugen Bleuler suggested symptoms (positive and negative) may be part of an elaborate psychological coping strategy:

> In part (possibly entirely) the overt symptomatology certainly represents the expression of a more or less unsuccessful attempt to find a way out of an intolerable situation ... The patient renders reality harmless by refusing to let it touch him (autism); he ignores it, isolates it, withdraws into his own thoughts. For these patients, autism has the same meaning as the walls of the monastery have for the monks, that the lonely desert has for some saints, and their studies for some scientists ... This type of reaction can only succeed completely if ... the isolation of reality is effected or if it has been transformed in accordance with the patient's wishes ... Thus the patients try to help themselves in the same way as the daydreamers or the poets.[5]

73

Autobiographical accounts of psychosis lend support to these suggestions. Thus, in a graphic description of her own experience of "madness", Lara Jefferson highlighted the fact that it had delivered her from unendurable pain:

> When a soul sails out on that unmarked sea called Madness they have gained release much greater than your loss – and more important. Though the need which brought it cannot well be known by those who have not felt it. For what the sane call "ruin" – because they do not know – those who have experienced what I am speaking of know the wild hysteria of Madness means salvation. Release. Escape. Salvation from a much greater pain than the stark pain of madness. Escape – from that which could not be endured. And that is why the Madness came. Deliverance; pure, simple, deliverance.[6]

In summarising the findings of his life-long research on schizophrenia, Professor Arieti emphasised the anxiety-alleviating function of this condition:

> Schizophrenia is an abnormal way of dealing with an extreme state of anxiety, which originated in childhood and was reactivated later in life by psychological factors.[7]

In the period immediately preceding the onset of psychosis some people may have reached a point of total despair about themselves and their prospects of future happiness. Innate sensitivity can intensify their anguish to an unbearable degree. As Professor Arieti explains, severely damaged self-esteem causes many in this situation to feel threatened by powerful feelings of self-condemnation:

> The patient feels threatened from all sides, as if he were in a jungle. It is not a jungle where lions, tigers, snakes, and spiders are to be found, but a jungle of concepts – in this case ideas about himself – where the threat is not to survival but to the self-image. The dangers are [feelings] such as that of not belonging, being unwanted, unloved, unlovable, inadequate, unacceptable, inferior, awkward, clumsy, peculiar, different, rejected, humiliated, guilty, unable to find his own way among the different paths of life, disgraced, discriminated against, kept at a distance, suspected, and so on … [he] feels not only that he is unacceptable to the segment of the world that is important to him, but also that he will be unacceptable to others

as long as he lives. He is excluded from the busy, relentless ways of the world. He does not fit; he is alone. He experiences ultimate aloneness; he becomes unacceptable even to himself.[8]

Feeling trapped, individuals in this situation may begin to panic. At this point an automatic psychological defence may be mobilised so that intolerable feelings are "split off" (dissociated) and projected into the surrounding environment. While the panicking individual initially felt their tormenting sense of personal failure and defeat was nobody's fault but their own, projection allows these feelings to be disowned and attributed to some *external* source or agency.[*] The world is transformed as a result:

> Before the patient became obviously [psychotic] he was not really well but had already developed serious psychological problems. He had very low self-esteem. He considered himself inadequate, worthless, unloved … He blamed himself for being inadequate and inherently inferior, for not having done what he should to improve himself. He thought people were justified in having a bad opinion of him. Although most of the time he tried to deny this vision of himself and even to suppress it from consciousness, the time comes when he can no longer do so. He externalises it in a way that is not supported by logic. No longer does he accuse himself; the accusation now comes from others … In order to make this shift, he has to resort to a primitive way of thinking that … appears to us to be exaggerations and distortions … Thus these mysterious, imaginary persons who accuse the patient do not call him "inadequate, unlovable, neglectful", but in the imagination of the patient they amplify the accusation to the point of calling him "pervert, spy, murderer, prostitute".[9]

This interpretation suggests that psychotic symptoms sometimes provide a means of escaping an intolerable emotional dilemma. They can thus be considered manifestations of a psychological coping strategy in which the mechanism of projection (in combination

---

[*] The unconscious psychological defence mechanism of *projection* results in a person's *own* characteristics, attitudes, feelings, or beliefs being unwittingly attributed to others. A similar process occurs quite normally in dreams so that the various characters encountered seem to have an existence outside and independent of the dreamer, even though they originate from within the dreamer's own mind.

with other unconscious processes such as non-rational dream-like thinking) creates a vivid alternate reality of hallucinatory experiences and delusional ideas. By such means feelings of self-reproach are externalised and attributed to others, e.g. people on TV or "voices" make critical and derogatory remarks.

On one level it may seem these developments make the affected person's situation even *worse* than it was previously. However, while it is true that some symptoms may be distressing (e.g. critical voices), their onset often coincides with a substantial reduction in extreme pre-psychotic anxiety. Professor Arieti explains how this occurs:

> If we go a little deeper into the matter, we are able to recognise that *the transformation of inner conflicts into symptoms that refer to the external world is advantageous to the patient.* As unpleasant as it is to be accused by others, it is not as unpleasant as to accuse oneself, to be unacceptable to oneself ... The patient who believes he is accused feels falsely accused. Thus, although the accusation is painful, it is not injurious to self-esteem. On the contrary, in comparison to the state he was in before ... the patient often experiences a rise in self-esteem, often accompanied by a feeling of martyrdom ... *The danger, which used to be an internal one, is now transformed [by psychosis] into an external one.*[10]

Because projection plays a prominent role in this type of psychosis the symptoms resulting often have a "paranoid" quality, e.g. delusions of persecution, ideas of reference, accusatory voices.[11] Grandiose beliefs may also be held – often in conjunction with those involving persecutory themes.

Manic episodes sometimes take the form of a frantic "flight" from painful reality into a superficial euphoria and exalted grandiosity. At the height of such episodes people may entertain beliefs about themselves which were formerly impossible. Although grossly exaggerated or distorted, such beliefs bolster a sense of personal worth and help protect a person from devastatingly low self-esteem. One young woman describes the gratifying aspects of her "grandiose delusions":

> Take this typical scenario of how I see myself in times of psychosis: I'm a big time hot-shot who conquers all evil doings committed by conspiring forces. I am the "White Angel of Victory" working for the good of the world, helping the down-and-out everywhere. I am

the people's hero, in fact. I can almost hear the crowds in the streets cheering me on! I know I have the support of millions, especially through the media via the cryptic messages they send all over the world in my support. When I'm high I am ecstatic, I feel I can do almost anything. Why, I could even be the "Second Coming" herself!

While psychosis is doubtless an *abnormal* way of coping with extreme anxiety and unbearable feelings of self-reproach, no other escape may have been possible at the time. As psychotherapists Murray Jackson and Paul Williams explain, "Psychosis originated as the best possible solution to intolerable psychological conditions."[12]

It is difficult to say why some people respond in a "psychotic" way to emotionally unbearable situations while others do not. Professor Arieti believes that a combination of biological and psychological factors may make some people prone to psychosis in highly stressful circumstances. It could be that certain combinations of these factors increase the likelihood that, if psychosis does occur, it will take a specifically "schizophrenic" form while others result in a tendency toward "bipolar" or some other type of symptomatology. In any event, the symptoms serve a vital purpose, as Arieti explains:

> The patient has a strong psychological need that he must satisfy: *He must solve his psychological problems. He attempts to do so through his symptoms.* However, he would probably not attempt to solve his problems in this abnormal way if he were not inclined to do so by a biological predisposition, or an unusual conglomeration of psychological factors, or a mixture of physical and psychological factors. At any rate, even if these factors are necessary, it is important to understand the psychological need for the symptoms.[13]

The fact that psychotic symptoms sometimes help to alleviate anxiety and satisfy pressing psychological needs raises questions about the wisdom, and likely effectiveness, of treatment strategies aimed solely at eradicating them.

Psychosis as a Psychological Irruption

Some acute psychotic episodes appear to primarily involve the dramatic emergence into awareness of mental contents previously confined to the unconscious realms of the mind. As Carl Jung explained:

When people lose their hold on the concrete values of life the unconscious contents become overwhelmingly real. Considered from the psychological standpoint, psychosis is a mental condition in which formerly unconscious elements take the place of reality.[14]

Something of this kind occurs quite naturally in dreams so that the dreamer has a vivid experience of memories, feelings, wishes or fantasies of which they might otherwise have remained totally unaware. This happens in dreams without causing problems since the dreamer is effectively in a state of suspended animation. However, if it should occur while a person is wide awake, the result may be the "waking dream" of psychosis.

Rather than being caused by a chemical imbalance in the brain, psychosis might sometimes be the result of a *psychological* imbalance between conscious and unconscious realms of the mind. A variety of influences might bring such a situation about − either by activating the unconscious, weakening the psychological barrier that prevents unconscious material from entering awareness, or having both effects simultaneously. In any event, the outcome is aptly described as a psychological *irruption* since unconscious contents may indeed "irrupt", i.e. invade or enter consciousness forcibly or violently. Jungian therapist John Sanford explains this notion as follows:

[Some types of acute psychosis] can be understood as an overwhelming of the ego by the forces of the unconscious. The unconscious expresses itself by exceedingly powerful images that are autonomous; that is, they have their own life and vitality. Ordinarily the ego is able to screen out these images of the unconscious sufficiently so that during waking hours we can function correctly, deal with the outer world, and keep a distinction between inner and outer reality. But in certain cases the inner images may be too strong, the defences of the ego too weak, and the threatened invasion takes place in the form of a psychosis. In this state the difference between inner and outer reality is obscured. It is like living in a dream when awake: the "dream reality" is so strong that the individual loses the common psychological perspective of his fellows and he becomes "crazy". This is especially likely to happen if the person is psychologically isolated from others.[15]

Psychological irruptions of this kind invariably have a profoundly disturbing effect on the conscious mind.* The ideas and images involved may appear bizarre and irrational and seem completely "un-understandable". However, similar material appears routinely in the dreams of entirely "normal" individuals. And, as Jung stressed, it existed – possibly for many years – in the unconscious of the affected individual before he or she became mentally disturbed:

> These unconscious forces and contents have long existed in him and he has wrestled with them successfully for years. As a matter of fact, these strange contents are not confined to the patient alone, they exist in the unconscious of normal people as well, who, however, are fortunate enough to be profoundly ignorant of them. These forces did not originate in our patient out of nowhere. They are most emphatically not the result of poisoned brain-cells, but are normal constituents of our unconscious psyche. They appeared in numberless dreams, in the same or a similar form, at a time of life when seemingly nothing was wrong. And they appear in the dreams of normal people who never get anywhere near a psychosis ... What happened was that our patient succumbed to an attack of weakness – in reality it is often just a sudden panic – it made him hopeless or desperate, and then all the suppressed material welled up and drowned him.[16]

Ordinarily unconscious mental contents might spontaneously enter consciousness in this way for a variety of reasons. Individuals experiencing psychosis or other types of severe psychiatric disorder are sometimes said to be "mentally unbalanced". Jung believed this is often a perfectly apt description of their psychological state:

> Hallucinations show very plainly how a part of the unconscious content can force itself across the threshold of consciousness. The same is true of a delusion whose appearance is at once strange

---

* According to the earliest beliefs about madness the disturbed person was *possessed* by some supernatural force or entity (a view still prevalent in certain quarters). The fact that people may change quite dramatically when psychotic – attracting comments like "He is not himself" – contribute to this anachronistic notion. However, Jung felt such changes were due to *psychological*, rather than demonic, possession: "Insanity is possession by an unconscious content which, as such, is not assimilated to consciousness." Wilhelm, R. (1984) *The Secret of the Golden Flower*. London: Arkana, p.112.

and unexpected by the patient. "Mental balance" is no mere figure of speech, for its disturbance is a real disturbance of the balance which – to a far higher degree than has been recognised – actually exists between the conscious and the unconscious contents. What happens is that the normal functioning of the unconscious processes breaks through into the conscious mind in an abnormal manner, and thereby disturbs the adaptation of the individual to the environment.[17]

Jung felt schizophrenia could often be explained in terms of this kind of disturbed mental balance. Indeed, he believed it appropriate to differentiate schizophrenia into two varieties according to the psychological processes involved:

> It may be that in schizophrenia a normal consciousness is confronted with an unusually strong unconscious; it may also be that the patient's consciousness is just weak and therefore unable to keep back the inrush of unconscious material. In practice I must allow for the existence of two groups of schizophrenia: one with a weak consciousness and the other with a strong unconscious.[18]

The preceding concepts help explain how illicit drugs – including amphetamines, marijuana, and psychedelics like LSD, mescaline, and psilocybin – can induce psychotic experiences, or even trigger full-blown psychotic episodes, in psychologically susceptible individuals. Psychiatrist Stanislav Grof's intensive research into the effects of psychedelic drugs led him to view these substances as *amplifiers of unconscious mental processes* that can facilitate the emergence of such contents into awareness. For this reason these drugs are sometimes used in shamanic and other traditional healing practices to induce altered states of consciousness in which non-ordinary experiences occur. However, indiscriminate use of potent psychoactive drugs could pose a risk to individuals with a history of mental disorder and anyone prone to becoming psychologically unbalanced (see *Chapters Seven* and *Eight*).

Psychiatrist Ronald Laing has described a particular type of acute psychosis which is a direct consequence of the irruption into awareness of previously hidden thoughts and feelings. In certain circumstances, Laing believed, the strain of maintaining a "false self" (*Chapter Three*) might become too great with the result that this complex

psychological structure collapses in dramatic fashion. In such cases
the ensuing psychosis involves the sudden emergence of the "true" self
from behind the façade of a "false" self constructed and maintained,
possibly for many years, as a self-protective measure:

> The observable behaviour that is the expression of the false self is
> often perfectly normal. We see a model child, an ideal husband, an
> industrious clerk ... *What is called psychosis is sometimes simply the
> sudden removal of the veil of the false self*, which had been serving to
> maintain an outer behavioural normality that may, long ago, have
> failed to be any reflection of the state of affairs in the secret self.
> Then the self will pour out accusations of persecution at the hands
> of that person with whom the false self has been complying for
> years. The individual will declare that this person (mother, father,
> husband, wife) has been trying to kill him; or that he or she has
> tried to steal his "soul" or his mind. That he/she is a tyrant, a
> torturer, an assassin, a child murderer, etc.[19]

Episodes of this kind could result in highly uncharacteristic
behaviour – possibly aggression or violent acting out directed at self
or others – on the part of an ordinarily docile individual. Family and
friends, greatly distressed to find that someone they thought they
knew well was capable of such outlandish conduct, may experience a
reflexive urge to curtail it as quickly as possible. However, psychotic
episodes that involve the dramatic irruption of previously unconscious
thoughts or hidden feelings can have constructive as well as destructive
potential. As Anton Boisen recognised, they sometimes herald the
start of a healing process:

> The favourable outcome which we have found in this group of cases
> may be explained by the fact that the acute disturbance serves to bring
> the cause of distress from the realm of evasion and concealment out
> into the realm of clear awareness. Such disturbances often serve as a
> sort of judgement day, the patient blurting out what before, for the
> life of him, he would not have dared to say. Just as inflammation in
> the physical organism is an attempt at repair or elimination, so the
> emotional disturbance serves to purge out accumulated poisons and
> break up malignant concealment devices which have been blocking
> development.[20]

At the very least, these dramatic crises provide all concerned with an opportunity to confront – and hopefully resolve – a range of long-standing issues.

Conclusion

The various kinds of psychosis described in this chapter highlight the fact that such events do not generally strike "out of the blue", as is often assumed, but are more often provoked by the accumulated pressure of a backlog of personal difficulties. Furthermore, rather than heralding the onset of a life-long "mental illness", such episodes may rightly be viewed as personal crises having constructive as well as destructive potential.

While psychotic symptoms sometimes serve a useful purpose – such as helping to reduce anxiety, counteract isolation or bolster self-esteem – their cost can be considerable. Thus, while "voices" originating in projection might alleviate self-condemnation, their presence might cause the hearer considerable discomfort. Even "good" voices could have untoward effects. For example, while they may provide welcome companionship at times, such voices could tend to become a substitute for relations with "real" people. Likewise, some delusional beliefs might alleviate anxiety or boost agonisingly low self-esteem but could result in greater frustration and isolation in the long term. As an old saying goes, "The house of delusions is cheap to build but draughty to live in". Thus, a clear distinction needs to be made between psychosis which serves as a temporary coping strategy, and psychosis as a limited and limiting way of life.

Symptoms occurring as part of a psychological coping strategy cause the affected person's world to change dramatically. While this may make life more bearable in certain ways, since a specifically *psychotic* solution has been resorted to the subject's perception of reality is invariably distorted to some degree. Psychosis creates a separate reality – a private world that can never be fully shared with others. Another possibility exists. Rather than attempting to change the world to accommodate one's needs, the wounded self could undergo a radical transformation. Some ways this might occur are described in the next chapter.

Chapter Six

Varieties Of Psychotic Experience II: Psychospiritual Crises

When the medical view of sanity and psychosis came to ascendance, a seemingly ageless understanding of insanity as a spiritual crisis was lost.

Edward Podvoll[1]

Although florid symptoms such as hallucinations, delusions, chaotic "bizarre" behaviour, and non-rational thinking readily create an impression of mental chaos and disorder, some psychotic episodes are not as negative or destructive as they may at first appear. Intensive study of the relationship between spirituality and mental health led psychiatrist Roberto Assagioli to conclude that, far from amounting to a catastrophic "nervous breakdown", some of the most dramatic crises could potentially facilitate significant psychological and spiritual growth:

> Man's spiritual development is a long and arduous journey, an adventure through strange lands full of surprises, difficulties, and even dangers. It involves a drastic transmutation of "normal" elements of the personality, an awakening of potentialities hitherto dormant, a raising of consciousness to new realms, and a functioning along a new inner dimension. We should not be surprised, therefore, to find that so great a change, so fundamental a transformation, is marked by several critical stages, which are not infrequently accompanied by various nervous, emotional, and mental troubles. *These may present to the objective clinical observation of a therapist the same symptoms as those due to more usual causes, but they have in reality quite another significance and function, and need very different treatment.* The incidence of disturbances having a spiritual origin is rapidly increasing nowadays, in step with the growing number of people who, consciously or unconsciously, are groping their way towards a fuller life.[2]

Some psychotic episodes may constitute a secretly hoped-for breakthrough which holds the promise of freeing a troubled individual from long-standing personal problems and difficulties. As Dr Podvoll has observed, for some people the psychotic experience carries with it "hopes of passing beyond, renouncing, or destroying the self that is felt to be incompetent and diseased by imperfections."[3] The successful resolution of this type of spontaneous *self-healing process* could result in enhanced self-esteem and a more flexible and resilient personality than existed beforehand. An allied group of psychospiritual crises often erroneously labelled psychotic are actually *spiritual emergencies* of various kinds. These dramatic episodes can assume a number of forms, some of which bear superficial resemblance to psychotic disorders familiar to *DSM*-trained clinicians. Lack of awareness of their true nature means they are often diagnosed incorrectly and treated inappropriately. With proper understanding and support these crises could facilitate profound healing and personal transformation.

Before proceeding it must be pointed out that the English language lacks a suitable word for the kinds of psychospiritual crises discussed in this chapter. Since the psychiatric term "psychosis" invariably implies a severe mental *illness* or *disease*, it is too narrow to encompass experiences conducive to growth and healing. The phrase "psychotic altered state of consciousness" has been used in reference to such phenomena.[4] Altered states of consciousness (ASCs) share a number of key features, the most important being that all involve a temporary period during which the subject's experience of self and outer world (consensual reality) is radically altered. This usage places psychosis alongside other ASCs such as mystical, psychedelic, and hypnotic states. In *Chapter Four* psychosis was likened to a waking dream state, dreams being the most familiar of the numerous ASCs to which human beings are prone. For the sake of clarity the familiar though manifestly inadequate term "psychosis" is used throughout this chapter. Readers are nevertheless urged to keep the foregoing comments in mind.

Psychosis as a Self-Healing Process

The fact that acute psychotic episodes sometimes facilitate positive psychological change has long been recognised by those who have studied the workings of the human mind in depth. Jungian psychiatrist

Dr John Perry believes that, to understand growth-promoting crises, it must be appreciated that human beings tend to grow and develop in fitful leaps rather than by gradual and steady improvement. Some of these transitional periods may be tumultuous:

> Contrary to our general expectations, growth and development do not proceed in a linear and upward fashion, smoothly advancing from point to point like grades in a school, however much we might wish for that. Rather, growth proceeds in a cyclic fashion, with alternating periods of calm and turbulence, progression and regression. Every few years there is an upset in one's experience of the world and a fresh start on a new footing begins. The acute episode we are considering here is another one of these highly charged upsets, but, of course, much more radical in the mode of change and more deeply disturbing ... [Nevertheless the] turmoil and disorder are anything but disastrous if we can actually look into the process giving rise to them ... Seen in this light, our fearsome "disorder" is merely nature's way of dismantling what was inadequate in the past, and in so doing allowing a new start.[5]

A number of the most eminent figures in the history of psychiatry acknowledged the possibility that some acute psychotic crises may be harbingers of personal growth and psychological reorganisation. Thus, in his seminal monograph on schizophrenia, Professor Eugen Bleuler stated "There are even patients who seem to be better off after an acute exacerbation than they were before".[6] Dr Karl Menninger, one of the towering figures of twentieth century American psychiatry, said "Some patients have a mental illness and then get well and then they get weller! I mean they get better than they were ... this is an extraordinary and little-realised truth."[7] Many other competent authorities have expressed similar views.[*]

---

[*] The therapeutic potential of certain acute psychotic episodes is occasionally acknowledged in mainstream professional publications, e.g. Silverman,J. (1970) When Schizophrenia Helps. *Psychology Today*, Vol.4, 63-65; Epstein,S. (1979) Natural Healing Processes of the Mind: I. Acute Schizophrenic Disorganisation. *Schizophrenia Bulletin*, Vol.5, No.2, 313-321. Professor John Strauss has expressed views consistent with those in this chapter: "A mechanism in schizophrenia, and perhaps also in other severe mental disorders, must be postulated to explain such massive realignments of psychological functioning from organisation through disorganisation to reorganisation with a new structure." Strauss,J. (1989) Mediating Processes in Schizophrenia. *British Journal of Psychiatry*, Vol.155 (suppl.5), 22-28.

One of the earliest proponents of this understanding was Anton Boisen, founder of the clinical pastoral education movement. A minister of religion and psychologist who endured several severe psychotic episodes early in his career, Boisen was uniquely qualified in this area. Galvanised by the insights he gained from his ordeals, Boisen subsequently carried out an intensive study of mental disturbances. He concluded that many of the more serious psychoses are essentially *problem-solving experiences*. Such episodes, he believed, were a natural process aimed at freeing a troubled individual from attitudes, beliefs and ingrained mental habits blocking personal growth and development. Boisen summarised these ideas as follows:

> Certain types of mental disorder are not in themselves evils but problem-solving experiences. They are attempts at reorganisation in which the entire personality, to its bottom-most depths, is aroused and its forces marshalled to meet the danger of personal failure and isolation … Even those whose beliefs have been warped in the effort to interpret some unhappy life situation in terms favourable to their self-respect may, through the disturbance, find release and emerge into new life and hope. The emotional disturbance thus serves to break up malignant sets and attitudes and to make possible a new synthesis ... even in definitely psychotic cases, emotional disturbances may be purposive and constructive. They may, and sometimes do, succeed in setting an individual free from what has been blocking his development, and in effecting a re-organisation of the personality.[8]

These views are based on two premises not recognised by conventional psychiatry. The first is that the maladaptive or dysfunctional state is not psychosis itself but the state existing *before* this disturbance occurred. Boisen noted, for example, that many people have endured extreme inner conflict and disharmony before the onset of psychosis:

> In all of our cases we find evidence of some *unsolved problem* relating to the patient's role in life – a problem which arouses intense emotion. Nearly always this problem involves some sense of personal failure and guilt. It has usually been on the patient's mind for many years as a source of distress and uneasiness until finally, in cases of this type, there comes a desperate attempt at solution.[9]

In some cases, Dr Perry believes, it is not simply an individual's conflict-ridden emotional state which is at the root of their problems but their basic personality structure. A second premise is that some acute psychotic episodes may be spontaneous attempts to bring about a fundamental reorganisation of a hitherto poorly-adapted or psychologically unbalanced personality. Dr Perry explains:

> It is justifiable to regard the term "sickness" as pertaining not to the acute turmoil [of psychosis] but to the *pre-psychotic personality*, standing as it does in need of profound reorganisation. In this case, the renewal process occurring in the acute psychotic episode may be considered nature's way of setting things right. Even though this compensatory process may become a massive turmoil, the turbulence is a step on the way toward the living of a more fulfilled emotional life.[10]

As explained in *Chapter Three*, from an early age individuals who later experience psychosis have sometimes developed a type of personality ("schizoid", "stormy") which, while it aided social adaptation for a time, eventually proved inadequate or unsatisfactory. Such cases might be likened to a structurally unsound or no longer adequate house which requires extensive alteration in order to meet current and future needs. In some instances an individual's personality might need to be "demolished" so it can be reassembled in a new way more in keeping with their true nature. Dr Podvoll has noted that in such cases, "The urge to transform is usually a motivating factor long before a predicament arises. This desire to become someone else has been 'cooking' since an early age."[11] Jungian psychotherapist Janet Dallett explains this notion as follows:

> My sense is that people often become psychotic because they have constructed a personality that is not congruent with who they really are. This happens because they are sensitive children who perceive things going on in their environment that are not confirmed by the people around them ... So the child builds up a personality for the sake of adaptation that is quite incongruent with his or her true nature. As life goes on, this discrepancy between the adaptation and the real person becomes greater and greater, so that a rather large split develops. Often in psychosis [it is] as if the ego dissolves – an ego that is brittle and not connected in a human way to what the

person *is* deeply ... this kind of psychotic episode is an opportunity for the person to heal in a deeper way.[12]

This view of psychosis is based on the assumption that, just as the physical body has an array of in-built mechanisms for healing illness or injury, the human psyche also possesses innate self-healing capacities. Anton Boisen acknowledged the vital role played by natural psychological self-healing mechanisms: "In the ailments of the mind no less than in those of the body we can see the manifestation of the healing power of nature so familiar to the physician".[13] Professor Eugen Bleuler appears to have shared this belief for, in his treatise on schizophrenia, he said "it is certain ... some psychic self-healing process must exist".[14] Natural therapy practitioners have long accepted the existence of an innate tendency toward healing and wholeness, as do adherents of Jungian psychology.

Dr Perry has made an in-depth study of psychotic episodes which eventually result in a constructive outcome.[15] He concluded that an innate healing impulse is responsible for initiating the psychosis (or "renewal process", as he calls it) and guiding its subsequent course toward wholeness and reorganisation of the personality. As John Sanford explains, in such episodes, "What looked like an illness is actually a cure; that is, the psychosis is really an attempt to cure that person of a maladjusted ego":

> The original illness was an inadequate conscious development; there was something wrong with that individual to begin with, some maladjustment or psychological inadequacy. The flood of images from the unconscious contains the cure. If correctly understood and integrated, the images result in a change of personality that can lead to greater health. So the flood of images that comes to someone in psychosis can be understood as an attempt on the part of the unconscious to cure him and set him on a path to wholeness.[16]

Since experiences of this kind originate in the depths of the psyche they tend to be expressed in the natural language of the unconscious: dream-like images and mythical archetypal symbols with a numinous, otherworldly character (see *Appendix: Archetypal Imagery in Acute Schizophrenia*). Boisen noted such episodes often have a profoundly spiritual quality: "Individuals who pass through them agree in feeling themselves in touch with some mighty personal force to which generally they give the name of God."[17]

Those experiencing a self-healing psychosis invariably feel they have been lifted from their usual mundane level of existence to one of great, even "cosmic", significance. Since the function of this type of psychosis is to break down a maladapted or inadequate personality and reorganise it into a more flexible, better-adapted form, ideas ("delusions") and visions ("hallucinations") experienced tend to involve grand mythic themes and awe-inspiring archetypal images. These often include a mixture of frightening or nightmarish aspects and lighter, more exalted imagery. The renewal process often begins abruptly:

> Such cases begin almost invariably with an eruption of the lower strata of consciousness which is interpreted as a manifestation of the superpersonal. To the individual concerned the effect is overwhelming. It shatters the foundations of his mental structure. It sweeps him away from his moorings out into the uncharted seas of the inner world. He is no longer concerned about the merely individual, but about the cosmic and universal. Very commonly he thinks of himself as in the central role in the cosmic drama. Such experiences are as old as the human race ... they are essentially attempts at reorganisation in which the entire personality is aroused and its forces marshalled to meet some serious obstacle to growth.[18]

At the beginning of such episodes people often feel as though they have embarked on a great journey or even been personally selected to fulfil an important spiritual mission. They may perceive themselves as being at the centre of a world process which is leading inexorably toward a radical personal and societal metamorphosis. At some stage people often feel they have returned to the beginning of time and are witnessing the creation of the universe and the origins of life. They may feel they are participating in a cosmic battle involving powerful forces of good and evil. A characteristic feature of these episodes is the theme of *death and rebirth*, and subjects often become engrossed in graphic images of death and destruction, preoccupations that eventually give way to a conviction of having been reborn or resurrected into a new life and more complete sense of personal identity. Some of key themes associated with the psychospiritual self-healing process are described overleaf.

(a) <u>World catastrophe</u>

Onset of the acute episode may be heralded by an overwhelming conviction that the world is about to be changed in some drastic and fundamental way, or even that it is about to be destroyed. People are sometimes convinced this has *already* occurred, in which case they may feel they are in a dead world or ghostly spirit realm. The following graphic account illustrates the emotional intensity of such experiences:

> Shortly after I was taken to the hospital for the first time … I was plunged into the horror of a world catastrophe. I was being caught up in a cataclysm and totally dislocated. I myself had been responsible for setting the destructive forces into motion, although I had acted with no intent to harm … If I had done something wrong, I certainly was suffering the consequences along with everyone else. Part of the time I was exploring a new planet (a marvellous and breath-taking adventure) but it was too lonely, I could persuade no one to settle there, and I had to get back to the earth somehow. The earth, however, had been devastated by atomic bombs and most of its inhabitants killed. Only a few people – myself and the dimly perceived nursing staff – had escaped. At other times, I felt totally alone on the new planet … At times when the universe was collapsing I was not sure that things would turn out all right. I thought I might have to stay in the endless hell-fire of atomic destruction.[19]

(b) <u>Return to the beginning of life</u>

People may feel they have returned to the beginning of existence and are experiencing the birth of the cosmos or witnessing the unfolding evolutionary process. Though self-healing psychoses usually only last a few weeks, a profoundly altered sense of time may make the duration of events seem infinitely longer. One of Anton Boisen's episodes continued for several weeks in real time, but he felt his inner journey spanned thousands of years:

> The experience … seemed to me that of passing through all the stages of individual development from the single cell onward. At the same time I seemed to be passing through all the stages in the evolution of the race. I was carried back to the period of the

deluge, back to the age of marshes and croaking frogs, back to the age of insects and also an age of birds. I also visited the sun and the moon [and] roamed all around the universe. My conscious self was indeed down in the lower regions at the mercy of all the strange and terrifying phantasms which were to me reality. It was a terrific life and death struggle in which all accepted beliefs and values were overturned, and I did not know what to believe.[20]

Some people may have a vivid experience of consciously reliving their own birth and personal developmental history. One woman felt she was required to repeat creation from the beginning:

That is, she had to go back to the beginning of the world and take part in its creation and evolution again. She was under the sea for a long time, in the presence of great primordial monsters. Then she came on land and saw the age of reptiles. Finally she lived among primitives and took part in their rituals and dances and chants. Also, she had to return to her own beginning, that is, her own birth, and repeat her childhood and growth up to her present age, and in this repetition of her life everything had to be done precisely and without error, otherwise she had to back to the beginning and start over again each time.[21]

(c) Cosmic conflict

People may feel they are caught up in a dramatic conflict of international, even cosmic, proportions involving powerful and mysterious forces. This battle may involve a struggle for world supremacy of polarised forces such as Good and Evil, Light and Dark, Order and Chaos, or Life and Death. Frequently it assumes a specific political or religious form, e.g. Democracy versus Totalitarianism, God versus Satan. An intense struggle may seem to be taking place between different aspects of a person's own being:

A cosmic struggle was going on. The Devil was hatching a plot to destroy the world by an explosion of radioactive substances that he was experimenting with. Opposing him was Christ, who was struggling against him to save the world. Each had followers, thus dividing the world into two camps, the communists in league with the devil to bring about the final disintegration of everything, and the democracies under the banner of Christ to keep the world intact. She said she felt these to be two sides also of her own nature, masculine and feminine sides in conflict. Both the Devil and God were speaking in her ear constantly, in conflict, and especially God's voice was always hilariously funny, cracking jokes and laughing. The Pope was possessed by the Devil, just as [she] was, and was in hell as she was. His hat, the threefold tiara, was torn into little triangular bits of paper which were scattered about the earth, and, at the same time, the Holy Trinity was separated and on earth in the same way, so work had to be done to reunite the Pope's hat and thus the Trinity.[22]

(d) Death and rebirth

Jungian psychology has long maintained that "The archetype of rebirth seems to represent a fundamental mechanism of psychic growth. Each step in the growth of personality requires the death of an old attitude before the new one can emerge."[23] Healing psychoses typically involve a stage during which subjects feel they have died and been reborn. The accompanying imagery is often extremely graphic, e.g. dismemberment (having limbs cut off, bones removed), crucifixion, torture, being poisoned, drowned, buried or cast into prison, or being in an afterlife like heaven or hell. This is eventually followed by a sense of being reborn into a new life, possibly accompanied by the feeling of having become a spiritual being of some kind. Some may be convinced they have given birth to a "royal" or "divine" child. Boisen describes one man's experience of these archetypal themes:

All through his first [psychosis] he was tremendously concerned about the problems of life and death, of survival and destruction ... For a time he thought he was dead and in hell, and in himself he saw diabolical features. Then he was translated into heaven. The trees took on a magnificent appearance. He recognised the work of the supernatural and he thought that the dawn of creation had come. He studied the formation of the clouds and the sky took on for him an appearance wonderful beyond expression. He heard an infinite voice say that six o'clock was the appointed time for the arrival of God's decrees. He visualised himself as passing from an earthly to a spiritual life ... At one time he felt a light within him as though he had touched the Holy Grail ... He identified himself with Jesus, with Augustine, with the martyrs of old. It came to him that the second coming of the Lord was at hand and that in this he himself was to have a most important role to play … He felt that through his disturbance he had found new life and new purpose.[24]

"A Great Cosmic Adventure"

The following case illustrates the characteristically tumultuous and awe-inspiring nature of self-healing psychoses. It also highlights the fact that, as arduous as they may be, such experiences can nevertheless result in substantial personal growth. The subject, a female social worker, underwent three psychotic episodes over a four-year period. For some time before her first episode she experienced mounting emotional distress. The strain of feeling she was failing to care adequately for her three young children led to an impasse in which she was tormented by the belief that she was an incompetent mother. Adding to her woes was the fact that long-standing marital difficulties forced her to make the difficult decision to end her marriage. This precipitated an intense crisis during which she experienced a sense of severe emotional deprivation. At the time, she said, "I seemed to be torn from my moorings and alienated from my former self". The prospect of imminent divorce stirred up intense feelings about childhood hurts which she felt "more keenly in retrospect than I had during my childhood". As she struggled to cope with deepening emotional isolation she felt herself succumbing to depression.

Her first acute psychotic episode began quite abruptly with what she described as "a sudden feeling of creative release". She believed she was rapidly attaining the height of her intellectual powers and that, for the first time in her life, she was finally about to fulfil her true potential. This exhilarating prospect was accompanied by an unshakeable belief she had penetrated the deepest mysteries of life:

> I was suddenly confronted with an overwhelming conviction that I had discovered the secrets of the universe, which were being rapidly made plain with incredible lucidity. The truths discovered seemed to be known immediately and directly, with absolute certainty. I had no sense of doubt or awareness of the possibility of doubt. In spite of former atheism and strong anti-religious sentiments, I was suddenly convinced that it was possible to prove rationally the existence of God.[25]

These realisations filled her entire being with an "audacious and unconquerable spirit". Sensing that she was embarking on a great "cosmic" adventure she began writing compulsively. Convinced she had been chosen to fulfil a vital mission she struggled with the idea that she may be the Messiah – a possibility accompanied by fear of the onerous responsibility of caring for the welfare of humanity. Soon thereafter she was engulfed by a horrifying feeling that a terrible catastrophe had befallen the world, leaving her embroiled in a cosmic struggle between the forces of good and evil for world peace and the salvation of the human species. She was certain her role in this struggle was paramount: "Though I seemed to be almost pulled apart in a disintegrating universe, I felt there must be some way I could hold things together. I was somehow an indispensable link in preventing total collapse".

She became convinced she possessed "cosmic powers" and began to feel she was able to influence the weather as it seemed to respond to her inner moods. She felt she had the ability to control the movements of the sun which had become for her "a mystical symbol of life and of truth". In an effort to prove that truth would not hurt her she stared at the sun for long periods, trying to see how long she could do so without blinking. Ideas about death and rebirth became an obsession: "I wanted to live again in another human life which would be less frustrating than my present one." The feeling she was fulfilling a predominantly maternal role toward the world led her to identify symbolically with Mary, the Mother of Christ.

At times she felt she was being persecuted for her beliefs and entertained paranoid ideas based on the conviction that her enemies were trying to interfere with her activities and wanted to harm or even kill her. She tried to convince people of the correctness of her beliefs but found it was difficult to get people to listen. Her lonely distress was relieved by periods during which she experienced a sense of creative excitement and what felt like moments of intense mystical inspiration.

Most of the experiences described above occurred during this woman's first acute psychotic episode which lasted approximately three weeks. While recovering from her second episode she reflected on the meaning of her psychological ordeals and concluded that what she had been through ultimately had a constructive purpose. She felt that certain personal problems lay at the core of this transformative process: "This was my problem in a nutshell. There was a part of myself that had not been trustworthy, attributes which I had not liked, and which had to be eradicated." She also recognised an intense confrontation with painful images of her mother's death during the psychosis had helped free her from a long-standing emotional dependency:

> During the terrifying first weeks of my illness I went through an experience of separation from my mother which was traumatic in intensity. The feeling I had was about as acute as it would have been had my mother died in the ordinary course of events. I had always dreaded the thought of my mother's death and during my illness I felt that I had lived through this event in advance. I would subsequently be able to react normally, but not to feel a terrible sense of loss for someone on whom I had leaned too heavily. The pain of the separation experience I attribute to the fact that my viewpoint was changing, my own ideas were developing, and that the area in which I could communicate with my mother in the future would be somewhat more restricted. I was also becoming more sharply aware of our dissimilarities in personality and temperament.[26]

It is noteworthy that this woman was given a diagnosis of catatonic schizophrenia, the same diagnosis Anton Boisen received. In-depth study of the various types of acute psychotic crises had led Boisen to conclude: "The *catatonic* type represents a desperate attempt at reorganisation following upon an awareness of danger, which tends either to make or break ... it bears a close relationship to the religious conversion experience."[27]

Psychotherapy formed a major component of the treatment this woman received during each of her three acute psychotic episodes. Looking back over a period of several years which included these episodes she concluded that the painful, at times terrifying, ordeals she underwent had helped bring about lasting improvements in her life. Among these were personality changes that included the loss of a long-standing feeling of chronic anxiety, greater self-confidence, increased independence, more relaxed relationships, less social competitiveness, heightened capacity for interpersonal warmth, enhanced sexual functioning, and development of a religious outlook on life.

Psychosis and Spiritual Emergency

Over the last few decades there has been a burgeoning of interest in spirituality throughout the Western world. This renaissance has made available a wide range of novel practices whose purpose is to foster personal growth by facilitating spiritual experiences of various kinds. Those desiring such experiences are now able to employ a bewildering variety of techniques such as yoga, meditation, guided imagery, experiential psychotherapy, dream work, hypnosis, biofeedback, sensory isolation, past life regression, channelling, trance dance and drumming, and shamanic practices, among many others. In pursuit of spiritual experiences many people have also experimented with illicit drugs – especially those with "mind expanding" properties, e.g. psychedelics such as LSD (see *Chapter Eight*).

Ordinarily, spiritual development is a subtle process in which progress occurs in a gradual, almost imperceptible fashion. Only after a relatively lengthy period of dedicated practice does spiritual awareness mature to the point of producing tangible effects in the practitioner's life. However, it is increasingly being recognised that spiritual phenomena can emerge in a far more rapid and dramatic manner. While this may involve experiences of tremendous spiritual value, the speed and intensity of this process sometimes gives rise to problems. As Dr Assagioli explains, this is especially likely in persons not adequately prepared for such an unanticipated – and possibly unwelcome – occurrence:

> But in some cases, not infrequent, the personality is inadequate in one or more respects and is therefore unable to rightly assimilate the inflow of light and strength. This happens, for instance, when the intellect is not balanced, or the emotions and imagination are uncontrolled; when the nervous system is too sensitive; or when the inrush of spiritual energy is overwhelming in its suddenness and intensity. An incapacity of the mind to stand the illumination, or a tendency to egotism or conceit, may cause the experience to be wrongly interpreted ... Instances of such confusion, more or less pronounced, are not uncommon among people dazzled by contact with truths which are too powerful for their mental capacities to grasp and assimilate ... In other cases the sudden influx of energies produces an emotional upheaval which expresses itself in uncontrolled, unbalanced and disordered behaviour.[28]

Though these dramatic experiences and unusual states of mind may be interpreted as symptoms of severe mental disorder by conventional psychiatry, they are in fact crises of personal transformation. Following intensive research on such phenomena, psychiatrist Stanislav Grof and his colleagues coined the term "spiritual emergency" in recognition of this possibility:

> Many difficult episodes of non-ordinary states of consciousness can be seen as crises of spiritual transformation and opening. Stormy experiences of this kind – or "spiritual emergencies", as we call them – have been repeatedly described in sacred literature of all ages … *Spiritual emergencies* can be defined as critical and experientially difficult stages of a profound psychological transformation that involves one's entire being. They take the form of non-ordinary states of consciousness and involve intense emotions, visions and other sensory changes, and unusual thoughts, as well as various physical manifestations. These episodes often revolve around spiritual themes; they include sequences of psychological death and rebirth, experiences that seem to be memories from previous lifetimes, feelings of oneness with the universe, encounters with various mythological beings, and other similar motifs.[29]

A wide range of circumstances could provoke psychospiritual crises of this kind. The triggering situation may be primarily physical such as an illness, serious accident or operation, extreme exhaustion, or prolonged sleep deprivation, all of which can result in a significant lowering of psychological defences. The extreme physical and emotional stress of childbirth may provoke a spontaneous transformational crisis. A spiritual emergency could be triggered by an overwhelming emotional experience, especially one that involves profound loss, e.g. death of a loved one, acrimonious divorce, financial catastrophe. Other possible triggers include intense inner experiences such as may occur in connection with use of potent mind-altering drugs or in the context of deep experiential psychotherapy. Although spiritual emergencies sometimes occur spontaneously, the single most important catalyst for such experiences is intensive involvement with spiritual practices – especially those which facilitate access to non-ordinary states of consciousness or which are intended to induce mystical experiences (examples of such techniques were listed at the beginning of this section).

Whatever the trigger happens to be, the ensuing psychospiritual crisis invariably entails a radical shift in the balance between conscious and unconscious mental processes with the result that previously unconscious material enters awareness. If this occurs in an intense and dramatic fashion to a person unprepared, it could significantly disrupt their psychological, emotional, and social functioning. While spiritual emergencies can take a wide variety of forms depending on the nature of the material flooding consciousness, the affected person is invariably preoccupied with deeply moving experiences arising from the depths of their being:

> When spiritual emergence is very rapid and dramatic ... this natural process can become a crisis, and *spiritual emergence becomes spiritual emergency*. People who are in such a crisis are bombarded with inner experiences that abruptly challenge their old beliefs and ways of existing, and their relationship with reality shifts very rapidly. Suddenly they feel uncomfortable in the formerly familiar world and may find it difficult to meet the demands of everyday life. They can have great problems distinguishing their inner visionary world from the external world of daily reality. Physically, they may experience forceful energies streaming through their bodies and causing uncontrollable tremors. Fearful and resistant, they might spend much time and effort trying to control what feels like an overwhelming inner event. And they may feel impelled to talk about their experiences and insights to anyone who is within range, sounding out of touch with reality, disjointed, or messianic.[30]

The various types of spiritual emergency identified by Dr Grof and his colleagues are described briefly below. (Since the boundaries between these are somewhat arbitrary experiences associated with more than one category may sometimes be evident.)

Episodes of unitive consciousness
This experience is characterised by a sense of stepping outside the boundaries of ordinary reality, transcending the limits of space and time, and entering a realm characterised by a feeling of complete inner unity and wholeness. The temporary melting away of personal boundaries ("ego dissolution") may be accompanied by a feeling of ecstatic oneness with nature, humankind, the universe, and God ("mystical union") that induces intense joy, bliss, serenity, and inner

peace. While in this state some may feel they have been granted access to ultimate knowledge and spiritual wisdom so that answers to perennial "meaning of life" questions seem absolutely obvious. Though mystical experiences may have lasting beneficial effects, problems sometimes arise as a result of failure to understand their true nature or difficulty integrating the profound insights gained.

Kundalini awakening
Hindu yogis believe a subtle energy called *kundalini* creates and sustains the cosmos and all life. Also referred to as the Serpent Power, this energy is believed to reside in latent form at the base of the human spine where it is depicted symbolically as a coiled serpent (kundalini literally means "she who is coiled"). When activated, kundalini changes into its fiery form, known as *Shakti*, which rises up the spine opening subtle spiritual centres called *chakras* as it moves towards the seventh or "crown" chakra at the top of the head. Awakened kundalini energy is believed to have the power to purify and heal the body and mind and to promote spiritual insight and awareness. The process of clearing the residue of old physical and mental traumas can be accompanied by a range of sometimes dramatic psychophysiological manifestations (*kriyas*). These include intense sensations of heat and energy streaming up the spine, waves of powerful emotions (both positive and negative), vivid memories of past traumatic experiences, spontaneous movements such as trembling, shaking, yogic postures and gestures, involuntary vocalisation (crying, laughing, speaking in tongues, making animal sounds), vivid sensory phenomena (visions, inner sounds and smells), and intense sexual arousal possibly involving orgasmic sensations. Though it is inherently beneficial and healing, a powerful kundalini awakening can cause considerable apprehension related to loss of control and fear of impending insanity or death.[*]

---

[*] Although the philosophy associated with kundalini originated in India this phenomenon is *not* the sole province of Hindu yoga practitioners. Psychiatrist Lee Sanella has found kundalini experiences are reported throughout modern industrial societies. Indeed, Dr Sanella believes many Western medical and psychiatric patients experience a syndrome closely matching ancient descriptions of kundalini awakening. Sanella, L. (1987) *The Kundalini Experience: Psychosis or Transcendence?* Lower Lake, Ca: Integral Publishing.

Near-death experience

The testimony of individuals who have come close to dying – some having experienced actual clinical death – but subsequently recovered has led to the realisation that many have had profound, intensely moving experiences while in the near-death state.[31] First person accounts have established that a typical near-death experience (NDE) involves a series of characteristic events: feelings of great peace, an out-of-body experience (consciousness detached from the stricken body), the sensation of travelling through a dark tunnel toward a brilliant light, an encounter with "spirits" of deceased relatives and friends or a "Being of Light", and an instantaneous life review. People who have had a powerful NDE may feel they have been given a precious opportunity to change their life so it is more in line with the spiritual insights afforded them. In such cases a near-death experience can serve as a powerful catalyst of spiritual awakening and personal transformation. However, the occurrence of an intense NDE could provoke great distress in some people, especially if it presents an unwelcome challenge to a rigidly held and highly materialistic world view and orientation.

Emergence of "past-life memories"

So-called "past-life memories" involve the vivid recollection of events which appear to be related to experiences from some former life. Such memories, which may entail detailed recollection of particular persons, circumstances, historical periods and cultural settings, are often centred on some emotionally-charged event or situation. Those who accept the idea of reincarnation may have little difficulty believing that these are "karmic memories" of a previous life. In any event, such experiences can have a deep psychological impact. Emergence of apparent past-life memories can have positive effects, e.g. providing insight into otherwise inexplicable aspects of behaviour such as irrational fears, difficulty relating to certain people or situations, obscure emotional problems, and intractable psychosomatic symptoms. Experiences of this kind could also cause problems. For example, if "past-life memories" are close to the surface but have not fully emerged into awareness they could provoke a range of psychological and physical effects, e.g. feelings, impulses, and bodily sensations with no obvious cause or explanation. In certain circumstances (e.g. childbirth, psychedelic drug states) a sequence of vivid "past-life memories" could surface abruptly and severely disturb the subject's mental state, behaviour, and reality-orientation.

Shamanic crisis

The term "shaman" refers to the traditional healers found in many non-Western cultures. Also known colloquially as "medicine men" or "witch doctors", shamans are specifically empowered to do their healing work by virtue of their ability to communicate with the "spirit world". In many cultures the process of becoming a shaman involves an initiatory crisis characterised by an involuntary period of severe physical, mental, and spiritual disturbance – the so-called "shamanic illness". There is growing evidence that people in Western cultures can sometimes have experiences strikingly similar to those of traditional shamans.[32] Such spontaneous shamanic experiences typically involve a "journey into the underworld" (realm of spirits) where people may experience themselves being attacked, dismembered, killed, and eaten by vicious demonic animals. This harrowing process of annihilation is typically followed by an experience of resurrection and rebirth and ascent to a heavenly realm ("Upper World") where animals previously encountered may reappear to serve as spirit guides, protectors, and wisdom teachers ("power animals"). Shamanic experiences such as these may be relatively brief (e.g. occurring while under the influence of a psychedelic drug), but sometimes last far longer, possibly many days. Their powerful, reality-shaking nature could provoke fear, psychological disorientation, and doubts about one's sanity.

Awakening of extrasensory perception ("psychic opening")

Spiritual emergence sometimes manifests in the form of heightened intuitive powers and the spontaneous acquisition of apparently paranormal or "psychic" abilities. Sometimes referred to collectively as "extrasensory perception" (ESP), the latter include phenomena such as precognition, telepathy, and remote viewing. In the course of a psychic opening some people appear to develop an inexplicable telepathic sensitivity such that they seem capable of "reading" minds and knowing what others are thinking. Some people may have seemingly accurate premonitions regarding future events. Another phenomenon that may occur in the context of psychic opening involves so-called "out-of-body" experiences in which consciousness is felt to detach itself from the body, so that the person concerned is able to watch him or herself from some vantage point outside their physical being. This disembodied consciousness might even "travel" to other locations – possibly including far distant ones – from where it is able to witness events without recourse to the physical senses. Psychic opening is often accompanied by a dramatic increase in the occurrence of remarkable coincidences such that people may feel their innermost thoughts, feelings, dreams, and intuitions have become attuned with outer reality in some inexplicable way, e.g. a person may have unexpected contact with a long lost acquaintance shortly after thinking about them for the first time in many years. (Jung coined the term *synchronicity* to refer to such meaningful coincidences, which he believed reflected the operation of a universal acausal connecting principle.[33]) Dr Grof has noted that genuine synchronicities can occur during *any* type of spiritual emergence but are especially frequent in the context of psychic opening. The sudden acquisition of apparently paranormal abilities together with the occurrence of inexplicable synchronicities could be disconcerting and confusing, especially to those unfamiliar with or sceptical about this realm of experience.

Communication with spirit guides and channelling
The philosophy of spiritualism rests on the belief that there exist departed human spirits with which it is possible to communicate. So-called "mediums" allegedly have the ability to contact such spirits during séances, with some claiming to be able to speak with them and hear their replies to questions. The phenomenon known as trance "channelling" is a contemporary form of mediumship in which various non-physical entities are alleged to speak through the chanel/medium using his or her vocal apparatus. While in non-ordinary states of consciousness some people may experience contact with what appear to be non-physical "entities" or "beings" of various kinds. Such beings, which are felt to be separate from and independent of the person encountering them, can manifest as discarnate human individuals, non-human entities, or various deities which supposedly inhabit higher planes of consciousness and possess knowledge far exceeding that of ordinary human beings. During intense psychospiritual crises some people feel they have come into direct contact with non-physical presences such as spirits of the deceased, astral entities, or supernatural beings. These sometimes serve beneficial functions such as teacher, guide, or protector. Unanticipated contact with apparently

autonomous non-physical entities could provoke considerable distress, especially in those committed to a materialistic world view.

Possession states

Possession refers to a state in which an individual's body and/or mind appears to have been invaded and possibly taken over by some kind of alien entity or energy with personal characteristics. When apparently malevolent entities or energies are involved the state is commonly referred to as *demonic* possession. This phenomenon also encompasses *benign* possession, i.e. by a benevolent influence exerting positive effects. In many non-Western cultures various beneficent spirits, deities, and energies are purposely invoked and invited to possess participants in healing rituals or sacred ceremonies. Many Christians consider possession by the Holy Spirit to be highly desirable. Possession states vary in intensity and generally occur only occasionally or intermittently, though they can become more persistent. Even when it involves benign influences, the loss of control associated with unanticipated onset of a state involving apparent possession by unfamiliar entities or energies can provoke fear and distress, both in the "possessed" individual and others.

Experiences of close encounters with UFOs

Many people report having had close encounters with what they believe were alien beings. Some even claim to have been taken on board extraterrestrial spacecraft (UFOs) by such beings and subjected to intimate physical examinations and other procedures against their will. While there is currently no scientific evidence to support the objective reality of such phenomena, individuals reporting these experiences are often deeply traumatised by what they believe happened to them. Psychiatrist Professor John Mack's in-depth research on the psychological impact of supposed "alien abduction" experiences found that they often provoke extreme emotional, intellectual, and spiritual crises in those undergoing them.[34] Many report that the experience shattered their former beliefs about the nature of reality, forcing them to question their identity and the place of human beings in the universe. For some, resolution of such a crisis may culminate in a personal transformation marked by a radically altered sense of their place in the cosmic design and a more respectful attitude toward the mystery of life.[35]

Psychological renewal through return to the centre

Dr John Perry has conducted pioneering research into the nature and dynamics of this type of autonomous transformational crisis. This phenomenon, which he considers a profound psychological "renewal process", typically centres around images of death and rebirth and the eventual merging and harmonisation of discordant aspects of the subject's personality. This type of profound healing crisis was described in detail earlier in this chapter under the heading "Psychosis as a Self-Healing Process".

Successful resolution of the crisis of spiritual emergence can help clear the deep-seated traumatic memories and psychological imprints responsible for a variety of mental and psychosomatic disorders. Dr Grof has also observed improved self-esteem, a reduction in anger and aggression, greater tolerance of other people, and enhancement in quality of life in many who have undergone these healing crises:

> Spiritual emergency takes many forms ... We have observed in countless cases that these conditions do not necessarily precipitate a plunge into insanity. When we treat such crises with respect and support, they can result in remarkable healing, a more positive and spiritual outlook, and a higher level of functioning in everyday life. For this reason, we must take spiritual emergencies seriously no matter how bizarre their manifestations may seem when viewed from the perspective of our traditional belief systems.[36]

> The concept of spiritual emergency is gradually being brought to the attention of mainstream mental health clinicians via the increasingly frequent appearance of erudite discussions of this phenomenon in orthodox professional publications.[37]*

A Meaningful Disturbance

A key principal emphasised by Dr Perry and others who follow Jung's lead is the notion that, like the physical body, *the human psyche is*

---

* In 1980 Dr Grof and his colleagues founded the *Spiritual Emergence Network* (SEN) to provide support, information, and referral to individuals experiencing spiritual emergencies and other psychospiritual crises. There is now a world-wide network of similar groups which can be contacted by following the links on the SEN website: www.spiritualemergence.info. An Australian affiliate of the Spiritual Emergence Network can be contacted at www.spiritualemergence.org.au.

a self-regulating system. As such it is has an innate ability to activate autonomous processes in the specific form needed to restore balance and promote healing. Dramatic psychospiritual crises of the kind described in this chapter may sometimes be absolutely *necessary* to overcome developmental constrictions, release untapped potentials, and impel a wounded soul on its journey toward wholeness. This sometimes entails the virtual dismantling of the ego and its repertoire of maladaptive defences (experienced as death or world destruction) and its subsequent reorganisation in a form better able to meet the demands of life (experienced as rebirth).

These ideas are congruent with the observations of such internationally recognised experts as psychiatrist Harry Stack Sullivan, who pioneered psychotherapeutic treatment of schizophrenia and other psychoses in the United States. Dr Sullivan found that some of his patients who had been excessively sensitive, self-conscious, and emotionally unstable emerged from psychotic crises with these difficulties overcome or greatly alleviated. He noted that, when they recovered, such persons had a more open and adaptable personality, enhanced self-esteem, and a greater capacity to discuss their problems frankly.[38]

Such observations are corroborated by the personal testimonies of those who have grown as a result of having experienced and successfully resolved a psychospiritual crisis. In spite of its extremely harrowing nature Maryanne Handel felt her own psychotic ordeal was a *meaningful disturbance* from which she learnt a great deal:

> Maybe there is a disturbance in your brain. But if that is so, then it must mean something about your brain, that it's indicating something about your emotional state. What is it indicating? What does it mean? My feeling was that the psychosis was there to teach me something. And it did teach me something! It did show me things and I did change through it and because of it I understood many things. Things I suppose that had always been wrong which perhaps I never would have come to understand if the psychosis had not happened to me, if I had not been through that absolute process. Maybe I would have gone on without ever really changing that much. It is a disturbance, of course, but it's a *meaningful* disturbance, and something that has to be understood before you can change and before it will go away.[39]

While he acknowledged that on one level they were undoubtedly mental disorders of a most severe kind, Anton Boisen was nevertheless certain psychospiritual crises hold tremendous healing potential. However, understanding and integrating the lessons of such crises is a task whose difficulty should not be underestimated. Indeed, it would be a grave error to assume healing occurs as an *automatic* result of undergoing such ordeals. On the contrary, Dr Perry emphasises that healing requires hard inner work and painstaking effort on the part of the person concerned and his or her helpers.

Sadly, it is still common for people experiencing potentially transformative crises to be diagnosed severely mentally ill and treated with potent "anti-psychotic" medications. Such responses are only likely to compound any fear the person in crisis (and others, such as relatives and friends) may have had about their sanity. Furthermore, by interfering with the operation of natural healing processes underlying such crises, conventional psychiatric treatment might inadvertently thwart healing and recovery.

Psychospiritual crises differ greatly in essential nature from psychoses described in the previous chapter as psychological crises. The responses appropriate to each are also significantly different. This raises a crucial issue: how can crises with a potentially healing purpose and outcome be distinguished from those of a more mundane kind? This question is discussed in detail in *Chapter Nine*. Meanwhile, it is timely to consider the increasingly common phenomenon of psychoses arising in the context of illicit drug use.

Chapter Seven

Varieties Of Psychotic Experience III: Drug-Induced Psychosis

Human beings will always want to suspend everyday reality, be it by legal means or otherwise, and they will always be at least curious about alternate states of consciousness.

Charles Hayes[1]

People who use illicit drugs sometimes have psychosis-like experiences or even become frankly psychotic. If hallucinations, delusions and allied phenomena are directly related to the effects of drugs, a diagnosis of Substance-Induced Psychotic Disorder is often given.[*] Commonly known as "drug-induced psychosis", such episodes can occur while people are under the influence of drugs or withdrawing from them.

Despite their illegal status a wide variety of illicit drugs are readily available and widely used and/or abused throughout contemporary Western societies. As a consequence, drug-induced psychosis is diagnosed with ever-increasing frequency. Widespread use of illicit drugs – particularly among young people – has helped fuel the belief that conditions like schizophrenia and bipolar disorder are sometimes directly or indirectly related to such use. If a person with a history of drug use develops a psychotic disorder, suspicion may arise that drugs have "triggered" the condition – a belief reflected in lay expressions such as "drug-induced schizophrenia". It might even be assumed that the drugs are responsible for *causing* the disorder.

This chapter examines the relationship between illicit drug use and certain types of psychosis. While in no way condoning abuse of such drugs, in keeping with the theme of preceding chapters it will be argued that, even if they occur in association with illicit drug

---

[*] The term "substance" is used formally to differentiate illicit drugs from prescription medications which many people also refer to as "drugs". This use also allows for the possibility that certain ingestible – and potentially abuseable – materials are, strictly-speaking, not drugs. Examples include inhalants such as petrol, glues, and aerosol paints. For the sake of clarity, the familiar term "drug" is used throughout this chapter.

use, psychotic episodes are never a *purely* biological phenomenon. It will be suggested, furthermore, that some states routinely diagnosed as "drug-induced psychosis" according to conventional psychiatric criteria may nevertheless involve experiences with profound personal and/or spiritual significance.

As noted at the beginning of the previous chapter, the clinical term "psychosis" is simply too narrow to encompass mental states of the kind alluded to above. In *Chapter Six*, "psychotic altered state of consciousness" was proposed as a possible alternative as it does not imply a state of illness or disease. In this chapter it might be appropriate to refer to "drug-induced psychotic altered states of consciousness" but since such expressions are extremely unwieldy the simplistic term "psychosis" will be used throughout the following discussion. Readers should understand that this term is not meant to imply the states under consideration necessarily involve "illness" in the usual medical sense.

Psychoactive Drugs

Modern scientific understanding of the way psychoactive drugs affect human behaviour generally, and the mind in particular, is still surprisingly limited. While this is partly due to the complexity of the phenomena involved, it is also a product of the fact that most research focuses on the *physical*, rather than *mental*, effects of these intriguing substances. As a result, far more is known about how drugs alter activity of the brain's neurons and neurotransmitters (chemical messengers) than is known about their multifarious subjective effects, such as on the user's sense of self, emotions, perceptual and thought processes, and state of consciousness. (This is analogous to psychiatry's approach to psychosis – and mental disorders generally – in that more attention is devoted to identifying neurological mechanisms than to understanding the lived experience of diagnosed individuals.)

This unsatisfactory state of affairs has not been helped by the fact that research on the effects of one of the most important and interesting classes of psychoactive drugs – the psychedelics – has been banned until very recently. In this context it is thought-provoking to realise that, while scientific understanding of the psychology of drug-induced states is extremely limited, traditional shamanic cultures have studied the effects of psychoactive substances on body, mind, and soul for thousands of years and applied this accumulated knowledge with great wisdom and skill. This important theme is revisited below and in *Chapter Eight*.

The huge variety of psychoactive drugs known to exist can, in the first instance, be divided into three broad groups:

Social Drugs: a number of quite potent psychoactive drugs are widely used and generally considered socially acceptable when consumed in moderation. Familiar examples include caffeine, alcohol, and nicotine (in tobacco).

Therapeutic Drugs: a wide range of medically-prescribed psychoactive drugs are used for the purposes of inducing desired changes in mood, thinking, perception, and behaviour. Members of this large group include common psychiatric medications such as hypnotics (sleep-inducing drugs), anxiolytics (anxiety-relieving), antidepressants, mood stabilisers, and neuroleptics (anti-psychotic).

Illicit Drugs: a wide variety of psychoactive drugs are outlawed in many countries. Those declared illegal include a large number of synthetically-produced drugs as well as many that occur naturally in various plants.[2]

Psychopharmacologists assign psychoactive drugs to various categories according to their principal behavioural effects.[3] Some drugs have such a broad range of effects it would be inappropriate to confine them to a single category, e.g. marijuana can have both sedative and psychedelic effects. For the purposes of this chapter the following classification has been used:

(1) Drugs that Depress Brain Function: Sedative-Hypnotics

A large number of psychoactive drugs lower the level of activity in specific areas of the brain and central nervous system (CNS). These CNS-depressant drugs reduce anxiety and induce feelings of calmness and relaxation, hence their use as "sedatives". Higher dosages induce drowsiness and sleep. Prominent members of this class include:

Alcohol: initial effects at low doses include physical and mental relaxation and euphoria (feeling of wellbeing). Higher doses produce disinhibition which could result in impulsive or uncharacteristic aggressive and/or violent behaviour. Heavy intoxication can provoke disinhibition, unpredictable emotional outbursts, hallucinations, delusions, and subsequent amnesia ("blackouts") for the period concerned. Prolonged consumption of large amounts of alcohol could culminate in psychosis. A withdrawal syndrome referred to as delirium tremens ("DTs") can occur shortly (within 48 hours) of reducing or stopping alcohol after a period of heavy drinking. This syndrome typically involves frightening hallucinations, confusion, agitation, tremulousness, disorientation, and sleep disturbance.

Benzodiazepines: sometimes known as "benzos" these medically prescribed Valium-type drugs alleviate anxiety (anxiolytic effect) and induce sleep (hypnotic effect). Prolonged use could result in physical and/or psychological dependence. Benzodiazepine withdrawal may lead to resurgence of anxiety for which the drug was originally prescribed ("rebound anxiety") possibly to an even more intense level, and to intensification of sleep problems ("rebound insomnia"). Periods of restless agitation with hallucinations or psychosis have been observed during benzodiazepine withdrawal.

Volatile inhalants: include a wide variety of organic solvents and other chemicals which readily vaporise when exposed to air. Commonly abused inhalants include petrol, aerosol (spray) paints, glues, paint thinners, nail polish remover, correction fluid, and marker pen solvent. Inhalation ("sniffing") induces light-headedness, euphoria, disinhibition, sedation, delirium, and mental changes similar to alcohol intoxication or light general anaesthesia. Severe intoxication can provoke hallucinations, impairment of higher cognitive functions, loss of co-ordination, and staggering gait. A so-called "inhalation psychosis" characterised by transient visual and auditory hallucinations and paranoid delusions sometimes occurs after prolonged use of these substances by susceptible individuals.[4]

Note: Although nitrous oxide is sometimes classified as an inhalant, its unique properties justify its inclusion among drugs possessing psychedelic effects – see heading (4) below.

(2) Drugs that Stimulate Brain Function: Psychostimulants
Psychostimulant drugs increase neuronal and metabolic activity in the brain resulting in heightened alertness, elevated mood, and greater physical and mental energy. These drugs reduce fatigue, suppress appetite and allay sleep. Prominent examples include:

Caffeine: undoubtedly the world's most popular psychoactive drug, caffeine is consumed in a multitude of forms including tea, coffee, cola drinks, and chocolate. Moderate doses result in increased mental alertness, wakefulness, and a heightened feeling of wellbeing. Excessive consumption can cause anxiety, agitation, tachycardia (accelerated heart rate), and insomnia. Persons with underlying anxiety or an established psychotic disorder may be particularly sensitive to caffeine and could experience physical and/or psychological distress when even small amounts are consumed ("caffeine intolerance").

Nicotine: nicotine is a potent psychoactive drug having numerous effects throughout the central nervous system. Users often claim smoking helps improve their concentration and mental capacity, but nicotine can cause nervousness and tremors at higher doses and is associated with an increased incidence of panic attacks and/or panic disorder. Nicotine is extremely addictive and regular users can experience craving and mental and physical withdrawal symptoms if they abstain even for short periods.

Amphetamines: referred to generically as "speed", these synthetic compounds are potent stimulants whose effects depend on the particular drug, dose, and route of administration.* Amphetamines have a range of physical and mental effects including heightened alertness and energy, excitement, feelings of power and self-confidence, exhilaration or euphoria, enhanced capacity for work, decreased need for sleep, and diminished appetite. Tolerance develops rapidly and ever-increasing doses may be required to achieve the desired effects. Regular users readily develop psychological dependence accompanied by intense craving. Abuse can provoke various adverse psychological effects including restlessness, tension, anxiety, and fear which may become so intense it leads to panic. A characteristic state of intense physical and mental letdown ("crash") occurs when regular consumption ceases (abstinence is sometimes undertaken voluntarily by users experiencing unpleasant effects after sustained heavy use). Amphetamine crashes are characterised by extreme lethargy, fatigue, bewilderment, anxiety, confusion, and terrifying nightmares. During periods of abstinence heavy users typically experience extreme

---

* Medically-prescribed amphetamines (e.g. dexamphetamine) and drugs with an amphetamine-like stimulant effect (e.g. methylphenidate) are commonly used to treat attention deficit hyperactivity disorder (ADHD).

irritability, possibly accompanied by demanding, aggressive, or violent behaviour. Prolonged consumption of high dosages can provoke a psychotic state ("amphetamine psychosis") characterised by anorexia (loss of appetite), continual, purposeless, repetitive behaviour, sudden outbursts of aggression, and paranoia. This state resembles paranoid schizophrenia and usually occurs during bouts of heavy amphetamine abuse but can also occur during withdrawal. Depression, which may persist for weeks and become so severe the affected individual becomes suicidal, can also occur as part of the withdrawal syndrome.

The recent advent of a potent, smokeable form of methamphetamine – commonly known as "ice" or "crystal meth" – has resulted in a significant increase in the incidence of amphetamine-induced psychotic reactions characterised by grandiosity, a reckless sense of invulnerability, paranoia, aggression and senseless violence. Symptoms provoked by "ice" may be transitory (minutes or hours) but prolonged use can induce a florid psychotic state that may persist for days or weeks *after* consumption stops. It is now believed heavy users of methamphetamine could incur potentially irreversible brain damage as a result of its toxic effects on neurons that manufacture dopamine and serotonin.[5]

MDMA ("**Ecstasy**"): methylene-dioxy-methamphetamine is a derivative of methamphetamine with amphetamine-like stimulant effects and mild LSD-like psychedelic effects. Favoured by participants in extended dance parties known as "raves", Ecstasy users describe experiencing heightened sensory awareness, an enhanced sense of wellbeing, and elevated mood which may reach the level of an intensely euphoric or even blissful "high" (hence the drug's street name). This drug is reputed to enhance emotional sensitivity and dissolve inner barriers to feeling and insight allowing users to experience a feeling of uninhibited connection with other people – hence its reputation as a "heart-opening" drug or *empathogen* ("engendering empathy"). Concerns have increasingly been expressed regarding possible toxic effects of Ecstasy on the human brain.[6] A recent Australian survey found many users had experienced psychological difficulties including confusion, depression, anxiety, auditory and visual hallucinations, paranoia, and panic attacks (though these experiences tend to be short-lived and mainly occur while using the drug or when its effect is wearing off).[7] A "comedown" during which people feel listless, melancholic, and emotionally burned out is well-known to regular users. There is growing concern some heavy Ecstasy users may be at risk of long-term cognitive impairment and disturbances of mood and personality.[8*]

Cocaine: a powerful psychostimulant obtained from leaves of *Erythroxylon coca*, a plant used in South America since ancient times for religious, medicinal, and social purposes. In relatively low doses cocaine produces increased energy and alertness, a heightened sense of wellbeing, exhilaration, and euphoria. While intoxicated users often become talkative, possibly to the point of incoherence, and may experience racing thoughts. The pleasurable effects of cocaine last for approximately 30 to 90 minutes, after which time the user may desire more of the drug in order to reproduce the enjoyable state. Tolerance develops with prolonged use so that increasing doses are required to obtain the original euphoric "high" and avoid withdrawal symptoms. Common modes of ingestion include "snorting" cocaine powder and intravenous administration. Highly concentrated smokeable preparations with a very rapid effect, e.g. so-called "crack" cocaine, encourage users to increase the dosage, frequency, and duration of use, thus greatly exacerbating the risk of toxicity and eventual dependency. Heavy cocaine users may experience rebound depression and an associated craving for the drug. Higher doses can have psychotoxic effects which include anxiety, impulsiveness, sleep disturbance, hypervigilance, suspiciousness, and paranoia. Sustained long-term use may intensify these negative effects until a vicious circle is established. High-dose, long-term use of cocaine can provoke a bizarre, violent psychotic state ("toxic paranoid psychosis") marked by anxiety, paranoia, impaired reality testing, compulsively repetitive behaviour, and vivid visual, auditory, and tactile hallucinations (the latter often involving the sensation of insects crawling under the skin, so-called "cocaine bugs"). This state can persist for days or weeks *after*

---

[*] There is ongoing debate regarding possible neurological toxicity of Ecstasy. Some authorities believe heavy use may result in lasting adverse effects such as sleep disturbance, anxiety, depression, impulsiveness, hostility, and memory impairment. Dehydration and hyperthermia (overheating) resulting from prolonged physical exertion in poorly-ventilated dance clubs may contribute to these adverse effects. In view of the many unanswered questions regarding potential hazards of this popular recreational drug, extreme caution is certainly warranted.

abuse of the drug ceases. Chronic heavy cocaine abuse is reputedly capable of inducing almost all known psychiatric syndromes including mood disorders (mania or depression), schizophrenia-like states, anxiety disorders, and personality disorders.[9] Prolonged heavy cocaine use may eventually result in damage to dopamine-sensitive cells in the brain's "pleasure centre".[10]

(3) Drugs that Alleviate Pain: Opioid Analgesics

Opiates are powerful analgesic (pain-relieving) and euphoriant drugs that occur naturally in exudate of the opium poppy *Papaver somniferum*. Morphine and codeine are the two main psychoactive compounds in raw opium. For thousands of years opium and various opium-based preparations have been employed for medicinal and recreational purposes. During the nineteenth and early twentieth centuries an alcoholic tincture of opium known as "laudanum" was legally available and widely used throughout the Western world for its pain-relieving and sleep-inducing effects. However, the euphoriant properties of opiates led to their widespread abuse and concern about the growing incidence of dependence led to prohibition of non-medical use of all opium products in 1914. Opioids are a large group of drugs, both naturally-occurring and synthetic, that mimic the effects of opiates. These drugs are extremely effective in alleviating emotional and physical pain. Prolonged use of opioids results in development of tolerance and, eventually, physical dependence. Opioid withdrawal is characterised by symptoms that are the opposite of the drugs' initial effects, i.e. anxiety, restlessness, irritability, insomnia, physical discomfort, and intense craving. Prominent members of the opioid group include morphine, codeine, and heroin.

Morphine: this potent analgesic compound makes up approximately 10% of the content of crude opium extract. Still the most effective analgesic known, morphine is used in the medical management of severe pain. Morphine induces intense analgesia and indifference to pain, sedation, relaxed euphoria (described by users as ecstatic or even sexual), feelings of contentment, tranquillity, and heightened wellbeing. The euphoric effects of morphine gradually diminish with repeated exposure and habitual users invariably develop physical dependence.

Codeine: codeine is often combined with aspirin or other analgesics in over-the-counter preparations used to relieve mild or moderate pain. Codeine is converted into morphine by metabolic processes in the liver. Abuse of codeine-containing medications is common.

Heroin: known medically as diacetyl morphine, this drug is a slightly modified form of naturally-occurring morphine which is three times more potent than its parent compound. Heroin induces an intensely pleasurable euphoric "high" when smoked or injected. Heroin is sometimes smoked in combination with "crack" cocaine, a practice that produces more intense euphoria and less anxiety and paranoia commonly associated with cocaine.

Psychosis is not usually associated with opioid abuse. However, a prolonged withdrawal syndrome characterised by mood disturbance and craving can continue for months or even longer after cessation of use.

(4) Drugs with Hallucinogenic/Psychedelic Properties

A large variety of substances, both naturally-occurring and synthetic, possess the ability to induce profound changes in the user's sense of self and perception of reality. These drugs are sometimes called "hallucinogens" because of their characteristic effects on perception, which can range from causing illusions and perceptual distortions to the induction of vivid hallucinations. Often classified as "psychedelic" because of their reputed ability to expand awareness and induce profound spiritual experiences (claims discussed in *Chapter Eight*). Psychedelic substances occur naturally in a host of indigenous herbs, fungi, vines, cacti, shrubs, and other plants. Although proscribed in most Western societies, an impressive variety of these potent psychoactive substances have long been employed for healing and ritual purposes in traditional shamanic cultures where they are regarded as sacraments and medicines.[11] Many psychedelics consumed for "recreational" purposes are manufactured synthetically.

The psychedelic group is so diverse it is difficult to describe specific drug effects. General effects include: induction of a dream-like state; intensification of feelings (both positive and negative); profound changes in sensation, perception, and sense of self; and altered sense of time. Important members of this large group include the following (the first three often being regarded as "classic" psychedelics):

LSD ("acid"): lysergic acid diethylamide is probably the most well-known psychedelic. Though its primary chemical constituent is a naturally-occurring substance derived from ergot (a parasitic rye fungus), the drug LSD is manufactured synthetically. Regarded by many as the quintessential psychedelic, LSD is an extraordinarily powerful psychoactive substance with effects lasting from 6 to 12 hours. During an LSD-induced "trip" users can experience a bewildering variety of extreme and unpredictable psychological phenomena which may include true synaesthesia (seeing sounds, hearing colours), arousal of intense emotions, vivid recollection of past events (possibly accompanied by a convincing sense of reliving them), and alteration or even temporary loss of self-boundaries. Many users feel that, by virtue of its unparalleled ability to induce profound spiritual experiences and insights, LSD can increase self-awareness and enhance self-understanding. Critics, on the other hand, consider it a dangerous drug whose users risk serious psychological harm.

Mescaline: the peyote cactus *Lophophora Williamsii* contains numerous psychoactive substances including the potent psychedelic, mescaline. Aztec and other Mexican Indians have used peyote since pre-Columbian times in their healing and religious ceremonies. Contemporary adherents of the Native American Church, whose use of peyote is legally sanctioned, regard it as a sacrament and employ it in their shamanic rituals. The subjective effects are similar to those of LSD, though mescaline tends to elicit characteristic visual phenomena including intense kaleidoscopic visions of brilliant lights, brightly-coloured geometric shapes and patterns, and visions of animals (which, in the context of ritual use, often have totemic significance to members of the user's tribe). A mescaline-induced "trip" lasts up to 10 hours.

Psilocybin ("magic mushrooms"): several species of mushrooms, particularly members of the *Psilocybe* genus, contain potent psychoactive substances. Like peyote, these plants have long been utilised for ritual purposes by various native cultures of North and Central America. So revered were these mushrooms by the Aztecs that they referred to them as "flesh of the gods". *Psilocybe* mushrooms grow wild in many regions of the world, users often referring to them by descriptive colloquial names such as "blue meanies" and "gold tops". The principle psychedelic in "magic mushrooms" is psilocybin, a compound with effects similar to LSD though far less potent. A psilocybin-induced experience typically lasts 4 to 6 hours.

DMT: (dimethyl tryptamine) this naturally-occurring psychedelic is found in a wide range of indigenous plants used in shamanic cultures throughout the world (e.g. it is one of the principal psychoactive ingredients in ayahuasca, the South American traditional medicine known as "vine of the soul"). Since it is readily manufactured in a laboratory illicit DMT is usually synthetic. A potent drug with LSD-like effects, DMT is possibly the strongest of all psychedelics. A distinguishing feature of the DMT experience is its extreme intensity and short duration: when snorted or smoked, mental effects begin rapidly with a powerful "rush" but are usually over within 30 minutes. Users report extremely bizarre experiences typically involving a vivid sense of being catapulted into an extraordinary otherworldly realm (sometimes described as "hyperspace") populated by strange non-human entities. Casual users often find the DMT experience so intense, overwhelming, and frightening they vow never to take the drug again.

Datura: many plants belonging to the *Datura* species contain psychoactive compounds, in particular the psychedelic scopolamine. Among plants containing scopolamine one of the most familiar is the "Angel's Trumpet", an ornamental shrub found in many public parks and household gardens. The flowers, seeds, and leaves of this plant are consumed for their psychoactive effects. Low doses cause mild euphoria, confusion, lethargy and drowsiness. Higher doses can induce a state of delirious intoxication (toxic psychosis) characterised by euphoria, excitement, restlessness, hallucinations, and disorientation. In contrast to other psychedelics, scopolamine does not foster heightened or expanded awareness but a dulling or clouding of consciousness. A characteristic of scopolamine-induced states is partial or complete amnesia for the experience.

Psychedelic Anaesthetics: a number of drugs originally developed for use as anaesthetics were subsequently found to have psychedelic properties. Two in particular, phencyclidine (PCP or "angel dust") and ketamine ("K" or "special K"), can induce a state of profound dissociation in which the user's awareness is temporarily separated ("split off") from their body and surrounding environment.

117

No longer administered to humans, phencyclidine is still employed as an anaesthetic in veterinary medicine. When smoked in low doses, PCP causes mild agitation, euphoria, disinhibition and excitement. Users may stare blankly and appear extremely drunk. Higher doses tend to induce stupor or coma. Ketamine produces similar though less intense effects to those of phencyclidine. People under the influence of these drugs may experience severe anxiety, paranoia, and panic which results in violent or aggressive behaviour. Repeated use of ketamine and phencyclidine can induce a persistent schizophrenia-like psychotic state characterised by hallucinations, delusions (particularly delusions of reference), flattened affect, and social withdrawal. This state may persist for weeks or months after consumption ceases.

Nitrous Oxide ("**laughing gas**"): nitrous oxide was the first compound to be employed as a general anaesthetic and it is still used in medical and dental procedures. Though it is a CNS depressant, the effects of nitrous oxide justify its inclusion among the psychedelics. Low doses (insufficient to bring about unconsciousness) induce mild euphoria, emotional exhilaration, and behavioural disinhibition often associated with an urge to laugh – hence the drug's common name. The most remarkable effects of nitrous oxide are related to its capacity to provoke what have been called "anaesthetic revelations": users have described a pleasurable trance in which they experienced a tremendously exciting sense of profound metaphysical illumination. The core of this experience is the subject's feeling of having entered a state of "mystical consciousness" in which sublime spiritual truths are revealed with total clarity. While under the drug's influence users may feel utterly convinced of the veracity of their insights. However, a characteristic of this experience is that memory of the contents of these revelations fades rapidly as the drug wears off. Nevertheless, those who have experienced a nitrous oxide-induced state are often left with an unshakeable feeling that, even if they cannot recall the details, they were indeed blessed with profound spiritual insights while under the drug's influence.

Marijuana (cannabis, "pot", "dope", "ganja"): The hemp plant (*Cannabis sativa*) has for thousands of years been a source of substances used throughout the world for healing, religious, and recreational purposes. The principal psychoactive ingredient in marijuana, tetrahydrocannabinol (THC), is present in varying concentrations in different parts of the plant. Hashish ("hash"), the dried resin from flowers of female hemp plants, contains the highest concentrations of THC while the flowers themselves ("heads") contain somewhat less, and leaves and stems ("grass") the least. Hydroponic cultivation techniques have led to development of marijuana strains (e.g. "skunk") which reputedly contain exceptionally high concentrations of THC. Marijuana can be eaten (e.g. "hash cookies") but is usually smoked, either in a cigarette ("joint") or water pipe known colloquially as a "bong". When smoked its effects begin rapidly and reach maximum intensity in about 15 to 30 minutes. The intoxicated state – known as being "stoned" – typically lasts around 2 to 4 hours, with specific effects varying according to the type of marijuana used, quantity consumed, and method of ingestion (e.g. smoking versus eating).

Small amounts of THC induce a mildly euphoric "high" accompanied by feelings of pleasant relaxation and enhanced wellbeing. Users often experience an enhancement of perceptual sensitivity, e.g. colours appear brighter, sounds seem richer and more complex. The user's temporal perception is often altered such that time seems to pass more slowly. Marijuana impairs short-term memory and stimulates appetite ("the munchies"). Higher doses can provoke anxiety attacks, confusion, disorientation, depersonalisation (feeling of not being oneself), paranoia, hallucinations and loss of insight. Even low doses of THC can cause negative reactions in individuals especially sensitive to its effects.

Continued use of marijuana results in development of tolerance so that increasing amounts are required to produce the desired effects. In time, prolonged heavy users can develop physical and psychological dependence and become entwined in compulsive and maladaptive patterns of consumption, e.g. continuing to use the drug despite being aware of its increasingly negative effects. If they stop abruptly, dependent users may experience a withdrawal syndrome characterised by anxiety, agitation, restlessness, irritability, sleep disturbance, insomnia, loss of appetite, nausea, and muscle cramps. The severity of these symptoms is related to level of use and the degree of tolerance a person has acquired. The marijuana withdrawal syndrome typically begins within 48 hours of ceasing use and lasts at least several days. Subsequent craving for the drug may become intense and lead to resumption of use despite an avowed desire to quit.

Marijuana has recently attracted a great deal of attention due to growing concerns about its potential to induce psychosis in susceptible individuals.[12] Since this drug is now so widely used, particularly by young people, a closer examination of scientific evidence relevant to this issue is warranted.

Abundant clinical experience has demonstrated that cannabis can exacerbate symptoms of a pre-existing psychotic disorder and inhibit recovery, especially if it is used heavily.[13] However, there is little good evidence that occasional, low-level cannabis use constitutes a significant risk to mental health for most people. Scientific investigation of claims that marijuana can cause psychosis has found there is no simple cause-and-effect relationship linking use of this drug with onset of severe mental disorder.[14] This is not really surprising given that the vast majority of people who smoke marijuana do not become psychotic or suffer any other lasting adverse effects. Nevertheless, there is growing evidence cannabis *can* increase the likelihood of psychosis in certain circumstances. Studies of young people (aged 14 to 24) have shown that, while cannabis only contributes to moderately increased risk of psychotic symptoms overall, it can have a far stronger effect on those predisposed to experiencing psychosis, especially if cannabis use begins early (by fifteen years of age) and is frequent (daily or near daily).[15] In view of these facts an authoritative report in the *British Journal of Psychiatry* included the following advice:

> Although the majority of young people are able to use cannabis in adolescence without harm, a vulnerable minority experience harmful outcomes. The epidemiological evidence suggests that cannabis use among psychologically vulnerable young adolescents should be strongly discouraged by parents, teachers and health practitioners alike. Findings also suggest that the youngest cannabis users are most at risk.[16]

The risk of harmful consequences is likely to be increased significantly if potent dopamine-stimulating drugs such as amphetamines ("speed"), "ice" (methamphetamine), and "crack" cocaine are used in addition to marijuana.

Psychoactive Drug Effects: The Importance of Set and Setting

The mental and physical effects of a psychoactive substance – be it a socially-sanctioned one like alcohol, a prescription medication, or an illicit drug – are influenced by a host of interrelated factors. The following are among the most important:

(a) Type of drug

While it is possible to make general statements about how a particular substance is likely to affect the user, idiosyncratic factors make it impossible to predict these with certainty. Different psychoactive drugs have different effects. Certain classes, such as psychedelics, tend to amplify psychological processes while others, such as the opioids, have almost the opposite effect, tending to slow or diminish mental activity ("narcotic" effect). The effects of some psychoactive drugs are notoriously unpredictable.

(b) Purity/concentration

Unlike medically-prescribed psychoactive drugs, the identity, purity, and concentration of many illicit substances tend to be uncertain and unpredictable. "Street drugs" vary greatly in purity and strength. While some may contain little if any of the nominated substance, others may contain much more than anticipated or even a completely different drug, e.g. tablets sold as Ecstasy are sometimes found to contain a mixture of amphetamines and various other substances. The synthetic derivatives of some naturally-occurring drugs may be far more potent than the natural form of the substance, e.g. the psychoactive effects of "crack" cocaine are very many times greater than those of raw coca leaf.

(c) Abuse potential

Psychoactive drugs vary greatly in this regard. Key variables include the extent to which continued use leads to development of tolerance to the drug's effects and its propensity to induce physical and psychological dependence. Since amphetamines, cocaine, opioids and marijuana have a stimulating effect on the brain's "pleasure centre" they are highly prone to abuse. Such abuse can readily become compulsive and eventually lead to dependence with continued use. This pattern is unlikely to occur with some classes of drug (such as psychedelics) which have a completely different mode of pharmacological action.

(d) Pattern of Use

How often a substance is consumed (e.g. rarely, occasionally, or frequently), whether use is intermittent or continuous, and the quantity ingested, all play a role in determining its effects. Users develop a tolerance to many drugs with continued exposure. The manner in which a drug is ingested can also influence its effects. Some methods (e.g. smoking potent forms of marijuana in a heavily-packed "bong", smoking "ice") result in larger quantities being ingested and ensure the drug's effects are felt more rapidly. Such highly efficient methods greatly increase both the psychoactive effects and potential toxicity of the drug concerned. Some illicit substances may be *more* harmful to the brain (neurotoxic) when consumed on a regular basis (e.g. daily) – even if only small amounts are used – compared to the effects of larger quantities consumed intermittently.[17] Regular use might overwhelm the brain's natural recuperative processes whereas periods of abstinence allow the nervous system an opportunity to recover from the drug's cumulative toxic effects.

(e) Physiological characteristics
These include the user's state of physical health together with his or her unique array of individual biochemical sensitivities (the latter being partly determined by genetic factors). Variations in innate sensitivity are partially responsible for the fact that some people are able to ingest large quantities of certain drugs with little obvious effect while others may be extremely sensitive to tiny amounts of the same drug.

(f) Psychological characteristics
A given person's responses to psychoactive drugs is strongly influenced by a range of highly individual variables such as their psychological makeup and stability, personality traits, repertoire of psychological coping mechanisms, and level of emotional and social maturity. Chronological age is obviously a major influence on many of these variables.

(g) Set and Setting
Of the various non-pharmacological factors that influence how psychoactive drugs affect human beings those known collectively as "set and setting" are among the most important. In this context "set" refers to an individual's attitude toward the drug in question, his or her reasons for using it, and expectations regarding its anticipated effects. Taken together these attitudinal variables may be said to represent the user's "mind set" about the drug. Also relevant is an individual's emotional state at the time they use the drug, e.g. relaxed, anxious, depressed, happy. "Setting" refers to the physical and interpersonal

environment in which drugs are taken. The importance of this factor is illustrated by imagining the difference between being under the influence of a powerful psychedelic like LSD while in the company of trusted friends in safe, aesthetically pleasing surroundings, compared to how it might feel while alone in a noxious or threatening environment.

The preceding considerations should make it abundantly clear that the effects of a given drug – including its propensity to induce psychosis – are determined by many factors in addition to its specific pharmacological characteristics.

The focus thus far has been on factors that influence the effects of a *single* drug taken on its own. However, people often consume more than one drug at a time, a practice referred to as "poly-drug use". A recent Australian survey of Ecstasy users found the vast majority also used other drugs including alcohol, cannabis, LSD, cocaine, amphetamines, nitrous oxide, and nicotine.[18] Ingesting a number of psychoactive drugs simultaneously or in close succession creates an extremely complex, inherently unpredictable situation. The possible interactions, additive effects, and combined toxicities of the various drugs – plus those of any unknown foreign substances they happen to contain – become extraordinarily complicated, so much so they are poorly understood by psychopharmacologists. It goes without saying that poly-drug use involving substances of dubious origin and unknown purity and potency is potentially extremely hazardous, both physically and mentally.

Drugs and Psychosis

Some drugs can provoke psychosis or at least increase the likelihood of its occurrence.[*] Individuals who have already been diagnosed with a psychotic condition such as bipolar disorder or schizophrenia may experience an exacerbation of symptoms or become more prone to relapse if they use illicit drugs. Symptoms typically associated

---

[*] This phenomenon is *not* confined to illicit drugs. Often overlooked is the fact that a range of common *prescription medications* have been known to evoke psychotic symptoms in certain individuals. Medications concerned comprise a formidable list and include anticonvulsants, antihistamines, antimalarial medications, corticosteroids, cardiovascular and antihypertensive drugs, antiparkinsonian medications, gastrointestinal medications, and anticholinergic agents. Source: *DSM-IV*, p.312.

with drug-induced psychoses include "paranoia" (delusions of persecution), ideas of reference, grandiosity, and manic behaviour (the latter typically being provoked by psychostimulants like cocaine and amphetamines). If hallucinations occur they often involve non-auditory experiences, e.g. seeing or smelling things, unusual physical sensations.

It is often assumed that the ability of certain drugs to induce psychosis is solely a result of their *physical* effects on the user's brain, i.e. their *neurological* effects. Indeed, *DSM-IV* asserts that symptoms of Substance-Induced Psychotic Disorder are "due to the direct physiological effects of a substance".[19] This view tacitly reinforces the notion that psychosis is a purely biological phenomenon and that drugs simply provoke or exacerbate some undesirable change or malfunction in the brain (e.g. a "chemical imbalance") which sends the unfortunate user over the edge into madness. The relationship between drug use and psychosis is actually far more complex than simplistic cause-and-effect biochemical hypotheses suggest. While illicit drugs obviously have a variety of physical effects on the brain, a complete account of their role *vis-à-vis* psychosis requires a sensitive appreciation of their *non-physical* effects. Indeed, it is impossible to understand how drugs can induce psychosis or psychosis-like experiences without considering their social, psychological, and spiritual effects.

Since a combination of physical and non-physical effects is certain to be involved in any given case it is difficult to ascertain the relative importance of each. How much of a particular drug can a person take before its neurological effects begin to exceed its subtle non-physical ones? Idiosyncratic psychological, social, and emotional factors are *always* important even if the physical effects of the drugs have played a major part. This may be illustrated by the fact that on one occasion a person might experience pleasurable feelings while drinking alcohol but become morose on another despite consuming exactly the same amount. Subjective factors *always* play a significant role in drug-induced psychoses.

Note: Though the physical and non-physical effects of psychoactive drugs are intertwined, for the sake of clarity they are dealt with separately in the following discussions.

Drugs and the Brain: Neurological Effects of Illicit Drugs

In their effort to unravel the mysteries of psychosis neuroscientists have concentrated on the extraordinarily complex biochemical processes which underlie the various functions of the human brain. Attention has focussed most intensively on a small number of the brain's numerous neurotransmitters – chemical substances responsible for transmitting electrical signals (and thus information) between brain cells. Two neurotransmitters in particular – dopamine and serotonin – have long occupied a central role in most medical hypotheses concerning the biochemical causation of psychosis. The so-called "dopamine hypothesis" was until recently the most widely accepted explanation for schizophrenia. Excess activity of dopamine receptors in certain parts of the brain was said to be responsible for causing the characteristic symptoms of this disorder. The various medications originally used to treat schizophrenia and other psychotic disorders – so-called neuroleptic drugs – worked by selectively blocking dopamine receptors. Reducing the hypothesised excess dopamine activity was thought to rectify the "chemical imbalance" underlying psychosis. A range of newer anti-psychotic medications, referred to as "atypical" neuroleptics, act in a similar way to the earlier drugs, though these agents also modulate activity of serotonin and other neurotransmitters.

On a neurological level psychoactive drugs alter the user's mental state as a result of their effects on the activity of brain neurotransmitter systems. Since illicit psychoactive drugs have a range of complex effects on the brain it would be simplistic to try to account for their actions in terms of *single* neurotransmitters. However, it is now known that many of these substances specifically affect dopamine activity. Cocaine and amphetamines have the net effect of markedly increasing dopamine levels in key brain areas. As a result of its effects on special cannabinoid receptors, cannabis stimulates activity of dopamine in the limbic system, the brain region that controls and modulates mood and motivation. These effects are amplified significantly if extremely potent forms of the drugs (such as "ice", "crack" cocaine, and hydroponic marijuana) are consumed in large amounts over extended periods. Since the "anti-psychotic" effects of neuroleptic medications are related to their ability to *reduce* dopamine activity in specific regions of the brain, drugs that cause it to *increase* could be expected have the opposite effect. Indeed, under certain circumstances these drugs could effectively function as *pro*-psychotic agents.*

Despite its awesome complexity the human brain is usually capable of maintaining a state of harmonious balance. Since its interconnected neurochemical systems function as a unified whole, altering the activity of any one neurotransmitter automatically results in adjustment of all the others so an overall balance is maintained. With these facts in mind it is not difficult to imagine how potent psychostimulants which provoke a serious excess of neurotransmitters such as dopamine can disrupt the entire network of delicately balanced chemical systems. Simultaneous ingestion of *several* drugs (poly-drug use) might result in complete neurological disarray. Such disturbances are usually temporary, lasting only until the drugs' effects wear off. However, it is possible that prolonged use of extremely potent drugs such as "crack" cocaine or "ice" (methamphetamine) might eventually result in *irreversible* changes. Commencing illicit drug use early in life may be especially risky since the human brain is still in a relatively immature state during adolescence and crucial neurodevelopmental processes are occurring which are not completed until adulthood. Even drugs which are perceived by many to be relatively harmless (e.g. marijuana) could have detrimental effects on the still-developing adolescent brain.

In some cases drug-induced psychotic symptoms only occur while the provoking substance is being used and quickly disappear when consumption stops. However, since the withdrawal process for some drugs is quite prolonged, psychotic symptoms may not begin until some time (possibly weeks) *after* use ceases. Furthermore, once it is initiated, a psychosis provoked by amphetamines, phencyclidine (angel dust), cocaine, and others may continue for weeks, months, or longer – even if the drugs are no longer being used. In such cases, symptoms may persist until neurotransmitter systems have gradually regained their natural state of balance. However, if substance abuse has been

---

* These facts throw light on some possible reasons for substance abuse among people receiving long-term treatment with "anti-psychotic" medications, common side effects of which include reduced energy, loss of spontaneity, and dampening of creativity. Illicit drug use (or even excessive consumption of stimulants such as caffeine) is sometimes motivated by a desire to overcome the "tranquillising" effects of neuroleptic drugs. Furthermore, people sometimes resort to illicit drug use in an attempt to rekindle the energy and excitement of their earlier psychotic or pre-psychotic experiences.

heavy and prolonged, or has involved potentially neurotoxic drugs (which could include "ice" and Ecstasy), it is possible a point could eventually be reached at which the brain's rebalancing mechanisms are no longer able to function properly.

Little is known about how a "chemical imbalance" in the brain – whether induced by illicit drugs or occurring spontaneously – could lead to psychosis. As a matter of fact, scientists are at a loss to explain how the brain's *normal* chemical activities result in the production of thoughts, emotions, and the host of other complex mental phenomena which distinguish human beings from lower animals. What has been called "the mysterious leap from brain to mind" remains shrouded in mystery. It does not seem too bold to suggest that philosophers and theologians are likely to make as much of a contribution to the task of unravelling this mystery as are neuroscientists and biochemists.

Drugs and the Mind: Psychological and Social Effects of Illicit Drugs

The human mind and body (including the brain) naturally function as a unified, superbly integrated whole. The science of *psychosomatics* evolved out of belated recognition of the fact that psychological (psycho) and physical (somatic) processes are inextricably linked. It is now well known that stimuli which affect the body also have mental effects, and vice versa. Consequently, anything that upsets the balance of the total mind/body system – be it a powerful emotion or a powerful drug – could result in a temporary loss of mental and emotional balance. This understanding helps explain how, while psychoactive drugs may act in the first instance on the physical level (i.e. altering brain neurotransmitter systems), their major impact may occur on the psychological and emotional level.

Young people start using drugs for a variety of reasons. Peer pressure is frequently a significant factor since the overarching adolescent desire to fit in, be accepted, and act "cool" may impel some to join group activities centred on drug taking (including social drugs such as alcohol and nicotine). Ironically, the temptation to experiment with illicit drugs is sometimes felt most keenly by individuals whose extreme psychological isolation makes them particularly vulnerable to psychosis.

As noted in *Chapter Three*, a person's first psychotic episode is often preceded by a prolonged period of psychological, emotional, and social marginalisation. Although the development of a "false self" may have been impelled by a desire to blend in and belong, elaboration of a "façade of normality" may result in an even deeper sense of alienation and estrangement in the long term. As psychological pressure builds some people may feel trapped in an intolerable dilemma from which escape seems impossible. Drugs, social and illicit, may grant temporary respite from pervasive emotional pain. They might even hold the promise of providing a way out of a seemingly interminable "no exit" situation. Dr Podvoll believes substance use is sometimes motivated by a (semi-conscious) hope it might provoke the longed-for transformation of a self felt to be deeply flawed:

> This desire to become someone else has been "cooking" since an early age. An ordinarily hidden hope and conviction grows that a transformation might come upon one suddenly, as can happen when falling in love … *The intention to transform awaits its catalyst … Usually, a substance is found that will fuel the momentum of the coming transformation.* Preferably, it is an "excitant", an accelerator. Alcohol and marijuana are the most popular (and the cheapest) these days. But every other kind of "street drug" is also used, the hallucinogens obviously being the most powerful. Very high dosages of caffeine even work when nothing else is available. So does nicotine … Increasingly, one hears about patients using their prescribed medications ("antipsychotic" or "antidepressant" drugs) in toxic amounts to imbalance the system and create "altered states".[20]

Some people may be familiar with the effects of drugs well before they reach this kind of desperate impasse. From an early age some – especially those with a "stormy" personality – may have felt an almost magnetic attraction to the excitement and dangerous thrill of drug-fuelled binges. Those with a more introverted "schizoid" disposition may have found that stimulating drugs can temporarily enliven their inner world or assuage the creeping numbness of "emotional shut-down". The consequences in either case depend on the type, amount, and way drugs are used, and – most importantly – on the psychological stability and emotional maturity of the user.

Despite what they may have once intended some people find themselves becoming increasingly involved in potentially hazardous drug-taking behaviour. Having enjoyed the sense of freedom and release that certain drugs so readily provide, the temptation to repeat the experience as often as possible may be hard to resist – especially for those who feel trapped by life. Since regular use inevitably results in gradual development of tolerance to the original effects of the drugs, increasing amounts may be required to evoke the desired response. Using more potent substances or combinations of drugs in the hope of obtaining stronger or longer-lasting effects may soon become an irresistible temptation. Before they even realise it is happening some people find they have become dependent on drugs which were once a matter of choice. A pattern of compulsive use may ensue which continues in spite of a steadily growing range of adverse psychological and social consequences for the user and others.

The specific attraction of mind-altering drugs for some is that they provide a quick and easy means of fleeing everyday reality. Adding to the allure is the promise of evoking experiences appealing to the user. Thus, the mind-numbing and analgesic ("pain killing") effects of opioids such as heroin make them an ideal choice for those wishing to escape emotional pain and conflict. By contrast, potent psychostimulants such as amphetamines and cocaine are "feel good" drugs *par excellence* with the ability to provoke a rapid, albeit short-lived, boost to the user's confidence and self-esteem. Excessive consumption soon begins to exact a terrible price, however. The emotional let down that inevitably follows a drug-induced high may leave the user craving more of the drug until a vicious circle is set in train. Those who habitually rely on drugs as a means of escape or to avoid dealing with personal issues eventually find their lives stagnating. Nowhere is this more evident than in those whose social networks are confined to others who collude with and reinforce their drug-centred lifestyle and increasing estrangement from reality.

Even if they are not physically or psychologically dependent, some people use drugs in potentially harmful ways – such as deliberately setting out to get "smashed" or "wasted" by ingesting the largest quantities possible of whatever drug or drugs happen to be available. These hedonistic binges often involve drugs of unknown potency and purity, or bizarre combinations of substances with totally incompatible or unpredictable effects. The possible long-term health consequences of such behaviour are impossible to foresee. Less extreme, and therefore more common, patterns of drug-taking have a range of more predictable effects. Even relatively "mild" drugs like cannabis (marijuana) can be used in ways that have significant negative consequences over time. Although use of such drugs often begins as a primarily social activity, with the occasional joint or pipe shared among friends, it sometimes devolves into a more solitary, self-centred, furtive pursuit. As French writer Charles Baudelaire recognised, with excessive use "Hashish, like all other solitary delights, makes the individual useless to mankind, and also makes society unnecessary to the individual."[21]

Those who are already isolated due to their introspective, somewhat pensive nature may find themselves drawn into a world where loneliness and frustration are replaced – if only for a short while – with drifting reverie and hypnotic otherworldly dreams. However, as drug use becomes heavier and more frequent, questions regarding identity and the need to find a place in the world may become even more burdensome than they were before. Depression, anxiety, and "paranoia", common accompaniments of prolonged drug abuse, may undermine a person's already shaky self-confidence, provoking further withdrawal into bleary solitude. Isolation, irregular sleep, poor diet, and lack of exercise all conspire in a self-perpetuating cycle of social deterioration and steady physical and mental decline. With work or school performance increasingly compromised by the combined effects of poor attendance and impaired concentration, the prospect of unemployment or academic failure may loom on the horizon like an unavoidable fate. Erratic moods and unpredictable behaviour may drive former friends away in search of more congenial company. Caught in a spiral of ever-deepening isolation, outcast users may feel ever more like the failures they have long suspected themselves to be. If drug use persists in spite of its increasingly negative consequences, the user's world may continue shrinking until it finally comes to revolve around the brief flare of the next freshly-packed pipe.

People in this situation are sometimes eventually able to pull themselves out of it with the help of others. Some are fortunate enough to do so before they suffer irreparable mental, social, and physical harm.

Drugs and the Soul: Spiritual and Existential Effects of Illicit Drugs

The drugs under consideration are classed as psychoactive specifically because they affect key aspects of mental functioning such as mood, perception, and thought processes. Often overlooked is the fact that a distinguishing characteristic of these drugs is their ability to induce mental states radically different from usual, these being referred to as *altered states of consciousness* (ASCs). Familiar ASCs include dreams, trance, meditative, mystical, and hypnotic states. The ability of certain drugs to profoundly alter consciousness provides the basis of some of their most constructive uses, such as in traditional healing practices and religious rituals and as tools for self-exploration. However, this same ability sometimes results in their misuse.

If used in a cautious and respectful way with appropriate guidance, some drugs can facilitate experiences that have a variety of beneficial consequences. The psychedelics, in particular, may enhance self-awareness and promote spiritual insight – as their continued use for thousands of years in traditional shamanic cultures attests (see *Chapter Eight*). On the other hand, indiscriminate use of these powerful drugs, or their employment as a form of hedonistic "spiritual thrill-seeking", could expose the user to a host of dangers. If they are used in a careless or cavalier manner, even the "milder" psychoactive drugs can have subtle detrimental consequences in addition to the possible neurological and social effects discussed previously.

Individuals who have had difficulty developing a stable identity and basic sense of psychological security – and those too young to have completed these vital developmental tasks – may be particularly susceptible to having their personal insecurities magnified by drugs. For these very reasons Dr Albert Hofmann, discoverer of the psychedelic properties of LSD, was strongly of the view that powerful mind-expanding drugs ought to be taboo for adolescents:

> Among persons with unstable personality structures, tending to psychotic reactions, LSD experimentation ought to be completely avoided. Here an LSD shock, by releasing a latent psychosis, can produce a lasting mental injury. The psyche of very young persons should also be considered as unstable, in the sense of not yet having matured. In any case, the shock of such a powerful stream of new and strange perceptions and feelings, such as is engendered by

LSD, endangers the sensitive, still-developing psycho-organism ... Juveniles for the most part still lack a secure, solid relationship to reality. Such a relationship is needed before the dramatic experience of new dimensions of reality can be meaningfully integrated into the world view. Instead of leading to a broadening and deepening of reality consciousness, such an experience in adolescents will lead to insecurity and a feeling of being lost.[22]

Powerful "mind-blowing" psychedelic experiences can have lasting psychological reverberations that further undermine an already tenuous adjustment. One man described how his first experience with LSD ("acid") left him feeling vulnerable and uncertain for a long time afterwards:

> I did not understand how one could come back from such mental vastness, and drop into one's identity again ... Over the following days [after his first acid trip], however, my ego boundaries hardened again, and my exposed psyche grew protective layers to insulate it from the world. But these layers were to be forever thinner than before.[23]

Far milder experiences might also have repercussions that contribute to insecurity. For example, under the influence of drugs people sometimes feel, see, or hear things not ordinarily perceived but which at the time seem absolutely real. Experienced psychedelic users describe a variety of extraordinary phenomena such as acquiring the ability to see auras, encountering "spirits" and other "cosmic" beings, or gaining insight into aspects of life about which they were previously ignorant. When the drug's effects wear off doubts often arise about the validity of such experiences: did they really occur or were they just drug-induced aberrations? Since such questions can be extremely difficult to answer with certainty the user may be left wondering what is real and what is not. Without some way to confidently evaluate them, repeated exposure to "way out" experiences might gradually undermine a person's ability to distinguish fantasy and reality. Those who *already* have problems in this regard could be susceptible to having their ability to "test reality" further compromised. Such people sometimes become prone to entertaining highly idiosyncratic explanations for their unusual experiences. This could result in the gradual development of a state of metaphysical confusion characterised by uncritical acceptance of a melange of fanciful and unprovable beliefs involving spirits, alien entities, magic, occult influences and conspiracies of various kinds – including supposedly "cosmic" ones. Such notions, if taken to an extreme and not subjected to critical evaluation, might gradually result in the elaboration of a world-view bordering on psychosis.

Some people use drugs in the hope of furthering their spiritual development. While this might be possible under certain circumstances, casual or recreational use of powerful mind-altering substances without appropriate guidance and safeguards is fraught with risk. For example, such drugs could initiate a spiritual emergence process (*Chapter Six*). While the ensuing experiences might ultimately prove beneficial they could be so overwhelming they constitute a "spiritual emergency" – a psychospiritual crisis that could be difficult to manage and for which adequate assistance may not be readily available.

Excessive drug use can facilitate a disengagement from the everyday world which users might perceive as reflective of their elevation to subtle realms beyond the limits of "mundane" reality, but which actually amounts to little more than growing self-absorption and ungroundedness. Avoiding illusion and self-deception calls for scrupulous honesty and sophisticated spiritual discernment. For those with a tendency to "space out", the task of keeping body, mind, and soul integrated and stably grounded in everyday reality may necessitate strict abstinence from all mind-altering substances.

Conclusion

For individuals whose mental and emotional state may have been rather fragile to begin with, combined physical, psychological, social and spiritual effects of drugs could further destabilise what was already a precarious situation. If mental balance is lost, one possible outcome is a psychotic episode. The form taken by such a "drug-induced psychosis" will be determined by the amount and type of drugs consumed, circumstances surrounding use, and psychological characteristics of the user.

Some drug-induced psychoses may be very brief. Psychotic symptoms induced by "ice" (methamphetamine), for example, sometimes only last for several minutes while the drug's effects are at peak intensity. On the other hand, drugs can provoke adverse changes in the user's mental state which are more persistent. Nevertheless, it is often the case that no specific treatment is required since most drug-related symptoms tend to abate as the drug's effects wear off. Individuals previously diagnosed with a psychotic condition such as schizophrenia or bipolar disorder may be an exception to this general rule, particularly those who have required treatment with anti-psychotic or mood stabilising medication to help them maintain stability and balance. Since illicit drugs with "pro-psychotic" effects can increase the intensity of symptoms and even provoke relapse, strict avoidance of these substances, and limited use of legal psychoactive drugs like caffeine and alcohol, is sound advice for anyone seriously intent on recovery.

Illicit drug abuse sometimes provokes psychotic symptoms or states that are both problematic and long-lasting. If drug use has been prolonged and heavy – and particularly if it has involved potent dopamine-stimulating agents like "ice" or "crack" – the ensuing psychosis may have a predominantly *neurological* basis, i.e. symptoms reflect the fact that drugs have affected the normal functioning of the user's brain. In such cases an extended period of strict abstinence from all drugs – social and illicit – provides natural self-healing mechanisms with the best opportunity to begin the process of repair.[24]

If substance use has been relatively minor, i.e. a person has only taken drugs very occasionally or intermittently, or the substances involved are of a kind not known to cause neurological impairment (e.g. psychedelics), it is reasonable to assume *psychological* and possibly *spiritual* factors have played the major role in provoking psychosis. In such cases symptoms sometimes persist until relevant underlying issues are identified and dealt with. If psychosis occurs in the context of a "no exit" situation, an opportunity may be provided to address long-standing personal problems (e.g. wounded self-image, poor self-esteem) once the crisis has subsided to a manageable level.

The central premise of this book – that acute psychoses are dramatic personal crises rather than mental illnesses – may still apply even if such episodes are catalysed by drugs. Nor does the fact that drugs may have played a triggering role negate the possibility that some tumultuous episodes inappropriately labelled "psychotic" may be potentially transformative psychospiritual crises. As the next chapter makes clear, such experiences often occur in altered states induced by drugs, psychedelics in particular.

Chapter Eight

Psychedelic Experience: Mysticism And Madness

The extraordinary phenomena of psychedelic experiences arouse a sense of wonder at the radiance and intricacy of the human mind.

Charles Hayes[1]

The large and diverse group of substances known collectively as "psychedelics" polarise opinion more than drugs of any other kind. Revered by some as divine gifts and a boon to humankind, these same substances are viewed by others as reality-distorting brain toxins capable of causing serious, possibly irreversible, mental disturbance. How could a single class of drugs give rise to such widely divergent views?

Misuse of psychedelics can have a range of negative consequences which include provoking acute psychosis-like states and possibly persistent psychological and emotional disturbances. However, the fact that these substances have played such a significant role in human affairs throughout history – and that they continue to do so – suggests they must possess some redeeming features. The first scientific treatise on mind-altering plants noted that the extraordinary subjective effects of certain species ensured their enduring appeal. As celebrated pharmacologist Louis Lewin observed in 1924, many of the drugs discussed in this chapter have long been employed in collective cultural and religious practices and private spiritual pursuits:

> This we can understand when we know their properties, the properties of evoking sense-illusions in a great variety of forms, of giving rise in the human soul as if by magic to apparitions whose brilliant, seductive, perpetually changing aspects produce a rapture which is incessantly renewed and in comparison with which the perceptions of consciousness are but pale shadows. Harmonious vibrations of sounds beyond all human belief are heard, phantasms appear before men's eyes as if they were real, always desired but never attained, offered to them as a gift from almighty God.

135

These properties explain why many of these substances have been and are used for illegal purposes.[2]

Many people feel psychedelics enabled them to have experiences which they count among the most significant of their lives. So profound are such experiences they are often described as life-changing. On the other hand, some people have undergone psychedelic ordeals so frightening they vow never to repeat the experience. Some feel they have been deeply wounded by these drugs. This chapter examines how it is possible for *both* kinds of experience to occur.

The Doors of Perception

Contrary to popular opinion, non-medical use of mind-altering substances in the West did not begin with the hippy movement in the 1960s – though it did undergo a tremendous surge in popularity during that era. Interest in such substances and their extraordinary effects dates back to at least the middle of the nineteenth century in European societies. It is noteworthy that some of the earliest experiments were conducted, not by disaffected social drop-outs, but by highly educated, psychologically sophisticated individuals who occupied prominent roles in their respective professions.

American journalist Fitz Hugh Ludlow was one of the first Western-ers to describe the effects of hashish (a potent form of marijuana). In *The Hasheesh Eater*, published in 1857, Ludlow described some of the extraordinary mental effects of this drug:

> A soul disenthralled, setting out for his flight beyond the farthest visible star, could not be more overwhelmed with his newly acquired conception of the sublimity of distance than I was at that moment. Solemnly I began my infinite journey. Before long I walked in entire unconsciousness of all around me. I dwelt in a marvellous inner world. I existed by turns in different places and various states of being. Now I swept my gondola through the moonlit lagoons of Venice. Now Alp on Alp towered above my view, and the glory of the coming sun placed purple light upon the topmost pinnacle. Now in the primeval silence of some unexplored tropical forest I spread my feathery leaves, a giant fern, and swayed and nodded in the spice gales over a river whose waves at once sent up clouds

of music and perfume. My soul changed to a vegetable essence, thrilled with a strange and unimagined ecstasy.[3]

One of the most influential pioneers was Harvard University academic Professor William James (1842-1910). The leading philosopher of his time and one the founders of modern psychology, James experimented with consciousness-altering anaesthetic agents, including nitrous oxide ("laughing gas"). He was struck by this drug's ability to induce a "tremendously exciting sense of an intense metaphysical illumination", a phenomenon he elaborated upon in his seminal treatise, *The Varieties of Religious Experience*:

> Nitrous oxide and ether, especially nitrous oxide, when sufficiently diluted with air, stimulate the mystical consciousness in an extraordinary degree. Depth beyond depth of truth seems revealed to the inhaler. This truth fades out, however, or escapes, at the moment of coming to; and if any words remain over in which it seemed to clothe itself, they prove to be the veriest nonsense. Nevertheless, the sense of a profound meaning having been there persists; and I know more than one person who is persuaded that in the nitrous oxide trance we have a genuine metaphysical revelation.[4]

The ability of nitrous oxide to stimulate mystical experiences so moved one early experimenter he declared: "The atmosphere of the highest of all possible heavens must be composed of this gas." Professor James's mind-altering experiences challenged his beliefs about the nature of consciousness:

> One conclusion was forced upon my mind at that time, and my impression of its truth has ever since remained unshaken. It is that our normal waking consciousness, rational consciousness as we call it, is but one special type of consciousness, whilst all about it, parted from it by the filmiest of screens, there lie potential forms of consciousness entirely different. We may go through life without suspecting their existence; but apply the requisite stimulus, and at a touch they are there in all their completeness, definite types of mentality which probably somewhere have their field of application and adaptation. No account of the universe in its totality can be final which leaves these other forms of consciousness quite disregarded.[5]

In 1954 the writer and religious philosopher Aldous Huxley published an account of his experiences with mescaline in a book called *The Doors of Perception* (a title he took from a statement by the visionary poet and artist William Blake: "If the doors of perception were cleansed, everything will appear to man as it is, infinite"). Huxley felt the drug granted him a glimpse of "the unfathomable mystery of pure being" and he was left with the unshakable sense he had seen a world transformed, "where everything shone with the Inner Light, and was infinite in its significance":

> Half an hour after swallowing the drug I became aware of a slow dance of golden lights ... An hour and a half later I was sitting in my study, looking intently at a small glass vase. The vase contained only three flowers ... At breakfast that morning I had been struck by the lively dissonance of its colours. But that was no longer the point. I was not looking now at an unusual flower arrangement. I was seeing what Adam had seen on the morning of his creation – the miracle, moment by moment, of naked existence ... I continued to look at the flowers, and in their living light I seemed to detect the qualitative equivalent of breathing ... a repeated flow from beauty to heightened beauty, from deeper to ever deeper meaning. Words like Grace and Transfiguration came to my mind ... When I got up and walked about, I could do so quite normally ... Space was still there; but it had lost its predominance. The mind was primarily concerned, not with measures and locations, but with being and meaning.[6]

The extraordinary effects of psilocybin-containing "magic mushrooms" were first brought to popular attention by an article in *Life* magazine in 1957.[7] The report focused on the experiences of Gordon Wasson, a former journalist researching the traditional use of vision-inducing fungi. Wasson's first encounter with psychoactive mushrooms took place in a remote Mexican village under the guidance of an esteemed local shaman. Called *teonanacatl* ("God's flesh") by the indigenous Indians, the mushrooms had a mesmerising effect:

> The mushroom seized possession of him completely, although he had tried to struggle against its effects, in order to be able to remain an objective observer. First he saw geometric, coloured patterns, which then took on architectural characteristics. Next followed visions of splendid colonnades, palaces of supernatural harmony

and magnificence embellished with precious gems, triumphal cars drawn by fabulous creatures as they are known only from mythology, and landscapes of fabulous lustre. Detached from the body, the spirit soared timelessly in a realm of fantasy among images of a higher reality and deeper meaning than those of the ordinary, everyday world. The essence of life, the ineffable, seemed to be on the verge of being unlocked ...[8]

While psilocybin-induced visions were awe-inspiring, more significant to Wasson was the power of the sacred mushrooms to free the human soul from its earthly bonds:

> It permits you to see more clearly than our perishing eye can see, vistas beyond the horizons of this life, to travel backwards and forwards in time, to enter other planes of existence, even to know God.[9]

Many of these pioneers were so impressed with the profound mental and spiritual effects of mind-altering substances they wrote glowing reports urging others to conduct similar experiments.

LSD: A New Magic Drug

Aldous Huxley's writings introduced many people to the idea that drugs might be used to enhance creativity, facilitate personal development, and heighten spiritual awareness. The serendipitous discovery of an extremely potent new drug – LSD – heralded the beginning of an era during which interest in these possibilities increased dramatically.

The first intentional LSD-induced experience occurred in 1943 when the drug's discoverer, biochemist Albert Hofmann, deliberately ingested a minute quantity in order to investigate its effects on human consciousness. At the time Dr Hofmann was a director of research at Sandoz Research Laboratories, a Swiss drug firm soon to become one of the rapidly growing number of multinational pharmaceutical companies.* The psychological impact of his courageous self-

---

* During subsequent decades Sandoz developed and marketed a range of psychiatric medications, including widely used neuroleptic ("anti-psychotic") drugs such as thioridazine (Mellaril). In 1990 Sandoz introduced clozapine (Clozaril), the first of the so-called "atypical" neuroleptics. It is one of history's ironies that the firm which gave the world the prototypical psychedelic LSD also produced Clozaril, the drug which ushered in the new wave of "second generation" neuroleptic medications.

experiment was profound. Initially, the drug only induced minor visual distortions, but as its effects intensified familiar objects assumed grotesque forms. Far more terrifying experiences were to come, however, as Dr Hofmann recounted in his autobiographical memoir:

> Even worse than these demonic transformations of the outer world were the alterations that I perceived in myself, in my inner being. Every exertion of my will, every attempt to put an end to the disintegration of the outer world and the dissolution of my ego, seemed to be a wasted effort. A demon had invaded my body, mind, and soul. I jumped up and screamed, trying to free myself from him, but then sank down again and lay helpless on the sofa. The substance, with which I had wanted to experiment, had vanquished me. It was the demon that scornfully triumphed over my will. I was seized by the dreadful fear of going insane. I was taken to another world, another place, another time. My body seemed to be without sensation, lifeless, strange. Was I dying? Was this the transition? At times I believed myself to be outside my body, and then perceived clearly, as an outside observer, the complete tragedy of my situation ... Slowly I came back from a weird, unfamiliar world to reassuring everyday reality. The horror softened and gave way to a feeling of good fortune and gratitude, the more normal perceptions and thoughts returned, and I became more confident that the danger of insanity was conclusively past.[10]

While comparable to other psychedelics, the effects of this new drug were much more intense. Dr Hofmann eventually determined that LSD is around 5,000–10,000 times more potent than mescaline, and 100 times more potent than psilocybin.[11]

Such were the extraordinary properties of this new drug that Sandoz decided to provide LSD free on request to bona fide researchers and physicians for experimental use. As clinicians started experimenting with LSD and related drugs debate arose as to the nature of their effects. The tendency of users to experience vivid sensory phenomena led to these drugs being described as "hallucinogenic" (hallucination inducing). Since many mental health professionals believed the LSD state was tantamount to a psychosis the drug was considered "psychotomimetic" (psychosis mimicking) or "psychotogenic" (psychosis inducing). Many researchers believed LSD made it possible to induce a psychotic state – a so-called "model psychosis" – in anyone taking it. The information Sandoz supplied with the drug claimed it could be used "to induce model psychoses of short duration in normal subjects" for the purposes of studying the nature of mental disorder. Furthermore it said, "By taking [LSD] himself, the psychiatrist is able to gain an insight into the world of ideas and sensations of mental patients".[12] In particular, it was thought this drug could provide a vivid sense of what it was like to experience schizophrenia.

While many clinicians continued to regard drugs like LSD as psychotomimetic or hallucinogenic, a view soon arose that such pathologising terminology was too narrow to encompass their full range of effects. Gordon Wasson's encounter with magic mushrooms led him to propose "entheogen" (generating god or divine within), but in 1957 Canadian psychiatrist Humphrey Osmond suggested that these substances be called "psychedelic" (mind-opening or consciousness-expanding), in view of the extremely broad spectrum of phenomena – positive as well as negative – they can induce. The term "psychedelic" was readily accepted by broad-minded investigators and remains the preferred designation in contemporary non-medical circles.*

LSD Psychotherapy

Early investigators noted that LSD "produces an upsurge of uncon-scious material into consciousness" so that "repressed memories are relived with remarkable clarity".[13] Many psychiatrists believed the drug's ability to bring long forgotten or repressed experiences to awareness, possibly allowing them to be relived in an extremely vivid manner, made it a potentially invaluable aid to psychotherapy.[14] However, it was soon understood that such treatment would not be suitable for everyone. As a safeguard it was recommended that LSD-assisted therapy should only be administered by specially trained therapists and that those undergoing treatment should receive intensive preparation for several weeks prior to their first LSD session and ongoing psychological support afterwards.

Many therapists reported remarkable results when carefully-selected subjects were given LSD in a setting that provided non-coercive

---

* Significantly, the word "psychedelic" is not used in *DSM-IV* which refers to these substances exclusively as "hallucinogens". This restrictive, pathology-focussed terminology continues psychiatry's long tradition of emphasising the drugs' negative aspects while failing to acknowledge their mind-expanding potential.

containment and adequate support. A range of techniques soon evolved. European practitioners favoured so-called *psycholytic therapy* that involved administration of relatively low doses of LSD in a series of sessions designed to lower the subject's defences, thus facilitating access to unconscious material. In the USA, by contrast, what became known as *psychedelic therapy* involved giving far higher doses in a single session in the belief that provoking a powerful psychospiritual experience would set in train a spontaneous process of emotional healing and personality restructuring. A man being treated for chronic alcoholism provided this graphic account of a life-changing experience induced by LSD:

> I found myself drifting into another world and saw that I was at the bottom of a set of stairs. At the very top of these stairs was a gleaming light like a star or jewel of exceptional brilliance. I ascended these stairs and upon reaching the top, I saw a gleaming, blinding light with a brilliance no man has ever known. It had no shape nor form, but I *knew* that I was looking at God himself. The magnificence, splendour and grandeur of this experience cannot be put into words. Neither can my innermost feelings, but it shall remain in my heart, soul, and mind forever. I never felt so clean inside in all my life. All the trash and garbage seemed to be washed out of my mind. In my heart, my mind, my soul, and my body, it seemed as if I were born all over again.[15]

Proponents claimed LSD made it possible to reach individuals who were resistant to conventional psychotherapy and that positive results could be achieved far more rapidly than with standard treatment.[16] However, it soon became obvious an appropriately trained and temperamentally suited therapist, whose role was to act as a supportive, non-intrusive "guide", was crucial to the success of LSD therapy:

> Mature, intelligent individuals with widely divergent interests and talents as well as different specific professional training will be needed if the psychedelic experience is ever to yield up all of the treasures it promises. Moreover, in addition to his specialties, it is highly desirable that each guide possess a broad background especially including knowledge of history, literature, philosophy, mythology, art, and religion … There exist, so far as we know, no psychiatric or other screening procedures for determining who will

make an effective guide – or who will make a poor or dangerous one … inept or exploitative management of a session may make it a painful and possibly damaging experience for the subject … this has resulted in guiding by psychiatrists and others who were eminently unsuited to the task and who inflicted some appalling experiences on their subjects.[17]

After a period of enthusiastic acceptance the use of LSD as a psychotherapeutic aid began to fall out of favour and the practice was gradually discontinued. Though some therapists claimed outstanding results, many who experimented with this approach were inadequately equipped to understand their clients' experiences and uncomfortable with the often extremely intense emotions many displayed under the drug's influence.

The Psychedelic Era

Since anecdotal reports often highlighted LSD's ability to induce ecstatic or blissful states many were eager to try it. Some believed LSD and other psychedelics made it possible to experience instant spiritual enlightenment ("God in a pill"), a gratuitous beatific state that would result in permanent inner freedom, happiness, and creativity. Many who took these drugs did indeed have profoundly moving experiences that they felt involved mystical or cosmic dimensions. One student given psilocybin reported the following:

Relatively soon after receiving the drug, I transcended my usual level of consciousness and became aware of fantastic dimensions of being, all of which possessed a profound sense of reality. It would seem more accurate to say that I existed "in" those dimensions … The feelings I experienced could best be described as cosmic tenderness, infinite love, penetrating peace, eternal blessing and unconditional acceptance [and as] unspeakable awe, overflowing joy, primeval humility, inexpressible gratitude and boundless devotion. Yet all of these words are hopelessly inadequate and can do little more than meekly point towards the genuine, inexpressible feelings actually experienced … It is misleading even to use the words "I experienced", since during the peak of the experience (which must have lasted at least an hour) there was no duality between myself and what I experienced. Rather, I *was* these feelings … In religious language, I was in "eternity" ... The dimensions of being I entered surpassed the wildest fantasies of my imagination and, as I have said, leave me with a profound sense of awe.[18]

Such accounts encouraged others to experiment with psychedelic drugs. After all, who would not want to have an experience such as this? Although LSD was at first only available to medical and research personnel, by the mid-1960s a flourishing black market in LSD and other psychedelics had developed and spread rapidly around the world.

The early popularity of psychedelics was spurred by vociferous advocates such as Timothy Leary, then a psychology professor at Harvard University, who said after his first encounter with psilocybin mushrooms: "I learned more in the six or seven hours of this experience than in all my years as a psychologist".[19] LSD and other psychedelics were still legal at this time and a growing coterie of intellectuals, artists, writers, and musicians experimented with them. Though Aldous Huxley felt the psychedelic experience ought to be reserved for an elite group of creative individuals, it was soon available to anyone who wanted it. In events reminiscent of contemporary Ecstasy-fuelled "rave" parties, groups of predominantly young people were soon gathering to dance, listen to music ("acid rock"), and watch dazzling light shows while under the influence of LSD and other psychedelics. Such activities were encouraged by influential figures like Leary, who attained notoriety for recommending that young people should take psychedelics in order to "Turn On, Tune In, and Drop Out".[20]

As use of psychedelics spread, concerns began to be expressed about their possible harmful effects. With more and more people taking these extremely potent drugs health workers began to encounter individuals suffering adverse reactions: so-called "bad trips". Hospital emergency departments frequently saw people experiencing drug-related panic, depersonalisation, depression, paranoia, acute psychotic episodes, and attempted suicide. Though most psychedelic crises resolved quickly – usually within 48 hours – prolonged adverse reactions sometimes occurred.[21] While most medical authorities acknowledged the relative safety of psychedelics when used by emotionally stable individuals receiving adequate supervision and support, concern was growing about the possible consequences of misuse, e.g. by immature or psychologically unstable persons in potentially hazardous circumstances. Such concerns were highlighted in Dr Sidney Cohen's research for the US National Institutes of Health:

> Reports on more than 25,000 LSD or mescaline ingestions by some 5,000 subjects or patients were obtained. My report says that in those instances where LSD is given to pre-selected individuals under proper controls with adequate screening and protection, that the evidence of side effects is indeed a rarity. It is not fair to use this report to state that LSD is, therefore, a safe drug. On the contrary this report must be sharply distinguished from the complications which follow its indiscriminate use. During the past three years I have seen seventy-eight people who have taken LSD under uncontrolled, random, frivolous conditions and who have had prolonged difficulties. During the past few months one in every seven admissions to one small ... Neuropsychiatric Hospital is for LSD-precipitated disturbances.[22]

Growing public and political concern about the potential negative consequences of "hallucinogen abuse" led the US government to pass legislation in 1966 proscribing LSD. A few years later the United Nations enacted the Convention on Psychotropic Substances making it an offence to produce, supply, or possess psychedelic drugs. In the eyes of the law these substances had effectively been lumped together with dangerous and potentially addictive "narcotics" like heroin, cocaine, and amphetamines.[*] These harshly restrictive measures were implemented against the objection of many reputable scientists, including some who believed psychedelics "afford the best access yet to the contents and processes of the human mind".[23]

Prohibition brought an end to legitimate scientific research on these extraordinary substances. Legal manufacture of LSD and other psychedelics was banned and researchers were required to return any remaining supplies. Political and economic pressures from the US-led

---

[*] As late as the mid-1980s publications whose nominal purpose was to educate the public about the hazards of illicit drugs warned that prolonged use of LSD could have a variety of "toxic" effects including induction of a so-called "psychedelic syndrome", defined as follows: "This syndrome is characterised by an interest in astrology, extrasensory perception, mental telepathy, mysticism, and magic. Long-time LSD users often become so preoccupied with these phenomena that they devote their full attention to them ..." Trulson, M. (1985) *LSD: Visions or Nightmares (Encyclopaedia of Psychoactive Drugs)*. London: Burke Publishing Company. p.74.

"war on drugs" ensured scientists worldwide were refused permission to conduct further investigations. After galvanising so much interest during the 1950s and '60s, from a scientific perspective it was effectively as if psychedelics ceased to exist. It was not until 1990 that the US Food and Drug Administration authorised new research on the human effects of these drugs.[24]

Legal restrictions on psychedelics led to the growth of a world-wide underground movement whose adherents do not consider these substances dangerous "hallucinogens" but unrivalled tools for self-exploration – or even sacraments. There now exist numerous groups and organisations whose purpose is to provide information about psychedelics and promote safe use. Their evangelical activities include publishing newsletters, magazines and books, hosting websites and chat-rooms, operating online libraries and bookstores, and organising conferences devoted to matters psychedelic.* (It is noteworthy that, despite their tremendous popularity, similar movements have not evolved among users of opioids or psychostimulants.) Given the fervour of the latter-day psychedelic renaissance, interest in these exceptional substances is unlikely to be curbed by shallow and censorious "tough on drugs" campaigns.

Safety of Psychedelics

Contrary to what many people – including many health professionals – have been led to believe, from a *physical* point of view most psychedelics are in fact extremely safe drugs. This statement applies, in particular, to the "classic" psychedelics – LSD, psilocybin, and mescaline – which in chemically pure form are renowned for their extremely low toxicity. (As noted in *Chapter Seven*, there is on-going debate about possible neurological toxicity of Ecstasy). There are no

---

* In January, 2006 an international symposium entitled "LSD: Problem Child and Wonder Drug" was held in Basel, Switzerland with over 2000 members of the global psychedelic fraternity in attendance. Among the participants were scientific researchers, therapists, writers, artists, doctors, academics, and survivors of the first psychedelic era. In addition to formal presentations the gathering celebrated the one hundredth birthday of Albert Hofmann who, as acknowledged "father of LSD", was greeted as honoured elder statesman of the psychedelic movement. The Multidisciplinary Association for Psychedelic Studies (MAPS) is a US-based non-profit research and educational organisation supporting psychedelic research (www.maps.org).

known fatalities associated with these drugs, even when ingested in amounts far larger than anyone would ordinarily use. Furthermore, tolerance develops rapidly so that their psychedelic effects become negligible after several consecutive daily doses. Prolonged use does not lead to craving or addiction, and no withdrawal syndrome occurs if consumption is stopped abruptly. In distinct contrast to commonly abused drugs such as alcohol, cocaine, heroin, and amphetamines, compulsive drug-seeking behaviour does not occur with psychedelics, nor do self-destructive, out-of-control patterns of use.

The preceding statements do *not* mean these substances are completely innocuous. However, if people suffer harm as a result of taking psychedelics it is more likely to be the manner and circumstances of use rather than the drugs themselves that are responsible. As Albert Hofmann has emphasised, the potential danger of these drugs lies in the inherent unpredictability of their *psychological* effects. Such risks are likely to be greatly increased if "street" drugs of unknown purity and potency are consumed, psychedelics are combined with alcohol and other drugs, or they are used in physically and psychologically adverse circumstances without appropriate safeguards.[25]

Heaven and Hell

While some consider psychedelics to be "psychotomimetic" drugs that induce a temporary psychotic state, others regard them as "entheogens" capable of revealing the divine within. Experiences like those of Aldous Huxley and Gordon Wasson concur with the latter view. However, the cumulative experience of numerous individuals has demonstrated that *both* effects can occur – often in the course of a single psychedelic session. When he coined the term psychedelic Dr Osmond composed a simple ditty in acknowledgement of this dual possibility: "To fathom hell or soar angelic, just take a pinch of psychedelic".[26] In-depth research has led some to attribute these seemingly contradictory properties to the capacity of the drugs to act as powerful amplifiers of unconscious mental processes.[*]

---

[*] This statement applies to the "classic" psychedelics but is *not* generally true of Ecstasy (MDMA). The latter is not hallucinogenic at usual doses and its amphetamine-like stimulant effects predominate over any psychedelic effects, which are generally mild at most. Ecstasy produces euphoria and a sense of emotional wellbeing, heightened capacity for empathy, feeling enhancement, and a sense of perceiving the

continued over page

Having personally supervised several thousand LSD sessions while he was Chief of Psychiatric Research at the Maryland Psychiatric Research Centre in Baltimore, USA, Czech psychiatrist Stanislav Grof is one of the foremost authorities on psychedelic altered states of consciousness in the world. Dr Grof (whose ground-breaking work on spiritual emergence was discussed in *Chapter Six*) augmented his own observations with reports of thousands of others – including "normal" volunteers and psychiatric patients – who had participated in supervised psychedelic sessions. Analysis of this vast body of data led him to the following conclusion:

> LSD does not produce a drug-specific state with certain stereo-typical characteristics; it can best be described as a *catalyst or amplifier of mental processes that mediates access to hidden recesses of the human mind*. As such, it activates deep repositories of unconscious material and brings their content to the surface, making it available for direct experience. A person taking the drug will not experience an "LSD state" but a fantastic journey into his or her own mind. All the phenomena encountered during this journey – images, emotions, thoughts and psychosomatic processes – should thus be seen as latent capacities in the experient's psyche rather than symptoms of a "toxic psychosis".[27]

In this view, rather than *causing* the experiences that occur while people are under their influence, psychedelics are seen as physical agents that possess the capacity to make certain types of experience possible. Dr Grof believes that, on a psychological level, drugs such as LSD act as a kind of "inner radar" that scans the unconscious, detects whatever has the strongest emotional charge, and facilitates its emergence into awareness. This may result in release of repressed unconscious material, including early childhood memories. Genuine age-regression phenomena may also occur such that these memories are not only recalled but relived in graphic detail.[28]

The ability of psychedelics to intensify and provoke the emergence of unconscious material makes them a two-edged sword. On the

---

world in a new way. Researcher Bruce Eisner believes Ecstasy is a "feeling enhancer" and "empathogen" rather than a psychedelic. "As a result of the differences between MDMA and its predecessors", he notes, "experiences catalysed by MDMA are nearly always positive." Eisner, B. (1994) *Ecstasy: The MDMA Story*. Berkeley, CA: Ronin Publishing. p.4.

one hand, it could make them a valuable aid to psychotherapy and a powerful tool for self-exploration if the subject's physical and psychological safety is assured and an experienced therapist or guide is on hand to provide support. However, it could be extremely hazardous in an uncontrolled, over-stimulating, or chaotic setting (e.g. a raucous party or frenzied rock concert), particularly if the subject is unable to handle extremely intense and highly volatile emotions.

Adding to the potential hazards is the fact that it is in the nature of psychedelics for their effects on any given occasion to be unpredictable. A complex array of factors related to the personality and psychological make-up of the user, his or her emotional state and expectations at the time of use, and the environment in which the drug is taken all play a part in influencing what occurs. Furthermore, variations in individual sensitivity mean some people could have an extreme response to a very small dose. As Dr Hofmann points out, these considerations mean there is some risk *every* time a psychedelic is taken:

> The advocates of uncontrolled, free use of LSD and other hallucinogens base their attitude on two claims: (1) this type of drug produces no addiction, and (2) until now no danger to health from moderate use of hallucinogens has been demonstrated. Both are true … Like the other hallucinogens, however, LSD is dangerous in an entirely different sense. While the psychic and physical dangers of the addicting narcotics, the opiates, amphetamines, and so forth, appear only with chronic use, *the possible danger of LSD exists in every single experiment.* This is because severe disoriented states can appear during any LSD inebriation. It is true that through careful preparation of the experiment and the experimenter such episodes can largely be avoided, but they cannot be excluded with certainty.[29]

Psychedelic states often involve disturbing as well as exhilarating aspects. Some unpleasant experiences reach such monumental proportions the subject may fear he or she will be overwhelmed or even annihilated. Expressions such as "spinning out" or "freaking out" are pale reflections of the awesome intensity of such "mind-blowing" experiences. Words like "nightmarish", "hellish", and "horrific" are frequently used by those who have endured the harrowing ordeal of a "bad trip". The terror of such experiences is often exacerbated by the certainty it will never end or will leave the subject permanently scarred and forever changed. The following account of an LSD experience graphically illustrates such an experience:

> My God, it was awful, like going to hell with no exit. I was dissolving, and there was nothing but an emptiness that had no end in time and space. I was sure I was dead, or at least permanently insane. Nothing was in any way familiar, and I was cut off from everyone and everything I cared about. I was spinning in space with no centre, nothing I could hold on to or trust. Later the hallucinations just kept coming and coming. There were mostly big spider-webs, and sometimes spiders would fall off and crawl around on my body. Then there were grinning faces that would melt and turn into other faces, like demons in a horror movie I saw once. For a while I felt that I was being punished for the sins of humanity, the way Jesus died on the cross. When my friends tried to comfort me, I was sure they were all laughing at me because they gave me poison and planned to kill me, but only after they tortured me for a while first.[30]

The sense of profound isolation typically associated with such experiences often provokes extreme fear – possibly to the point of panic. Suspicion and distrust may become so intense the person's mental state resembles clinical paranoia. Escalating anxiety could drive some into a state of frenzied excitement reminiscent of mania.

Psychedelic experiences are often so extreme and so different to everyday reality they leave a lasting impression on the subject's mind. Such impressions encompass both positive and negative experiences. For example, long after a powerful psychedelic trip is over people may recall intense feelings of bliss, ecstasy, serenity, and "cosmic oneness" which rank among the most important and cherished experiences of their lives. On the other hand, some experiences might have been so frightening or disconcerting they leave dark traces that are difficult to eradicate. First-hand reports, traditional and contemporary, are filled with stories of people undergoing terrifying ordeals while in psychedelic altered states. Vivid experiences of death (so-called "ego death") are common, as are encounters with threatening non-human or demonic beings, a sense of having been cast into hell or condemned to a ghostly underworld, or the feeling of being totally alone in an infinite and eternal "cosmic void".[31] The capacity of psychedelic states to encompass both ecstatic and agonising aspects was recognised by the first Europeans to take mescaline:

Vague terrors and the sense of impending disaster often mingle with the cosmic experiences. The immensity of the new realms perceived may frighten more than they enlighten … the experiences in the mescal state are not easily forgotten. One looks "beyond the horizon" of the normal world, and this "beyond" is often so impressive or even shocking that its after-effects linger for years in one's memory. No wonder some subjects are disinclined to repeat the experiment.[32]

Even seemingly positive experiences sometimes have unanticipated repercussions. Thus, one young woman described a powerful psychedelic experience as "an explosion that lit up my being and then sent a shadow through it".[33] After many intense experiences another person opined that "A trip can function as a crack of lightning, an explosion of light so brilliant that it scorches the emotional flesh and casts deep saturnine shadows in the cavern of the soul."[34]

Fear of insanity often arises in psychedelic states. As the drug's effects intensify some may become convinced this dreaded possibility is about to occur. With strange ideas looming out of nowhere and trains of thought changing direction without conscious intent people may feel they are losing control of their mind. Paradoxically, struggling to regain control might *exacerbate* incipient mental chaos. After taking a large dose of mescaline one man became enmeshed in such a self-perpetuating spiral:

> My intellect was so affected that every time it produced a thought, it would automatically think about the thought, think about thinking about the thought, and so on down a tunnel of mirrors. The more I tried to use my intellect to get me out of expanding confusion, the more dimensions the confusion assumed.[35]

Apparently trivial stimuli – such as a bystander's insensitive remarks or ill-timed actions – could be sufficient to propel a person into a vicious circle of excruciating doubt. One person described having such an experience toward the end of a long trip:

> I'd become depressed and scared by now. Someone had whispered the word "paranoid" and I became more so than I already was. I began to realise that I was losing my mind. The hallucinations had stopped long before [but] my mind became ambiguous and disconnected. The more I tried to be logical, the more my

thoughts raced wildly around, first this way and then that, in terrible confusion, scuffling their way along in the endless winding labyrinth of mental darkness. Definitions had lost their grasp. I simply could not connect one thing with another. Could I ever climb out of this chaos? No, I concluded. Of course not. How can one lose knowledge? How can one forget naked horror? … I couldn't organise my thoughts and so I began to believe that I wouldn't even be able to solve the most elementary problems … I honestly thought I was ready for the insane asylum.[36]

Although they are almost always transitory, such experiences could contribute to a persistent sense of insecurity. Thus, one man explained how psychedelic experiences had undermined his confidence: "I realised how fragile sanity was, like a layer of thin ice over a seething sea of passions and appetites."[37] Once such seeds of doubt are sown, a lingering doubt may remain: could it happen again?

Psychedelic-induced fear and disorientation can often be allayed relatively quickly with non-coercive support and skilful guidance. In the optimal circumstances of a benign, low-stimulus setting a skilled and experienced guide can usually "talk down" a person in a frightening psychedelic impasse and help them move through it to a state of inner peace. Dr Grof has noted that the most dramatic psychedelic crises often culminate in the most profound personal breakthroughs. However, positive outcomes are far from assured when such crises occur during unsupervised experimentation, especially if it occurs in a noxious setting and those involved are psychologically fragile.

Psychedelics and Psychosis

The fact that psychedelic altered states sometimes resemble acute psychosis has long been recognised. In *The Doors of Perception* Aldous Huxley suggested that "The schizophrenic is like a man permanently under the influence of mescaline." Although the widely held assumption that *all* psychedelic states are instances of drug-induced psychosis is incorrect, these drugs can induce mental states in which the affected individual is temporarily out of touch with consensual reality. If such a person has prominent hallucinatory experiences, holds unconventional ideas with delusion-like intensity, appears "thought disordered", and exhibits seemingly erratic or "bizarre" behaviour, they may be deemed to be in the throes of a drug-induced psychosis.[*]

Indiscriminate use of psychedelics can have a shattering impact on psychologically troubled or emotionally insecure individuals. Pre-existing problems related to self-image, self-esteem, and trust (of self and others) could be amplified to an extreme degree. As one experienced user explained, "On psychedelics, there was no hiding from who you were. If you were worried or scared about something, that would be intensified."[38]

While he never doubted the potential value of psychedelics, Huxley's mescaline experiments alerted him to their darker side. He believed certain qualities in a person's psychological and emotional disposition – including some they might not even be aware of – could instigate horrific rather than blissful experiences: "Fear and anger bar the way to the heavenly Other World and plunge the mescaline taker into hell". As Huxley saw, the "unremitting strangeness" of the world perceived though the eyes of someone under the spell of a psychedelic, the immensity of a universe "at once beautiful and appalling", could readily evoke a malevolent interpretation. The consequences could be dire:

> Once embarked upon the downward, the infernal road, one would never be able to stop. That, now, was only too obvious. "If you started in the wrong way," I said in answer to the investigator's questions, "everything would be a proof of the conspiracy against you. It would all be self-validating. You couldn't draw a breath without knowing it was part of the plot." "So you think you know where madness lies?" My answer was a convinced and heartfelt, "Yes". "And you couldn't control it?" "No, I couldn't control it. If one began with fear and hate as the major premise, one would have to go on to the conclusion."[39]

---

[*] The discovery that psychedelics sometimes induce states resembling psychosis led some early researchers to speculate that schizophrenia might be a result of intoxication by a psychedelic-like substance (a so-called "endogenous hallucinogen") produced within the body, possibly by some faulty metabolic process. Though never widely accepted in medical circles, this notion is the basis of orthomolecular psychiatry which uses nutritional measures to prevent and/or remedy such hypothetical intoxication. See Hoffer, A. and Walker, M. (1978) *Orthomolecular Nutrition*. Connecticut: Keats Publishing.

Even if they involve extremely harrowing aspects, substance-induced psychotic episodes usually resolve spontaneously within a few hours as the drug's effects gradually wear off. However, some episodes may *not* come to an end so quickly or necessarily have a benign outcome. People have been known to struggle for weeks or months – far longer in some cases – with the aftermath of unsettling psychedelic experiences.

Conventional psychiatric explanations for such negative eventualities are usually based on the idea that a "predisposition" towards psychosis must have already existed and that drugs have triggered a latent psychotic disorder by disrupting normal neurotransmitter activity in the unfortunate user's brain. A more sophisticated explanation acknowledges that certain individuals may be prone to psychosis as a result of complex combinations of social, psychological, and spiritual factors, such as outlined earlier in this book. For some persons, exposure to potent psychedelics could be tantamount to dropping a lighted match into a barrel of gunpowder.

Even relatively stable individuals could succumb to psychosis-like episodes in the course of an intense "trip". However, researchers believe such developments are often largely a result of the psychedelic experience being misunderstood and responded to in an inappropriate or insensitive manner. The following remarks, focusing on LSD, are equally applicable to other psychedelics:

> The widely held belief that "LSD makes you crazy" is primarily derived from both medical and lay misinterpretation of the psychiatric hypothesis that the "hallucinogenic" drug-state is a psychotic or psychotomimetic one, resembling if not identical with schizophrenia. This hypothesis, since much modified, and by many or most abandoned as erroneous, emerges repeatedly in the press and elsewhere as a flat declaration that the LSD subject becomes temporarily insane ... That almost any LSD subject may experience, under certain conditions, a transient psychosis or psychosis-like state, is a fact. However, it is also a fact that a "psychosis" rarely ever will occur in a reasonably healthy subject who has not been led to expect it and who has not been exposed to stresses precipitating the "psychotic" episode. *Not LSD, but mishandling of the session, is with few exceptions the key factor when an LSD subject experiences an LSD "psychosis"*... As this has come to be generally understood, and as

session-guiding techniques have improved, the occurrence of drug-state "psychoses" has diminished accordingly.[40]

Though unsupervised experimentation with psychedelics is potentially hazardous, crises arising in this context may eventually be resolved without the user suffering serious harm. Such benign outcomes are most likely if the person concerned is psychologically well-adjusted, has the support of trusted friends, and is able to spend time re-orienting in a safe place. As well as facilitating recovery, such circumstances increase the likelihood of profiting from the ordeal. Dr Grof has found that, if handled skilfully, psychedelic crises – including those with psychosis-like aspects – can result in psychological and emotional healing and personality transformation:

> Unpleasant experiences are caused by the emergence of highly-charged emotionally traumatic unconscious material. Since this material is the source of the patient's difficulties in life, negative episodes in LSD sessions, if properly approached and handled, represent great opportunities for therapeutic change.[41]

On the other hand, Dr Grof has warned, "an insensitive and ignorant approach can cause psychological damage and lead to chronic psychotic states and years of psychiatric hospitalisation."[42]

Quiet, low-stimulus surroundings, non-judgemental empathic support, patience and positive expectations on the part of helpers, are sufficient to facilitate resolution of most psychedelic crises. If these simple measures prove ineffective, Dr Grof recommends judicious use of benzodiazepines (Valium-type drugs) as these relatively mild medications can alleviate anxiety without impeding natural healing processes.[43]

Individuals in the throes of a psychedelic crisis who find themselves in the mental health system do not always receive support of the kind outlined above. In Dr Grof's view "the approach of mental health professionals to complications of the non-medical use of psychedelics is generally ineffective and often harmful."[44] Most psychiatric responses are based on the belief that psychedelic drugs are psychotomimetic and the state they induce is a psychosis. This limiting perception results in the common practice of endeavouring to suppress the crisis with tranquillising "anti-psychotic" medications.

In an emergency, conventional medical treatment can have the beneficial effects of alleviating extreme distress and ensuring physical safety. However, if not administered with great skill and sensitivity, such treatment could hamper self-healing processes which facilitate natural resolution of psychedelic crises. As Dr Grof explains, heavy-handed use of tranquillising drugs could inadvertently result in lasting psychological harm:

> The most dramatically negative LSD experiences have a very strong tendency toward positive resolution; if they are well resolved they are extremely beneficial for the subject in the long run. If tranquillizers are administered in the middle of a difficult psychedelic state they tend to prevent its natural resolution and positive integration. They "freeze" the subject in a negative psychological frame and thus contribute to the incidence of prolonged reactions, negative after-effects, and "flashbacks". The routine administration of tranquillizers in the middle of negative psychedelic experiences is therefore a harmful practice that should be discontinued ... If we terminate an unpleasant experience by administering tranquillizers, the unresolved material will continue to surface in future sessions till the patient reaches the point where he or she is capable of confronting and resolving it.[45]

Inappropriate use of suppressive techniques can result in a wide range of persistent psychosomatic symptoms and psychological difficulties. Common after-effects of poorly resolved psychedelic crises include anxiety, depression, guilt, emotional instability, anger, persecutory feelings (paranoia), altered body image, and perplexing physical sensations, e.g. feeling disconnected from one's body. The principal ongoing difficulty in some cases is a pervasive feeling of being emotionally "stuck".

So-called "flashbacks" involve the recurrence, possibly long after the initial effects of a psychedelic wear off, of unusual experiences, perceptions, or mental states similar to those that occurred under its influence.* These phenomena are *not* due to traces of drugs lingering in the body, as is widely believed, nor to residual neurotoxic effects.[46]

---

* *DSM-IV* classifies flashbacks under "Hallucinogen Persisting Perception Disorder" (HPPD), defined as the transient recurrence, in a person not presently using drugs, of one or more perceptual disturbances that first occurred while under the influence of a hallucinogenic (psychedelic) substance. For this diagnosis to apply flashbacks must cause significant distress or impairment, and the affected individual must recognise that the experiences are drug-related and not objectively real.

Rather, they reflect the continuing influence of poorly integrated psychedelic phenomena due to incomplete resolution of the initial experiences.

Individuals who have had extremely frightening experiences sometimes vow never to touch psychedelics again for fear of another "freak out". However, some people look on such experiences as having something valuable to show or teach them. This attitude was epitomised by a young person who said: "It's so far out, so weird, so out of control, you have to learn something".[47] In collecting first-person accounts of psychedelic experiences researchers Robert Masters and Jean Houston were surprised at how common this attitude was: "After describing in hair-raising detail the most harrowing sort of experience, the person will go on to say that it was valuable, and claims of consequent enhancement of self-esteem and specific therapeutic benefits may be made."[48] A striking illustration of this is found in the case of a man who experienced a psychotic episode that continued for six months after he took a high dose of mescaline. Though at times extremely disturbing, this man felt the experience ultimately helped transform his life and lead him toward a more rewarding career:

Even during the worst of it, I felt it was a price I was willing to pay to come out the other end as the person I was hoping to be. In fact, that's what happened. When I became a professional writer, I actually created the life I was looking for ... I feel very lucky that I was able to live through this psychotic episode and emerge from it without being destroyed. My circuits had been fried and so profoundly modified that people around me didn't know whether I'd ever rejoin the ranks of the normal. But I came out of it actually treasuring the experience. Somehow I got through this extended strangeness relatively unscathed. I didn't get killed or maimed or go permanently insane. Instead of the devastating breakdown it could have been, the psychosis became a breakthrough into the life I wanted to live.[49]

It is noteworthy that, having become depressed as his experiences finally abated, this man undertook a year of intensive psychotherapy to help him better understand why he became psychotic. This process of self-exploration, he feels, played an important role in bringing an extremely tumultuous period of his life to a satisfactory conclusion.

Sacrament or Party Drug?

Use of naturally-occurring materials to induce altered states of consciousness is a common practice in many traditional cultures. For thousands of years indigenous tribal groups have utilised plants containing psychedelic substances in ceremonial and ritual contexts and for various spiritual, divinatory, medicinal, and healing purposes. In discussing psychedelics it is instructive to compare the attitudes and behaviours characteristically associated with traditional use of these powerful substances with those widely prevalent in contemporary Western culture.

Humility and respect are the hallmarks of traditional practices that involve use of psychedelic substances. Respect – for the "magical" properties of the drugs, the gods that are believed to empower them, and the truths they are capable of revealing – is reflected in many of the traditional names given to sacred plants. For example, the Kechua Indians of South America attribute the awesome power of their psychedelic ayahuasca brew to its principle ingredient which they call "vine of the soul", while the Aztecs referred to their psilocybin mushrooms as "divine flesh".[50]

So great is the respect traditionally accorded sacred plants that the act of gathering and preparing them for ceremonial use often entails elaborate rituals and observances. The Mexican Indians who use the mescaline-containing peyote cactus (*peyotl*) as a sacrament believe it is a "divine food" capable of nourishing the human soul. Since it is revered as a gift of the gods, the task of collecting the plant is treated as a sacred undertaking for those involved and the community as a whole:

> So holy a plant is not to be dragged from the earth without proper respect and those who go forth to gather the *peyotl* do so with awareness of the sacred nature of their mission. For several weeks before the expedition starts those who are to take part prepare themselves with prayers and fasting. Abstinence from sexual intercourse is imposed upon them, as both strength and purity are required for the success of the expedition. Chanting prayers and reciting sacred verses, the leaders of the party proceed over the rocky mesas, followed by the pack animals which will bring back the harvest. Before reaching the holy place the members of the expedition perform a public penance. Then, displaying every sign of veneration, they approach the plants, uncovering their heads,

bowing to the ground, and censing themselves with copal incense ... Then, having discharged arrows to right and left of the plant to ward off evil spirits, they dig the cacti with care so as not to hurt them, brush off the soil from the roots, and place the plants in jars. As the expedition returns there is great rejoicing in all the villages through which it passes. *Peyotl* is offered on the altars and fragments given to every person met.[51]

Respect for consciousness-altering plants is invariably marked by keen awareness of the limits of the user's knowledge and the vulnerability of the human body and mind. Traditional cultures often consider it unacceptable – and unwise – to ingest sacramental substances without undergoing the physical and spiritual preparations stipulated by tribal lore. For example, before partaking in the peyote ritual, members of the Native American Church are expected to be physically clean, spiritually pure, psychologically humble, and in a meditative state. Before using their sacramental mushrooms the Mazatec Indians also undertake a process of ritual cleansing:

The Indians' reverence for the sacred mushrooms is also evident in their belief that they can only be eaten by a "clean" person. "Clean" here means ceremonially clean, and that term among other things includes sexual abstinence at least four days before and after ingestion of the mushrooms. Certain rules must also be observed in gathering the mushrooms. With non-observance of these commandments, the mushrooms can make the person who eats it insane, or even kill.[52]

As the first European to participate in the Mazatec ritual, Gordon Wasson noted the strict prohibitions against casual or recreational use of the revered mushrooms by any of the tribe's members:

The mushrooms are sacred and never the butt of vulgar jocularity that is often the way of white men with alcohol ... Among the Indians, their use is hedged about with restrictions of many kinds. Unlike ordinary edible mushrooms, these are never sold in the marketplace, and no Indian dares to eat them frivolously, for excitement. The Indians themselves speak of their use as *muy delicado*, that is, perilous ... The Indians who eat them do not become addicts: when the rainy season is over and the mushrooms disappear, there seems to be no physiological craving for them.[53]

In traditional cultures sacred plants are thought to allow the soul to leave the body and enter the spirit world where it can commune with departed ancestors and supernatural beings and powers. Because this journey is fraught with danger, knowledgeable guides are needed to ensure smooth passage through this otherworldly realm and safe return home. Certain individuals are recognised as having the ability to navigate the often treacherous path between the two worlds. Anthropologists use the term "shaman" for such individuals. The power of these singular persons (who are sometimes known as "medicine men") is such that they are accorded revered status within their communities.[54] In many traditional cultures it is understood that only spiritually and morally elevated individuals can become true guides and healers.[55] Thus, the female Mazatec shaman who gave sacred mushrooms to Gordon Wasson was reputedly "a woman without stain".

As "technicians of the sacred" shamans employ a variety of methods to induce the trance-like state which enables them to perform their role. In many cultures prayer, fasting (water and food), sensory deprivation, extreme pain, breathing techniques, meditation, and ritual dancing and drumming are the preferred methods for inducing the requisite altered states of consciousness. If sacred plants are used, often it is only the shaman who ingests them in order to use insights gained via drug-induced revelations to help sick or troubled individuals seeking assistance. Sometimes a shaman administers sacred medicine to others then serves as guide and overseer of their spirit journey.[56]

Traditional cultures sometimes permit sacred plants to be consumed by the entire tribe on important ceremonial occasions. However, such events are strictly controlled by cultural norms, taboos, and circumscriptions. Children, in particular, are rarely allowed to participate. Any breach of these conditions is considered disrespectful to the sacred nature of the plant and potentially harmful to the individual user and the community as a whole. Gordon Wasson's sojourn with the Mazatec instilled in him a reverential attitude toward their psychedelic ritual:

> I have often taken the sacred mushrooms ... but never for a "kick" or for "recreation". Knowing as I did from the outset the lofty regard in which they are held by those who believe in them, I would not, could not, so profane them.[57]

160

Traditional attitudes and practices contrast sharply with those prevalent throughout the Western world where casual "recreational" consumption of psychedelic drugs is rife. In his memoir, tellingly entitled *LSD: My Problem Child*, Albert Hofmann lamented the fact that his discovery had led, not to the creative outcomes he originally envisaged, but to a worldwide epidemic of "inebriant mania". Assailed by doubts about whether the drug's potential value would be outweighed by the harm caused by its misuse, he asked himself if LSD was a blessing for humanity or a curse. Dr Hofmann was gravely concerned about the risks associated with frivolous use of powerful mind-altering drugs:

> Deliberate provocation of mystical experience, particularly by LSD and related hallucinogens, in contrast to spontaneous visionary experiences, entails dangers that must not be underestimated. Practitioners must take into account the peculiar effects of these substances, namely their ability to influence our consciousness, the innermost essence of our being. The history of LSD to date amply demonstrates the catastrophic consequences that can ensue when its profound effect is misjudged and the substance is mistaken for a pleasure drug. Special internal and external advance preparations are required; with them, an LSD experiment can become a meaningful experience. Wrong and inappropriate use has caused LSD to become my problem child.[58]

Many people use psychedelics in a duly respectful manner and with appropriate precautions.* However, there are many for whom such substances represent nothing more than a means of getting "high" or another way of experiencing a pleasurable "buzz". Such hedonistic consumption often involves behaviours that would be totally unthinkable in a traditional shamanic culture. The very idea of someone "scoring" from a drug dealer in the toilets of a seedy nightclub, or of using psychedelics while intoxicated with alcohol or

---

* Various groups now exist whose specific purpose is to provide sincerely motivated individuals with an opportunity to experience sacred plants under conditions approximating those pertaining during traditional sacramental use. In the USA, for example, it is possible to participate in a guided Indian *peyotl* ceremony, and there are native South American shamans who permit Westerners to partake in traditional ayahuasca rituals. The Council on Spiritual Practices (www.csp.org) is a US-based, non-profit organisation advocating responsible use of psychedelics/entheogens.

161

to intensify the violent thrill of a heavy metal rock concert, would be anathema to the gentle *peyotl* gatherers whose deeply reverential attitude was described earlier.

As well as helping to expand the minds and open the hearts of many people, wildly cavalier experimentation and unrestrained indulgence during the psychedelic Sixties left a trail of psychic damage (though its extent has been much exaggerated). Sadly, the ranks of the so-called "acid casualties" of the free-wheeling hippy era may yet be joined by a new generation of hedonistic users who have remained oblivious to the risks that necessarily attend use of these extraordinarily powerful substances.

From LSD to DSM and CBT

Recent research has provided scientific support for the age-old contention that, when used wisely, psychedelics can facilitate profound spiritual experiences. In a 2006 report entitled "Psilocybin Can Occasion Mystical-Type Experiences Having Substantial and Sustained Personal Meaning and Spiritual Significance", the journal *Psychopharmacology* published results of a double-blind study conducted at Johns Hopkins University School of Medicine in which mature (average age 46 years), psychologically stable volunteers ingested a high dose of psilocybin, the active ingredient of "magic" mushrooms. Of 36 volunteers, 22 had a "complete" mystical experience which many (33%) rated the most spiritually significant event of their life. A majority (67%) said taking psilocybin had been the most meaningful experience of their life or among the top five such experiences and all attributed to it sustained positive changes in their attitudes and behaviour. These findings are similar to those of the 1962 "Good Friday Experiment" in which volunteer theology students took the same drug during a religious service in a Boston University chapel. Many (30%–40%) involved in this pioneer research also reported mystical experiences.[59]

Some participants in the more recent research alluded to above experienced mild to moderate anticipatory anxiety at the start of the session. These feelings were generally transient but four volunteers said the entire experience had been dominated by anxiety and other unpleasant feelings. Several experienced mild, transient paranoid thinking or ideas of reference sometime during the session, two compared it to "being in a war", and three said they would not want to repeat the experience. While readily managed with simple reassurance, these issues highlight the importance of safeguards such as careful selection of participants and adequate supervision during and after psychedelic sessions:

> It is important that the risks of hallucinogen use not be under-estimated. Even in the present study in which the conditions of volunteer preparation and psilocybin administration were carefully designed to minimise adverse effects, with a high dose of psilocybin 31% of the group of carefully screened volunteers experienced significant fear and 17% had transient ideas of reference/paranoia. Under unmonitored conditions, it is not difficult to imagine such effects escalating to panic and dangerous behaviour. Also, the role of hallucinogens in precipitating or exacerbating enduring psychiatric conditions and long-lasting perceptual disturbances should remain a topic of research.[60]

Like all powerful tools psychedelics have the potential to do harm as well as good. (Something similar might be said regarding the seemingly ever-expanding range of potent mind-altering drugs now routinely used in psychiatry.) Unfortunately, concerns about the negative consequences of irresponsible, unsupervised use of psychedelics led not only to the drugs themselves being outlawed but also to a ban on legitimate scientific research. As a result, findings such as those of the "Good Friday Experiment" have been ignored by medical, psychiatric and religious fraternities for over forty years. While the decades-long prohibition on research has recently been eased, it has had significant consequences, not the least of which is widespread ignorance about psychedelic drugs. Dr Rick Strassman, one of the first psychiatrists to conduct new research, notes the medical profession has not been spared this unfortunate legacy:

> With the new drug laws in place, interest in human psychedelic research died off almost as rapidly as it had begun. It was as if the psychedelic drugs became "un-discovered". Considering the intense pace of human research with psychedelics just thirty years ago, it is amazing how little today's medical and psychiatric training programs teach about them. Psychedelics were *the* growth area in psychiatry for over twenty years. Now young physicians and

psychiatrists know almost nothing about them. By the time I was a medical student in the mid-1970s … psychedelics were the topic of just two lectures in my four years of study. Even this may have been more information than students received at most other medical schools.[61]

In this context it is interesting to recall that psychiatrists and other mental health clinicians were once expected to not only have a theoretical understanding of the effects of psychedelics, but advised that actually *taking* drugs such as LSD could help them gain insight into themselves and the experiences of their clients.

Perhaps even more important than the value psychedelics may have for individual users is what they reveal about the human condition – the nature of the mind in particular. One of the most valuable characteristics of these drugs is that they enable observation and study of ordinarily unconscious mental processes. If used responsibly, Dr Grof believes, "It does not seem inappropriate and exaggerated to compare their potential significance for psychiatry and psychology to that of the microscope for medicine or the telescope for astronomy."[62] Sadly, use of this powerful tool for the purpose of exploring the mysteries of the human psyche has been prevented by the social and medical conservatism that was responsible for outlawing psychedelic research in the first place. Nevertheless, Grof has amalgamated his own observations and those of others to devise an "extended cartography of psyche" – a revolutionary new view of the human mind integrating traditional spiritual wisdom with the findings of modern consciousness research.[63]

Paradoxically, rather than fostering development of a more expansive view of the human mind, psychedelics have in some ways had the opposite effect on conventional psychiatry. The realisation that miniscule amounts of substances like LSD can profoundly affect the mind galvanised attempts to explain psychosis and other mental disorders in terms of anomalies in the brain's neurochemical functioning. According to proponents of this view, psychedelics trigger psychosis by disrupting normal biochemical activity of the brain so, by analogy, spontaneous psychoses such as schizophrenia and bipolar disorder must also be due to a biochemical abnormality in the brain.

Many phenomena evoked by psychedelics also occur in other experiential states described in this book. Thus, dreams, spiritual emergencies, and psychoses involving a psychospiritual self-healing process can entail unusual perceptual experiences (including hallucinations); novel ideas and beliefs (at times reaching delusional intensity); altered perception of time, space, body-image, identity, and outer reality; and intense emotions.[64] It is noteworthy that all of these states may entail vivid sequences of death and rebirth, a sense of reliving personal or collective evolutionary history, out-of-body experiences, and a variety of phenomena with apparently "cosmic" or transpersonal characteristics. These similarities lend support to the view, outlined in *Chapter Six*, that the states in question are appropriately seen, not as intractable mental disorders, but as potentially transformative or healing altered states of consciousness.

Psychedelic phenomena represent a profound challenge to conventional notions of reality and personal identity. They raise fundamental questions about the human mind and the nature of sanity and madness. Under the spell of a psychedelic many people have had experiences which seemed *more* real than everyday reality. These often involve radically altered perceptions of self, the world, and other people. Are such phenomena invaluable glimpses into the *true* nature of reality or simply the bizarre fabrications of a drug-addled brain? Should they be honoured as precious visions or dismissed as reality-distorting hallucinations? Experiences with seemingly deep metaphysical or spiritual significance often occur in psychedelic states. Should they be accepted as genuine revelations or treated as delusional misinterpretations of reality? These complex questions – as pertinent to psychosis as they are to psychedelics – are the subject of the next chapter.

Chapter Nine

Psychosis: Breakdown or Breakthrough?

Current psychiatric practice does not attempt to distinguish between psychotic episodes with growth potential and those which indicate a mental disorder.

David Lukoff[1]

Toward the end of the preceding chapter a carefully-conducted experiment was described in which individuals given psilocybin reported profound spiritual experiences. While such responses are consistent with anecdotal accounts and traditional shamanic practices, when scientific peers of the American researchers performed a similar trial in Switzerland they declared the drug had induced a "schizophrenia-like psychosis" in the participants.[2] Such radically divergent interpretations highlight the extent to which the meaning attributed to extreme or unusual experiences is often strongly influenced by the observer's background, beliefs, and preconceptions. If one observer perceives a spiritual experience where another sees only psychosis, it is clear a great deal lies in the eye of the beholder!

When they diagnose individuals experiencing a psychotic "illness", psychiatrists assign labels such as bipolar disorder, schizophrenia, schizoaffective disorder, substance-induced psychotic disorder, delusional disorder and so on according to standard clinical criteria. However, lumping together all psychotic episodes as various forms of "mental breakdown" fails to acknowledge the possibility that some could be manifestations of a psychological coping strategy, spontaneous self-healing process, tumultuous spiritual emergency, or psychedelic altered state of consciousness.

This chapter discusses how acute psychoses can be differentiated from one another so their real nature and meaning becomes clearer. It must be acknowledged that this is no simple matter – which is why these questions are generally ignored or consigned to the too-hard basket. The fact that it is rarely a clear case of one variety of psychosis or another makes the task all the more challenging. Nevertheless, the questions involved are far too important to gloss over: providing appropriate care and support depends on how they are answered.

Drifting, Concealment, Panic

Anton Boisen, founder of the clinical pastoral education movement, was one of the first to stress the importance of looking beyond diagnostic labels in order to discern the real meaning of psychotic experience. Though Boisen's pioneering ideas have since been much refined his original concepts remain fundamentally sound and inform the approach outlined below.

As explained in *Chapter Three*, a state of inner conflict and disharmony centred on deep-seated feelings of inadequacy, guilt, and failure often precede the onset of psychosis. If the resulting emotional distress becomes unbearable a breaking point may finally be reached which catalyses an acute psychotic episode. The particular form this takes will be partly determined by the way the affected person reacts to the crisis. Among a multitude of possibilities Boisen identified three common reactions he termed *drifting*, *concealment*, and *panic*.

1) The Drifting Reaction

One way of responding to overwhelming despair is to simply give up. Some people make no effort to face their problems, choosing instead to follow the "line of least resistance" in their lives. While surrendering in the face of what seems like a losing battle may alleviate anxiety and inner turmoil, it is a costly strategy. As Boisen explains, the lack of "fighting spirit" which characterises this reaction may result in a downhill slide into ever-deepening isolation and deterioration:

> A considerable number make little or no resistance. They do not fight. They do not attempt to turn over a new leaf. They do not try to do anything about it. They merely shut their eyes and drift. Very commonly they resort to easy modes of satisfaction. They withdraw into a world of fantasy, often hastening the process by a resort to drink or to drugs. Eventually they reach the point where the dream world has become for them the real world. The drive for self-realisation is thus short-circuited and the individual becomes more and more listless and ineffective and unable to take care of himself. He thus becomes so peculiar and so much of a burden on his family or friends that they find it necessary to have him committed to the hospital. Such patients seldom show any great emotional disturbance. They have no marked hallucinations and their ideation is not particularly bizarre. But they drift down toward dissolution and destruction.[3]

Such persons would be described clinically as suffering predominantly "negative" symptoms, i.e. social withdrawal, loss of motivation, reduced emotional expressiveness (blunt or flat affect), impaired social functioning, and poor self-care. Earlier psychiatric classifications referred to this state as "simple" schizophrenia, a diagnosis once frequently applied to socially and emotionally withdrawn, apathetic, and aloof individuals who were not overtly psychotic. The following description refers to more extreme cases:

> The simple schizophrenic's principal disorder is a gradual, insidious loss of drive, interest, ambition, and initiative. He is usually not hallucinating or delusional, and, if these symptoms do occur, they do not persist. He withdraws from contact with other people, tends to stay in his room, avoids meeting or eating with other members of the family, stops working, and stops seeing his friends. If he is still in school, his marks drop to a low level, even if they were consistently high in the past. The patient avoids going into the street during the day, but may go for long walks by himself at 2:00 and 3:00 in the morning. He tends to sleep until noon or later, after staying up alone most of the night. During the early stages of his illness, the patient may have many somatic complaints, variously diagnosed as fatigue, nervousness, neurosis, psychosomatic disease, and laziness … He becomes increasingly shallow in his emotional responses and is quite content to drift aimlessly through life as long as he is left alone. Although he appears to be indifferent to his environment, he may react with sudden rage to persistent nagging by members of his family.[4]

Simple schizophrenia is not included in *DSM-IV*. Such individuals would now be diagnosed as having a Schizoid Personality Disorder (characterised by a lifelong pattern of extreme social withdrawal) or Schizotypal Personality Disorder (characterised by social isolation and strikingly odd or strange behaviour, e.g. magical thinking, ideas of reference, highly idiosyncratic or odd speech and communication, excessive interpersonal anxiety). *DSM-IV* states that such personality disorders are sometimes evident before schizophrenia symptoms appear, but that it is unclear whether they are prodromal syndromes or separate diagnostic entities.[5]

Tragically, some on the downward path Boisen described may deteriorate to such an extent they eventually require full time care.

Once diagnosed as having "hebephrenic" schizophrenia, those in the later stages of a drifting reaction would now be diagnosed with schizophrenia of the Disorganised or Residual type according to *DSM-IV*.

Since "drifting reactions" entail severe mental and social disability they are most appropriately considered a specific variety of "Psychosis as a Psychological Breakdown", as described in *Chapter Five*. Boisen stressed that while drifting may become a habitual way of life for some, it is *not* necessarily permanent or irreversible.

2) The Concealment Reaction

Carl Jung long ago recognised that the common human tendency to deny or conceal from oneself personal problems and difficulties could play an important role in the development of certain kinds of psychosis:

> Anyone who observes himself, carefully and unsparingly, will know that there is something within him which would gladly hide and cover up all that is difficult and questionable in life, in order to smooth a path for itself. Insanity gives it a free hand. And once it has gained ascendency, reality is veiled, more quickly or less; it becomes a distant dream, but the dream becomes a reality which holds the patient enchained, wholly or in part, often for the rest of his life.[6]

In the face of intolerable inner conflict various psychological defence mechanisms may be invoked which serve the common purpose of reducing emotional distress. Boisen noted how the effort to construct a more acceptable self-image might result in adoption of unrealistic beliefs and distorted perceptions:

> There are many others who meet the threatening failure by trying to "save their face". They refuse to admit defeat or error and resort to distortion of belief in order to escape the sense of failure and guilt ... In delusional misinterpretation of the psychotic type we see this process carried to such an extreme that the individual is isolated from his fellows. These delusions are many and varied but they generally centre around the problem of the relationship of the individual to his environment. Even though a delusional system may separate an individual from his group and cause him to be

169

looked upon as queer, it serves to keep him from going to pieces and enables him to maintain a certain degree of integration and poise.[7]

Concealment reactions foster development of "paranoid" beliefs and behaviours. Among those resorting to concealment are persons who seek refuge in a fictitious sense of self-importance, a strategy which might ultimately give rise to "grandiose" delusions. This reaction also encompasses individuals who habitually blame others for their difficulties, a tendency which could culminate in development of "persecutory delusions". In Boisen's view, hearing accusatory voices or believing one is being talked about or laughed at are often the result of an "externalisation" of conscience. A deep-seated sense of guilt might reveal itself in a person's belief that his or her mind is being read or thoughts broadcast, while an "uneasy conscience" might underlie a fear of being followed, spied on, poisoned, or conspired against. It could also manifest in the form of "bizarre" persecutory beliefs, such as that electric currents or other ethereal forces are acting upon a person's body or that unseen enemies are hypnotising them or employing mysterious invisible influences to control their mind. These ideas are in accord with Professor Eugen Bleuler's suggestion regarding schizophrenia that the overt symptoms "represent the expression of a more or less unsuccessful attempt to find a way out of an intolerable situation".

Those who resort to concealment frequently demonstrate an exaggerated sense of self-importance ("grandiosity"). This may provide sufficient protection against emotional insecurity the person concerned is freed of incapacitating anxiety and thus able to function adequately. As Boisen observed "The paranoic who succeeds in achieving some sort of systematisation in his misinterpretations may be socially isolated but he does manage to keep his head above water".[8] While concealment could enhance psychological stability it is likely to compromise social and emotional development if it becomes a habitual coping strategy.

Individuals demonstrating beliefs and behaviours such as described above would probably receive a diagnosis of Paranoid Schizophrenia or Delusional Disorder according to *DSM-IV*. Concealment reactions were considered to be a specific type of "Psychosis as a Psychological Coping Strategy" in *Chapter Five*.

3) The Panic Reaction

In-depth study of the antecedents of psychosis led Carl Jung (*Chapter Three*) and Silvano Arieti (*Chapter Five*) to note that many acute episodes are preceded by severe emotional panic. In some instances this may instigate an autonomous transformative process whose purpose is to bring about complete reorganisation of the affected individual's personality, beliefs, values, and life-orientation. (Boisen noted that attitudes and behaviour associated with concealment reactions may have been prominent prior to such upheavals.)

Psychospiritual crises of this kind – which Boisen termed "panic reactions" – often begin abruptly with an overpowering sense something momentous is occurring. Suddenly being flooded with extraordinary ideas, emotions, and impulses is a common though often extremely disconcerting characteristic of such crises:

> They begin generally with some eruption of the subconscious which is interpreted as a manifestation of the supernatural. The impact of such an experience is apt to be terrific. It may destroy the foundations of the mental organisation and upset the structure upon which the judgements and reasoning processes are based. We have then that bewildered state which is called "schizophrenia" … The sufferer finds himself in a strange new world in which previous experience and accepted standards of value do not apply. He sees strange meanings in everything about him and he is sure of only one thing, that things are not what they seem.[9]

Affected individuals often feel as though they are being inundated with ideas and images from some other dimension of reality and that hitherto unknown aspects of life are being revealed to them with great clarity (Boisen took such phenomena as confirmation of Jung's notion of the collective unconscious – see *Appendix: Archetypal Imagery in Acute Schizophrenia*):

> The deeper levels of the mind are tapped and in many cases the mental processes are quickened. Ideas and pictures flash into the mind as if from an outside source and constitute the "voices" and "visions" which loom so large in psychiatric examinations. Very commonly it is as if the conscious self had descended to some lower region where it is no longer in control but at the mercy of the primitive and terrifying ideas and imagery which throng in upon it. The eyes are opened so that one seems to see back to the beginning

171

of creation. One seems to have lived perhaps in many previous existences. Such ideas we find with striking frequency in cases after case. To the individual concerned they carry conviction because they seem so utterly new, so completely apart from all his previous thinking and reading.[10]

Early in such episodes people might be struck by fear of impending death. This is frequently accompanied by an inexplicable sense that the world is about to be transformed or that a major catastrophe is imminent and matters of universal significance are at stake. The person concerned may feel he or she has been selected for a special role or mission, possibly that the fate of the world or humanity depends on them. In this context some may feel they have taken on a "cosmic" identity such as saviour or world teacher. Such ideas and feelings are the hallmarks of psychospiritual crises:

> The presence of ideas of death, of cosmic catastrophe, or of cosmic identification may be taken as the mark of the profounder panic reactions. The ideas of cosmic catastrophe and cosmic identification tend to occur together as part of a constellation of ideas which includes also ideas of rebirth, previous existence, mission, and so forth … The presence of any one of these ideas means the others of this constellation are also likely to be present.[11]

Individuals experiencing psychospiritual crises often become greatly interested in religious and spiritual matters. Indeed, Boisen noted that shortly before such crises begin people who may have previously been indifferent to such things sometimes begin praying or meditating, reading the Bible or other scriptures, and pondering the deepest "meaning of life" questions.

A diagnosis of Catatonic Schizophrenia is likely if an individual experiencing this type of crisis displays psychomotor disturbances such as prolonged physical immobility or significantly diminished responsiveness to environmental stimuli ("catatonic stupor"), or excessive and apparently purposeless activity ("catatonic excite-ment").* If the duration of the disturbance is less than six months

---

* *DSM-IV* provides the following important clarification regarding catatonic states: "Although catatonia has historically been associated with schizophrenia, the clinician should keep in mind that catatonic symptoms are non-specific and may occur in other mental disorders" (p.276). The latter could include Mood Disorders with Catatonic Features.

possible *DSM-IV* diagnoses include Brief Psychotic Disorder or Schizophreniform Disorder. Individuals who become elated and hyperactive might be diagnosed with Schizoaffective Disorder or Bipolar Disorder (Manic Episode). Acute psychospiritual crises were discussed in *Chapter Six* under the heading "Psychosis as a Self-Healing Process" as well as in the context of phenomena referred to collectively as "Spiritual Emergencies".

Many Ways of Being Psychotic

Acute psychotic episodes can take various forms and involve different causative factors, symptoms, subjective responses, and trajectories. Differentiating the major types can be difficult due to the fact that they may involve superficially similar overt symptoms and behaviour. The following cases highlight characteristic features of each type.

Anton Boisen: *"A terrific life and death struggle"*

Early in his career Boisen experienced several severe psychotic episodes which led to him being diagnosed with catatonic schizophrenia. Though considered incapable of pursuing his chosen vocation – "my people were told there was no hope of recovery" – Boisen's harrowing ordeals galvanised his interest in the connection between mental disorder and religious experience. His seminal book, *The Exploration of the Inner World* and various other writings contain vivid descriptions of the potentially transformative crises he termed "panic reactions".

Boisen's first psychotic episode came on very suddenly and was extremely severe. It began with a thought that shook him to the core: "There came surging in upon me with overpowering force a terrifying idea about a coming world catastrophe". The idea that the Earth was about to undergo a metamorphosis flashed into his mind as if from a source outside himself. His mood fluctuated between exaltation and despair in keeping with his rapidly changing sense of identity: "I myself was more important than I had ever dreamed of being; I was also a zero quantity". He felt his inner world had come crashing down, revealing mysterious evil forces whose existence he had never suspected. At times, he says, "I was terrified beyond measure". Though the episode was relatively brief he felt he had journeyed thousands of years and relived every stage of development from the single cell through the entire process of human evolution. The end came suddenly: "I came out of it much as one awakens out of a bad dream". The experience felt like "a terrific life and death struggle", he later recalled. Though in excellent physical health his weight dropped thirty pounds during the three week episode. His diagnosis was catatonic schizophrenia. A few months after the first episode he went through another upheaval "quite as severe as the first" which lasted ten weeks. It, too, began suddenly and ended abruptly.

Boisen was admitted to hospital soon after the first episode started, whereupon his experiences intensified. Though frequently tormented by outrageous thoughts – "Many of the ideas that came to me were shocking, horrifying in the extreme" – there were times he was overjoyed by what he experienced, such as when he heard what sounded like a choir of angels, "the most beautiful music I had ever heard". The emotional atmosphere often changed abruptly: "The next night I was visited, not by angels but by a lot of witches." His room seemed to fill with the odour of brimstone, confirming his belief that witches were around. Hearing a constant tapping along the walls he feared he was in grave danger: "This was due to the detectives in the employ of evil powers who were out to locate the exact place where I was". As his anxiety mounted Boisen made a discovery that brought great comfort: "I found that by lying flat on the floor near the ventilator shaft, I could hear the most beautiful voice I had ever heard. It was the celebration of the Last Supper". With his imagination running wild he was finally placed in seclusion:

> I had now come to the place where I no longer distinguished day from night. I had become an old stallion who had remained behind at the time of the Flood in order to help his friends escape and had been forgotten by them. He was now imprisoned and exploited by a lot of unprincipled medical men and nurses. The only way of escaping was by having my head cut off. I was locked in my room now and I kept getting wilder and wilder, singing and shouting and pounding the glass on the door with fists and elbows. I was ordered to be quiet but this only made me pound the more violently.[12]

Though confined to a locked room Boisen felt he was free to roam the universe, at one time believing he had reached the moon:

> The idea of being in the moon had been present almost from the beginning of the week. Now this became an outstanding feature.

The Moon seemed ordinarily quite far away, but really it was very near. The medical men knew about it and they had perfected a way of spiriting people away and burying them alive in a cell in the Moon, while in the meantime some designing person, a sort of double, would take their place in this world. Everything was run in a very strange way in the Moon. It was done in the most scientific manner. It seemed that it was the abode of departed spirits and all the interests were frankly and openly concerned with the problem of reproduction and of sex … It was very important to be on one's guard, for it seemed that they had a peculiar custom of chopping off one's head and sending one down an invisible chute to the lower regions. This was done in a matter of fact, scientific manner, just as they slaughter cattle in Chicago.[13]

In his imaginative journeying Boisen also visited the sun where he feared he had inadvertently caused a terrible catastrophe:

At one time I succeeded in climbing into the sun, but through some clumsiness, I managed to destroy the balance of things and my friends and relatives in the sun suffered heavily in consequence. Thousands and thousands of them lost their lives. Their blood seemed to gush into my throat and I was nearly strangled with it. I kept groaning, "My friends, my friends, my friends". But I kept struggling in the effort to restore the balance and keep the floor of my room from tipping up and sending everything down to the lower regions.[14]

Boisen's graphic account illustrates the broad range of experiences his episodes entailed. Whereas some had overtly "cosmic" and spiritual themes (metamorphosis, death and dying, angelic presences) others were distinctly "paranoid", e.g. pursuit by detectives employed by evil powers. Some could even be described as bizarre, e.g. feeling he was in the sun being strangled by the blood of his friends, fearing his head would be chopped off on the moon. Though he would probably be given a diagnosis of catatonic schizophrenia according to contemporary psychiatric criteria, Boisen felt the crises were of great benefit: "To be plunged as a patient into a hospital for the insane may be a tragedy or it may be an opportunity. For me it has been an opportunity."[15] He believed the dramatic upheavals had been problem-solving experiences which had answered important personal questions and introduced him to exciting possibilities: "They have opened up, as by powerful flashes of insight, new avenues of service and new vistas into the great unknown."[16] When released from hospital Boisen embarked on a new path. Following his graduation from Harvard Divinity School he became the first full-time psychiatric hospital chaplain in America, a position that enabled him to conduct ground-breaking research on spirituality and mental health.

Paul Noble: *"Spy satellites are controlling my thoughts"*

Paul Noble did not look unusual but police were concerned the twenty-four year old could pose a risk to others as he was convinced his next-door neighbour was using sophisticated electronic equipment linked to satellites to manipulate his thoughts and control his mood. He was extremely angry about this and had confronted his neighbour many times. He was admitted to hospital as an involuntary patient after trying to break into his neighbour's house while he was out. He believed voices he heard were those of renegade government spies plotting with his neighbour against him. He would not accept there was anything wrong with him and refused psychiatric treatment. He insisted his story was true and that spy satellites really were disrupting his thinking. He also claimed his neighbour was making him sick by pumping toxic gas through a pipeline he secretly constructed under Paul's house.

Paul's diagnosis was paranoid schizophrenia. He became extremely angry when told his odd experiences were due to a chemical imbalance in his brain. He admitted he had not been able to locate the underground pipe but said he knew it was there because he could smell poison gas. He also insisted he could feel the negative mental effects of the electronic interference and made a special silver-foil lining for a hat he wore at all times to protect him from mind-controlling rays beamed at him from the orbiting satellites. When asked why anyone would want to control his thoughts Paul explained it was because he possessed secret knowledge which could bring down the government. "They are paranoid about what I know", he insisted. Paul's life was centred on these ideas and his efforts to escape the satellites. His family and friends did not share his beliefs.

Paul often asked the police to arrest his neighbour and investigate his surreptitious activities but they always refused and when the hospital staff also declined to intervene he became extremely irate and accused them of conspiring with his neighbour. He threatened to sue the hospital and the police as soon as he was released – after he had "taken care of" his neighbour. Paul was discharged on a Community Order because of concerns about his behaviour and his refusal to cooperate with treatment. He reluctantly attended outpatient appointments for one year before absconding. Though friendless, unemployed, and living on the streets he remains determined to get someone to help him investigate his former neighbour.

From a psychiatric perspective Paul is a textbook case of paranoid schizophrenia. His thinking encompasses delusional beliefs which are both grandiose (claiming to have special knowledge that could topple the government) and persecutory (believing satellites are interfering with his thoughts and that poisonous gas is being pumped into his house). He also hears hallucinatory voices of unseen enemies plotting against him. Paul would be described as "lacking insight" into his mental condition as a result of his apparent inability to appreciate the illusory nature of his experiences.

Elizabeth Farr: *"Some kind of horrible Enlightenment"*

In *Chapter Four* Elizabeth Farr told how her interest in religion and the occult began as an attempt to explain her experiences, including the voices she heard from an early age:

> I do not know when it was that I first started hearing voices – they were just there and I think they had probably been going on for some time before I was consciously aware of them. Sometimes I heard the voices speaking my thoughts. They would often think my thoughts before I even thought them. Many times I could hear them speaking about me as if I were at a cocktail party and I could hear them in the next room ... Many times the voices were harsh with me; they called me obscene names and criticised me unreasonably. Sometimes they yelled and screamed at me and occasionally would wake me up in the middle of the night with such tirades. The voices made it hard for me to concentrate on the things I wanted to do. Another disturbing phenomenon was that sometimes my thoughts were audibly loud and I began to think that other people could hear what I was thinking. I used to think that I could hear my thought waves being broadcast over speakers ... I had absolutely no sense of privacy. My innermost thoughts were broadcast to the world.[17]

She had unusual visual experiences which she assumed were real but only visible to exceptionally sensitive individuals such as her. Certain experiences made possible by this innate hypersensitivity could at times be quite frightening:

I used to see what I called "interference patterns". These were colourful designs that danced around in the air and on surfaces, on walls, and on people's faces ... I thought these interference patterns were leakage from parts of parallel systems which were similar to our own, but which we here on earth generally were unable to perceive. I thought that I was a particularly sensitive person and was thus able to perceive these things of which no one else was apparently aware ... There were times when I could see the room breathing, the walls expanding and contracting. I had a word for this very special feeling that came over me when I had these perceptual experiences: I called it the "Super Real" ... a sinister feeling of meanings locked behind meanings. A lamp was not just a lamp; it had a personality and was trying to communicate with me. A chair was not just a chair; it seemed more real than reality itself. It scared me.[18]

At times Elizabeth was so overwhelmed by her experiences she tried to escape by isolating herself and going into a state of mental and emotional shut-down:

There were times when I did not function at all. It seemed as if there was no point in moving. Movement was beyond reality – it was an absurdity. When I walked I wasted no movement. I did not swing my arms and when I turned I turned my body as a unit. In conversation I sometimes noticed that after I gestured my hand would stay suspended in the air, forgotten, and it would not occur to me to move it for a long time. I used to sit in the corner of my apartment for days at a time, motionless, petrified. These were usually times when I was perceptually overstimulated, times when the voices might be having a war with each other, yelling and screaming at me, or when I was hallucinating helicopters flying over my apartment. Not moving came naturally. It was the way things had to be. It was almost as if this were a compensation to help de-stimulate me, like a way to subtract the lack of physical movement from the excessive sensory stimulation I experienced.[19]

Elizabeth's odd experiences continued for years and she eventually came to feel she was being led toward a state of spiritual enlightenment. The voices convinced her she had to perform a dangerous act to bring her journey to a fitting conclusion:

I thought I was approaching some kind of horrible Enlightenment about which I felt quite ambivalent. I walked around feeling as if I was exposing the bareness of my soul before God; the fact that everyone could hear all my most private thoughts did not help either … I was susceptible to kooky ideas. I thought the voices came from other worlds. I explained away my strange perceptual phenomena as leakage from parallel dimensions. I believed I was approaching an Enlightened state. The voices told me that in order to reach this Enlightened state I would have, at the appropriate moment, to jump from the seventh floor of a building and land on my head in a certain way. This would put me in a cosmic junction whereupon my spirit would be taken up from my body and transported to the parallel world where I would receive the ultimate Enlightenment. This would allow me to integrate my discordant experiences and perceptions into the everyday world and understand it all in terms of a greater system. I would be able to enlighten mankind to all the full scope of reality that lay beyond and … would have enough knowledge to overcome the conflict that I had experienced between reality and the parallel systems.[20]

Her ordeal continued for eight years and involved many hospital admissions and numerous medications, none of which were truly effective. Eventually, a combination of counselling and personal effort led to renewed confidence and psychological stability:

During my hospitalisations I tried numerous methods of treatment … Some of the medications produced intolerable side-effects [and] I was not able to tolerate high enough doses of the medicines to get any benefit from them. Since then, my schizophrenia has gone into remission. I was ill for eight years, and now I have been well for two and a half years. I am so mentally healthy now that I have been able to return to my career which had been disrupted because of the severity of my symptoms. Although my illness was unpleasant, I cannot say that I completely regret that it happened. The psychosis was an experience in learning, problem-solving, and perceptual broadening that is an opportunity available to few. It has undoubtedly increased my sensitivity to other people … I have a greater appreciation of art and music because of my strange perceptual experiences. And I still have a strong belief in the beyond, although it is no longer of delusional proportions … No matter what I do officially with my life, unofficially it will always be affected by my eight years of psychosis … The experience seemed profound at the time it happened, and it seems profound now as I reflect on it. But I would not go back to it. It is over.[21]

Elizabeth Farr's diagnosis was catatonic schizophrenia. Her experiences included a number of textbook schizophrenia symptoms including auditory hallucinations in the form of derogatory voices and "command" hallucinations, e.g. voices telling her to jump from a tall building. She also experienced persecutory and grandiose delusions (it was her role to enlighten mankind) and bizarre delusions, e.g. "thought broadcasting" (she felt her inner thoughts were broadcast over loudspeakers). The fact that she exhibited unusual gestures ("my hand would stay suspended in the air") and was at times extremely withdrawn and immobile ("I used to sit in the corner of my apartment for days at a time, motionless") would justify a diagnosis of catatonia according to *DSM-IV* criteria. After years of severe mental disturbance Elizabeth Farr recovered fully and now feels the ordeal enriched her life in various ways.

Jeanette Keil: *"I felt a part of God"*

Though Jeanette Keil's episode involved many ecstatic experiences it was so sudden and intense it totally disrupted her life. The episode began abruptly, as if she had woken from a dream:

The affliction came upon me suddenly. Up until the day I was hospitalised I was carrying on the active life of a wife and mother with two pre-school children. However, for several days prior to hospitalisation, the world I experienced was changed even though my actions and speech remained normal. It was as if a light had come on in a dark room and everything which was always there, now became clear. I puzzled. Had I suddenly acquired greater intelligence?[22]

She was soon admitted to a hospital but was so engrossed in her inner experiences she erroneously assumed it was a place of sacred initiation:

Ideas flew through my mind as the doors of a San Diego psychiatric hospital's locked ward clicked behind me. There lay the lounge of the Intensive Care Unit. Was it, I wondered, a chamber for initiations into new levels of awareness … Or was the large, oblong room a launching pad for spaceships to unknown places in the universe? That day, May 18, 1972, I embarked on an incredulous journey into my mind. Shortly after being admitted, I was diagnosed as suffering from an acute schizophrenic episode.[23]

Jeanette was swept into a transformed reality and felt herself to be at the centre of the universe. Overcome with excitement at recognising her own innate perfection and that of all human beings, she lost interest in the mundane world around her:

> In the beginning of my journey into a schizophrenic state, I was euphoric, carried away by the creation of a universe within my own mind. I believed I was a significant part of an all-encompassing plan. Everything evolved around my existence. The reason was simple. After nearly thirty years of living, I had finally found completeness within. Before the schizophrenic experience, I tended to look to people and things outside myself for satisfaction and reinforcement. In the excitement of my discovery that all I needed was within, my mind buzzed. It raced on and on, making seemingly unrelated associations between events and memories. If I was, indeed, the person I had always hoped to be (intelligent, successful, unique), then all people had the same potential to recognise their own perfection and completeness. I was content to sit on my hospital bed and let my mind fling itself from one insight to another. Food didn't interest me. Hospital activities which I was encouraged to participate in were, at the time, aggravating interruptions.[24]

At the height of her inner journey Jeanette experienced mystical identification with God and the whole of creation:

> I knew magnificence! My own place within this universal master plan was so secure that I not only thought I experienced God, but I felt a part of God. This God was not limited to a figurehead somewhere out in ethereal space. It was a force, a power, a momentum which activated (always for good) life on earth. Even inanimate objects were part of this motivating agent which reigned

supreme and with perfection over the entire universe. The feeling was one of an incredible oneness with all creation.[25]

Within a few weeks the intensity of her experiences had subsided considerably and she was subsequently discharged from hospital with a diagnosis of schizophrenia. She felt nobody really understood what had happened to her:

> I was convinced that no one understood or could understand what I was going through. Why was I a totally changed individual? Nothing I was told about the illness made sense with what I was experiencing.[26]

No longer sure what to believe about her experiences, Jeanette was consumed by doubt and uncertainty and eventually succumbed to depression:

> I was dismissed from the hospital in a state of absolute confusion. In terms of what I had experienced, nothing now made sense. What I had believed was good, was bad. What I had thought was real, was fantasy. What I had *known* was true, was crazy. My mind reeled with unresolved problems … In my confusion I agonised over what to write on my shopping list, which dish to pick up next in the process of clearing the table, and dreaded getting out of bed because it meant another meaningless day had begun. The universe had been in the palm of my hand, only to be snatched away … As reality became clearer I experienced confusion's stepchild, depression. Life, even with family and friends, was empty. I wondered if life was really worth all the effort it required of me.[27]

Jeanette's long and painful struggle to make sense of her experiences eventually paid off as her self-confidence gradually returned and she began to enjoy life again:

> Working towards comprehension of my schizophrenic episode was the only thing that made day to day living bearable for a time … I no longer experience days on end when I feel barely able to cope. I have found meaning and enjoyment from the ordinary things of life: family, friends, the beauty of the ocean's changing moods, the warmth of the afternoon sun. I have found meaning in my search to comprehend what happened to me those fateful days back in 1972. I have grown. I have known heaven on earth, and hell. I have come

to better understand myself and can better accept the devastating illness which rocketed me to dazzling heights, abandoned me – psychotic, confused and depressed – and from which I now emerge, a more complete person.[28]

"Journey Within", the title Jeanette Keil gave her account of this difficult period, reflects her feeling that the experience – which centred on a feeling of oneness with God and all creation – held deep personal significance. Though diagnosed with schizophrenia, the episode appears to have had the characteristics of a spiritual emergency ("Episode of Unitive Consciousness") as described in *Chapter Six*.

Frederick Frese: *"My mission was a sacred one"*

Frederick Frese refers to the experiences that occurred during his three psychotic episodes as "cosmic adventures". His second episode began a few months after he started working as a management trainee devising a new problem-solving system for a large business firm:

I started to "understand" that all decisions could be made by translating the decision-making process into numerical codes. I decoded many of the problems I knew the corporation was having, but unfortunately in the process, I myself started turning into various animals, in an evolutionary descending manner. I spent brief periods of time as an ape, a dog, a dragon or snake, a fish, an insect, and an amoeba; finally, I was turned into an atom in the inside of a nuclear explosive device that was on its way to destroy the Soviet Union and the rest of the world as well.[29]

Six months after leaving hospital Frederick was having difficulty finding a job due to the stigma of his recent psychotic episode. He worked for a few months as a real estate agent but left without making any sales. He felt increasingly despondent after attending many interviews without success and began to fear he might never again be productively employed. Then one day, as he was getting ready to go to a party, his outlook suddenly changed:

In readying myself for the party, for some reason I got it in my mind that I should dress my very best. Something was telling me that this was going to be a very special day ... Now I was feeling very good. I was dressed in my best, I was making people laugh, and I knew it was going to be a very special day. It was going to be a special day because I started to realise that all human beings were related in one big family of mankind, and realising the joy of this fact made all other considerations unimportant, less than trivial. We were all family, and I was at peace in the wonderment of this one great truth.[30]

This startling revelation filled him with such joy he longed to share it with others, but he needed a tangible way of convincing people of its truth:

I realised that one of the things that got in the way of our remembering that we were all family was money. Yes, that was it. I had to demonstrate to myself and to the world that money meant nothing to me. Joyfully, I went to my room and gathered all my money together. It could not have been more than a few hundred dollars. I then took it to the living room where some fellows were playing cards. I told them that we are all family members and should love one another, and that money was not important. I began throwing the money about the room, saying something like "Take this money. Take all my money. It means nothing." It was wonderful. We were all family and, for whatever reason, I had become a very rich "uncle" who could make people happy by giving them everything I had.[31]

Frederick felt his identity had undergone a complete transformation and that it was his personal mission to proclaim a great new message to humanity:

I was the uncle and everyone in the world was related to me. They were all my cousins, nieces, and nephews. Happiness was here. The world was one. People of all races and religions, of all ages, and of both genders were happily joined in family bonds, and I was "Uncle Fred". It was so wonderful. I had a message that must be shared with all mankind. Just like Mohammed, I had a message and the message must be shared. There was such joy in my heart as I went from person to person, joyfully greeting each of them as my niece or nephew. I started with the people at the party ... we were all being freed, freed from our blindness. We had not been able to see that we were all one in spirit and in family. How wonderful! I must sing it out to all. I had a mission. I had a job. And it was such a joy to sing out the good news to all.[32]

Having greeted with joy all his newfound "nieces" and "nephews" at the party he felt the time had come to go forth and spread his joyous message to everyone he met:

> I went into the street to proclaim to all the great truth that we were all one wonderful family and that we could now be as one in goodness and joy. And I danced and sang out the great news for all to hear. There were people all around. They were on the sidewalks, they were in the streets, they were in the cars passing by. I must sing, I must dance. All for the wonderment of the spirit of man. I hailed people in cars. Everyone was smiling. Their troubles were leaving them. It was Independence Day at last. People were free. Such wonderful joy.[33]

As he was dancing in the street some of his friends at the party became concerned and phoned for assistance. However, Frederick was so overwhelmed with joy that he was not in the least concerned when the police arrived:

> They seemed very serious. Clearly, they needed the message very badly. I held up my arms and joyfully yelled, "Nephews, your Uncle Fred is here! We are all in the family of mankind!" They suggested I get in the back of their car. How wonderful it could be that the police were now going to help me, Uncle Fred, spread the joyous message. It certainly seemed appropriate, but something did not seem quite right. But I did not worry. I was still quite confident that joy was here at last and that my mission was a sacred one.[34]

The police took him to hospital to be psychiatrically assessed. Frederick continued to spread his joyous message on the ward but found people were not responding as he had expected:

> The physician I talked with was a very serious man. He did not seem to appreciate at all that I had a joyous message. Most people smiled when I gave them my message. The doctor did not smile … On the ward were many "nephews". I began greeting them with joy. I told them I was Uncle Fred and that everything would be all right now. Most of my nephews seemed to like me, but for some reason I was placed in a seclusion room … I stayed in the seclusion room for some time. I could see some of my nephews in the day hall … I yelled that we were all one family and that the time for joy had

come. They did not seem to react at all … I became confused. My metaphor was so joyful. But maybe spreading the joy of the family of man was not going to be quite so easy as I first felt it might be.[35]

During the years following this episode Frederick Frese returned to study, earned a doctoral degree and then served for many years as the director of psychology services at a large American psychiatric hospital. In accordance with *DSM-IV* criteria his psychotic experiences would likely be considered symptoms of the manic phase of Bipolar Disorder. Nevertheless, he says that every day when he speaks to his patients, "I know I am talking to the nieces and nephews of Uncle Fred".[36]

David Lukoff: *"Become a healer"*

In the early 1970s, at the age of twenty three, David Lukoff had a psychotic episode which turned out to be positively life-transforming. Having dropped out of a doctoral programme in anthropology, he was hitchhiking around the USA and experimenting with psychedelic drugs as part of his search for the "meaning of life". One day he had the sudden revelation that he had uncovered the secrets of the cosmos and was the reincarnation of both Buddha and Christ. He felt he was in direct contact with guiding spirits who were assisting him in his mission to write and disseminate a "Holy Book" which would unite humankind and bring into being a loving, conflict-free world:

> What followed was an exciting time for me. I needed little sleep …
> While writing my "new Bible" I held internal conversations with the
> "spirits" of eminent thinkers in the social sciences and humanities.
> I had discussions with contemporary persons, including R.D. Laing,
> Margaret Mead, and Bob Dylan, as well as individuals no longer
> living, such as Rosseau, Freud, Jung, and – of course – Buddha
> and Christ. I talked with them about the design of a new society
> that would herald a return to tribal living and I recorded brief
> summaries of the "messages" I obtained from each of them. While
> writing, the apparent clarity of my thoughts and beauty of my
> vision sometimes brought tears to my eyes. After initially assuming
> "The Scholar" as a pen name alluding to the erudite origins of this
> project, I soon adopted "The Scholar" as my new reincarnated
> identity. In five days I produced a forty-seven-page book that
> contained a combination of parables, poems, and instructions for
> organising the new society.[37]

Lukoff sent copies of his writings to various friends and family members but soon discovered they did not share his messianic vision. During the following months he was homeless and unemployed and, though still preoccupied with his mission, gradually began to see that his "Holy Book" was little more than a semi-coherent collection of unoriginal ideas. Filled with embarrassment and self-reproach over his grandiose beliefs and actions, and grieving the loss of the role that had given his life meaning, he became depressed and suicidal. But his journey suddenly took an unexpected turn:

> The book had been my raison d'etre for the previous several months, and now it seemed worthless. I felt totally lost and confused ... I began to consider the possibility of committing suicide. The image of my skeleton spontaneously appeared to me on several sleepless nights. During the height of these difficulties I went for a walk near the bay, ruminating about events of the last six months. Suddenly I heard a voice say, "Become a healer". I was startled. At that time, lost in self-recrimination, I didn't even think of myself as having a future. However, this voice – the only disembodied voice I've ever heard emanate from outside of myself – set a whole new sequence of events in motion. Prior to this episode the healing arts had never interested me. Yet this voice set me on the path towards my own healing – and a new career.[38]

For several years after receiving this vocational call Lukoff made an intensive study of holistic healing practices, though the true nature of his psychotic crisis remained hidden until nine years later when he began studying shamanism. Contact with indigenous shamans reassured him of his sanity, particularly as he was told by one highly respected Cheyenne medicine man that his temporary psychosis was brought on by spirits to convey teachings. Now a professor of clinical psychology, Lukoff believes his psychotic episode was a "shamanistic initiatory crisis" similar to the "Shamanic Crisis" type of spiritual emergency described in *Chapter Six*.

Differential Diagnosis

In all the cases described above the subjects' experience of themselves and the world was radically altered. This was sometimes accompanied by dramatic intensification of sensory and emotional experience with feelings of release, exhilaration, or revelation and a sense of having stepped beyond the bounds of everyday reality. In some cases the entire episode was marked by fear, anxiety, and bewilderment. Although many subjects initially felt their unusual experiences were a result of something being done *to* them, many later realised they were subjective phenomena that had occurred entirely within their own mind. While the episode was relatively short-lasting in many cases, and sometimes had positive effects, in others the experiences continued in some form for years on end and left the individual concerned severely incapacitated.

From a diagnostic perspective these tumultuous experiences would all be classified as acute psychotic episodes, their principle difference being the symptoms and behaviours most prominent during the disturbance. *DSM*-oriented practitioners place great emphasis on identifying such symptoms because of their alleged diagnostic significance. However, closer scrutiny reveals important differences between psychotic experiences – even if they appear superficially similar. These differences, which are at times quite subtle, are crucial to the task of differentiating psychoses on the basis of their meaning and purpose.

The guidelines below can help differentiate a *psychospiritual crisis* from *psychosis* that manifests as a psychological breakdown, coping strategy, or irruption (as described in *Chapter Five*). Note that these are general principles not rigid diagnostic rules.

(a) Physical Health

A wide variety of medical disorders and conditions can affect the normal functioning of the brain and central nervous system in ways that facilitate psychosis or psychosis-like phenomena. Physical disorders that can provoke psychosis include infections such as viral encephalitis (e.g. herpes, HIV), meningitis, and syphilis; endocrine imbalances associated with adrenal and thyroid dysfunction; metabolic disorders such as porphyria, electrolyte imbalances, kidney or liver failure; space-occupying lesions (tumours); allergies; fever; nutritional deficiencies; vascular abnormalities (aneurism, intracranial haemorrhage); head trauma (especially right-sided injury); cerebral hypoxia secondary to decreased cardiac or respiratory output or severe blood loss; and epilepsy, in particular involving the temporal lobe of the brain.[39]

Clinical indications that physical abnormalities may be contributing to a psychosis include: intellectual impairment (e.g. the person has difficulty with ordinarily manageable mental tasks), clouding of consciousness (reduced mental clarity and alertness), memory impairment, confusion, disorientation (person is unsure of time, date, or where they are). Non-auditory hallucinations (e.g. seeing or smelling things, unusual physical sensations) tend to be more common than hearing things (e.g. "voices") in mental disorders associated with impairment of brain functioning. If these features are prominent a *DSM-IV* diagnosis of Psychotic Disorder Due to a General Medical Condition may be applicable.

Biological factors which have played a role in causing psychosis are often readily identified by physical examinations and laboratory tests. Psychological tests can also help identify abnormalities of brain functioning. Since illnesses or injuries affecting the brain may require specialised treatment a thorough medical examination should be performed at the earliest opportunity. Only after physical causes have been ruled out is it safe to assume the psychosis is primarily a result of psychosocial and/or spiritual factors.

(b) Substance Use

Some psychotic episodes may be associated with substance use and/or withdrawal. Since issues requiring specific therapeutic management may be involved, careful assessment is essential. Clues that can help identify Substance-Induced Psychotic Disorder include:[40]

1. A history of recent substance use (physical tests, e.g. urine screening, may be required). Due to the protracted withdrawal process associated with certain drugs, onset of psychotic symptoms can occur up to four weeks after cessation of use.
2. Symptoms and/or course of the episode are different to those usually associated with psychotic disorders such as Schizophrenia or Bipolar Disorder, e.g. atypical age of onset, prominent non-auditory hallucinations.
3. Sudden appearance of psychotic symptoms in a person over 35 years of age with no prior history of psychotic disorder.

(c) Consciousness and Orientation

Psychospiritual crisis: In general subjects remain alert, in a state of clear consciousness, well-oriented to their surroundings, with no impairment of intellect or memory. Especially intense episodes could possibly entail temporary loss of awareness of the environment due to person becoming totally absorbed in their inner world (e.g. catatonic stupor).

Psychosis: Some drug-induced episodes, and those resulting from illnesses or injuries that affect brain function, could involve clouding of consciousness, disorientation (time, place, person), and impairment of memory and intellect.

(d) Onset and Pre-Episode Functioning
Psychospiritual crisis: Often begins abruptly over the course of hours, days or weeks, i.e. onset is *acute* (e.g. the Boisen and Keil cases above). The subject may have functioned adequately before the episode was "triggered" by an intense emotionally charged situation or experience. In Boisen's opinion, "The more sudden the onset and the more acute the disturbance, the more likely the patient is to recover".[41]

Psychosis: Possibly preceded by a long period (months or years) of gradually deteriorating functioning and deepening social isolation, i.e. *insidious* onset. Subjects sometimes have a history of problematic social adjustment, few close relationships, and limited academic or vocational achievement, possibly coupled with a long pattern of psychiatric problems and associated treatment.

(e) General Behaviour
Psychospiritual crisis: Though they may at times be totally absorbed in their inner world subjects generally remain responsive to their environment and are capable of relating with others and able to trust and cooperate with them. Except during the most intense phases behaviour tends to conform to accepted social norms. Willingly seek help in dealing with disturbing inner experiences and are amenable to sensible suggestions and advice.

Psychosis: Subject's thinking, emotions and behaviour may have a fragmented, chaotic or erratic quality. Disinhibition and diminished self-control may result in flouting of social norms and expectations. Psychoses involving strategies of avoidance or defence are often characterised by isolative behaviour, social and emotional withdrawal, and controlling or manipulative tendencies (e.g. Noble). The lack of trust underlying concealment reactions may result in secretiveness, a tendency to blame or find fault with others, suspiciousness (e.g. seeing others as potential enemies), overt or covert hostility and aggression directed at self or others, and "paranoid" beliefs and behaviour. Self-destructive impulsivity may occur in extreme cases, possibly in response to hallucinatory commands and/or delusional misinterpretations.

(f) Feelings and Mood

Psychospiritual crisis: Emotional state may be elevated, e.g. joyful or ecstatic, though fear and anxiety could be prominent if subject is undergoing extremely intense or frightening inner experiences. Early stages may entail profound emotional turmoil marked by extreme and dramatically fluctuating emotions (e.g. Boisen, Keil). Perplexity and bewilderment may occur at the beginning of episodes whose sudden onset leaves the subject struggling to make sense of a flood of peculiar new experiences.

Psychosis: Subjects may demonstrate pronounced emotional instability ("labile affect") or become excessively elevated with hyperactivity, irritability, pressure of speech, and flight of ideas (manic episode). Hallucinatory phenomena and delusional ideas often develop on a background of pervasive anxiety or despair. Some psychotic episodes are characterised by inappropriate emotional behaviour (e.g. uncharacteristic displays of sexuality, anger, or aggression). Concealment reactions may involve extreme emotions such as unbounded excitement in those who have become "grandiose" (e.g. Frese) or anger and argumentative attitudes in "paranoid" individuals (e.g. Noble). Drifting reactions are characterised by a gradual diminution in the range and intensity of emotional expressiveness ("blunt or flat affect").

(g) Thought Processes

Psychospiritual crisis: Thought processes (as reflected in speech) are essentially normal, i.e. no gross disorganisation with minimal disturbance of flow and continuity, allowing for clear and coherent expression of ideas and feelings. Delusional ideas, if present, tend to be coherent and involve prominent spiritual, religious, and mythological themes (see below). While such beliefs may be strongly held during the episode the subject often remains open to the possibility of doubt ("I might be wrong").

191

Psychosis: Thought processes may possess a fragmented, uncoordinated, or contradictory quality, sometimes to such a degree the subject's train of thought is difficult or impossible for others to follow. Various kinds of formal thought disorder may occur, e.g. loosening of associations, thought blocking, thought insertion or withdrawal, thought broadcasting (all associated with schizophrenia), and "flight of ideas" (manic episodes). Delusional beliefs tend to centre on worldly matters, e.g. grandiosity, persecution, self-reference ("ideas of reference"). Such beliefs may be highly idiosyncratic or bizarre and are often incorrigible, i.e. rigidly held with no possibility of doubt.

(h) Sensory Phenomena

Psychospiritual crisis: Visual experiences (seeing things) tend to be more common than auditory phenomena (hearing things) and may involve perceiving divine or mythic beings and other numinous imagery. Such "visions" often evoke intense feelings of awe, wonder, and reverence. Auditory phenomena may involve transcendental sounds and/or music, e.g. heavenly choir. If voices are heard they may appear to emanate from some supernatural or celestial source (e.g. God, angels, spirits), have benevolent qualities (wisdom, gentleness), and exert a soothing and spiritually uplifting effect. Such voices generally entail complete sentences and may occasionally involve longer monologues or extended discourses which provide spiritual guidance and/or teachings ("revelations").[*]

Psychosis: Auditory phenomena – hearing "voices" and/or other sounds – tend to be more common than visual (drug-induced episodes are a possible exception to this general rule). Hallucinatory voices are often terse, e.g. repeating single words or short phrases, and may be extremely negative. Such voices sometimes issue commands, possibly accompanied by threats of dire punishment for non-compliance. Some make a running commentary on the hearer's thoughts, feelings or behaviour. According to *DSM-IV* criteria two or more voices speaking among themselves about the hearer ("third person voices") is considered to be diagnostic of schizophrenia.

[*] For a comprehensive account of the voice hearing phenomenon see Watkins, J. (2008) *Hearing Voices: A Common Human Experience*. Melbourne: Michelle Anderson Publishing. This book discusses voices which occur in the context of mental disorder as well as those occurring as part of spiritual experience and includes a section on "discernment of spirits".

(i) Predominant Experiential Themes

Psychospiritual crisis: The hallmark of these episodes is a preponderance of spiritual, "cosmic" and/or archetypal themes and marked concern with "meaning of life" questions. Common themes include death and rebirth, a special journey or mission, cosmic conflict, encounters with supernatural forces or beings, and a sense of having acquired a new role and/or spiritual identity. Subjects often feel the experience is deeply spiritual and some are convinced they have been granted access to profound knowledge and/or esoteric wisdom. If hallucinatory phenomena occur they often entail spiritual content such as seeing visions of sacred images or divine personages or hearing the voice of God or other supernatural entities. A vivid sense of imminent world destruction sometimes heralds the beginning of such crises (e.g. Boisen). Subjects sometimes feel certain they are personally responsible for preventing this terrible event, an awesome burden which may induce total mental and physical paralysis (catatonic stupor) or provoke seemingly bizarre behaviours intended to avert the looming apocalypse. Psychologist Louis Sass provides these examples:

> One catatonic patient felt he was obliged to keep "the wheel of the world" in motion by making circular movements with his body; another stood in an uncomfortable position for hours, up on her toes with one arm upraised, for fear of upsetting the universe: "If I succeed in remaining in a perfect state of suspension," she explained, "I will suspend the movement of the earth and stop the march of the world to destruction."[42]

Psychosis: Concealment reactions typically entail more mundane themes, often centred on ongoing issues related to the subject's identity, social role, and relationships. Phenomena with a paranoid quality are common, e.g. persecutory delusions and/or hostile, accusatory voices. If grandiose beliefs occur they sometimes co-exist with those of a paranoid nature. Since ostensibly spiritual experiences can occur in this context the task of differentiating genuine and illusory phenomena is extremely important (see *Chapter Ten*).

(j) Progress and Trajectory

Psychospiritual crisis: Though the subject's hour-to-hour experiences may appear chaotic and directionless, a broader perspective – e.g. observing what takes place over the course of several days or weeks

– often reveals the unfolding of a dynamic, potentially growth-promoting, healing, or transformative process.

Psychosis: Concealment fosters development of a restricted outlook and limited repertoire of rigidly held beliefs which tend to block growth and contribute to emotional "stuckness" and social stagnation. Ever-increasing mental deterioration and social dysfunction are the hallmarks of drifting reactions.

(k) Insight & Reality Testing
Psychospiritual crisis: Except when the episode is at peak intensity subjects are generally able to distinguish inner and outer reality and realise that their experiences are subjective phenomena rich in symbolic meaning and personal significance. Successful resolution of these crises is facilitated by a willingness to "own" the transformative process and keep it internalised.

Psychosis: Concealment reactions typically entail a relatively limited ability to recognise the subjective nature of idiosyncratic ideas and beliefs and consequent confusion of inner and outer reality. Subjects tend to take inner experiences literally rather than as symbolic or metaphorical (so-called "concrete thinking"). This may be accompanied by a habitual tendency to disown inner experiences and project them onto the surrounding environment and/or other people (e.g. Noble and Farr), resulting in impaired "reality testing", distorted or frankly erroneous beliefs (delusions), unshared perceptual experiences (hallucinations), and a tendency to blame others and "act out" unresolved inner conflicts.

(l) Duration
Psychospiritual crisis: These crises are inherently transient. In general they tend to begin abruptly, rapidly reach peak intensity, and – in ideal circumstances – continue a relatively short time (days or weeks) before reaching a natural conclusion. Dr Perry noted that the process of inner transformation in self-healing psychoses seems to take around six weeks ("forty days in the wilderness") to be completed. Though these episodes sometimes end as suddenly as they began ("I came out of it much as one awakens out of a bad dream", said Boisen of his first episode), it could take considerable time for some people to process and fully integrate the experience.

Psychosis: Drifting and concealment reactions tend to be enduring. Since they can provide a degree of stability and a means of containing overwhelming anxiety these reactions can readily become deeply entrenched. For this reason Anton Boisen drew a sharp distinction between psychotic crises which are dramatic attempts at reorganisation and psychosis as a restrictive way of life.

(m) Prognosis and Outcome

Psychospiritual crisis: Though their ability to perform everyday activities may have been impaired temporarily, in optimal circumstances subjects tend to return to their generally good pre-episode level of functioning when the episode comes to an end. Dr Perry notes that the most severe crises often have the best outcomes: "Episodes characterised by the richest outpouring of imagery, while appearing most disturbed, were the most favourable of good outcomes".[43] He elaborates as follows:

> Our experience indicates that in the acute episode the more floridly disturbed the persons are, the more rapidly they move through it. Intensity seems to correlate directly with brevity of time, and with favourable outcome. The persons who are frightened, overwhelmed with imagery, and engrossed in their preoccupations are the ones most likely to have a favourable inner experience, from which they emerge with significant change.[44]

Successful resolution of such crises can result in improved psychological, social, and occupational functioning. Abiding calmness and serenity are the hallmarks of genuine spiritual growth.

Psychosis: Outcome is extremely varied. While some people may only experience a single episode from which they recover fully, others could have multiple episodes that culminate in an enduring state of severe psychosocial disability ("chronic mental illness"). Bipolar disorder and schizophrenia often follow an episodic pattern with intermittent psychotic episodes ("relapse") separated by stable periods ("remission") of variable duration. Some people have persistent positive and negative symptoms during periods of relative stability.

Beyond Symptoms

While the guidelines outlined above are broadly correct it is vital they not be applied in a rigid or inflexible way, as though some episodes were *invariably* constructive or "benign" and others *invariably* destructive or "malignant". A combination of different facets of the three reaction types (drifting, concealment, and panic in Boisen's terminology) will often be evident. For example, while Boisen's psychosis was undoubtedly a healing crisis which ultimately proved beneficial, some phenomena occurring during the upheaval resembled those associated with concealment, e.g. at times he was tormented by frankly paranoid ideas and feared he was being pursued by "detectives in the employ of evil powers"). A mixture of exhilarating and disturbing aspects was evident in the ordeals of Elizabeth Farr, Frederick Frese and David Lukoff. Of the episodes described above only Jeanette Keil's appears to have been predominantly positive – though its protracted aftermath was painful and difficult. Tragically, Paul Noble's ongoing paranoid nightmare seems to have had an entirely negative impact on his life.

Since acute psychotic crises typically entail complex mixtures of highly subjective elements the conventional diagnostic check-list approach is clearly inadequate. Boisen felt it was necessary to look *beyond overt symptoms* to correctly evaluate such crises: "Great caution must be exercised in passing judgement on the basis of objective behaviour alone. What we need to know is the meaning of the particular behaviour to the patient and its relationship to his accepted objectives."[45] He stressed that attention should be paid to the overall pattern of experiences and behaviours occurring in connection with an episode: "Classifications must be made more upon the basis of *dominant mood and attitude* rather than upon that of sporadic ideas which may at one time or another be expressed."[46]

The feelings an acutely psychotic individual elicits in others can provide valuable clues as to what they might be experiencing on a subjective level. For instance, even if a person in the grip of threatening hallucinations or anxiety-provoking persecutory beliefs does not disclose their existence to others, a perceptive observer may experience a sense of fear, wariness, or aloofness which is suggestive of the "paranoid" or "grandiose" stance often associated with psychoses of the coping strategy type. By contrast, individuals in the throes of crises involving profound spiritual or "cosmic" aspects are sometimes subject to such sublime inner experiences their emotional state has an infectious quality that may induce (if only briefly) joyfulness, excitement, awe or other numinous feelings in persons closely involved. In some cases an observer might simply experience an intuitive sense that something of extraordinary significance is occurring.

Breakdown and Breakthrough

It is impossible to predict how a psychotic crisis is likely to affect a person's life over the long-term since a host of inner and outer variables can influence the outcome for better or worse. In this context the following considerations should be born in mind.

Although psychospiritual crises can potentially facilitate growth and healing on the deepest level it would be naïve to assume that every upheaval of this kind will *necessarily* have beneficial effects. Such desirable outcomes are by no means automatic – indeed, they are unlikely in the absence of adequate support and much painstaking effort on the part of the affected individual and others. Boisen noted that people often return to their previous state following such disturbances:

> First of all, there may be no particular change. The individual may come out of his disturbed condition and become normal again without solving his problem. He may stick his head in the sand and try to forget. He may go back to his former manner of life and to his customary reaction modes. He may continue to compromise or "pull the wool over his eyes" or "pass the buck" or seek escape from responsibility.[47]

In contemporary terminology this outcome reflects a coping style referred to as "sealing-over", characterised by active avoidance of all reminders of the psychosis and an effort, on the part of persons concerned, to put the experience behind them as quickly as possible (*Chapter Eleven*). In Boisen's view, such individuals may remain susceptible to further crises:

> Most of the patients discharged from our mental hospitals are probably of this type, and because their problem is still unsolved, and because the sense of personal failure and isolation is aggravated by the

discouragement and humiliation incident to the hospital experience, there is soon a recurrence and perhaps repeated recurrences.[48]

The cases described in this chapter underscore the fact that psychotic crises often involve potentially constructive *and* potentially destructive aspects. Even psychospiritual crises are not without their dangers. This type of crisis, Boisen cautioned, "tends either to make or to break the patient and to produce change either for better or for worse."[49] While acknowledging that the outcome of such crises is sometimes negative, Boisen remained of the opinion that "the disturbance itself is none the less constructive in purpose".[50]

Psychospiritual Recovery

In distinct contrast to the perspective of biomedical psychiatry, this book holds that some varieties of psychotic experience are essentially benign. However, it is in the nature of *all* psychotic crises – including those referred to as "breakdowns" – to force a momentous confrontation with basic life issues. Everybody experiencing psychosis will at some time feel their identity, beliefs, and assumptions about reality have been totally undermined. In a very real sense psychosis involves nothing less than a profound identity crisis. And, as they struggle to rebuild a stable identity and find their place in the world again, diagnosed individuals will repeatedly encounter their deepest fears and insecurities.

The outcome of such a shattering crisis will be influenced by the way the person concerned and others respond to its numerous challenges. Some people reconstruct their lives on an illusory basis, e.g. clinging to a grossly inflated sense of their identity and abilities ("grandiosity") or developing a fearfully distorted view of the world ("paranoia"). Boisen warned of the danger of such strategies becoming deeply ingrained habits.

Another possibility exists. Breakdowns which involve collapse of an outmoded or maladaptive identity and limiting belief systems might create a space for positive change and personal growth. Allan Pinches alludes to such a prospect:

A breakdown, far from being the "end of the road" it may seem in the darkest days, can be a catalyst for change and development in our lives, possibly opening out to new ways of being in the world, insight into the human condition, and profound wisdom. A key message I want to convey is that far from being some meaningless "mishap", a breakdown is intrinsically bound to the whole questions of meaning, purpose, and identity ... While my departure from what could be called "consensus reality" propelled me into devastating highs and lows, and considerable downward social mobility, I can honestly say I have learnt a lot and have grown from the experiences. In many ways it has been a journey of discovery. I believe I have learnt things about life and human nature I could probably not have learnt any other way ... A breakdown can add greater urgency and direction to one's self-exploration. It can be a very powerful catalyst in one's search for self-realisation ... Our experiences and struggles have given us a rare education.[51]

In this view some "breakdowns" may hold the potential to become *breakthroughs* to a more harmonious and fulfilling way of life. Before such change occurs some people may feel as though they have "hit bottom", that "the only way left to go was up". Sadly, many who feel this way succumb to hopelessness and despair and are subsequently mired in gloomy prognoses and stigmatising labels. But such feelings seem to galvanise in some the determination to find a new direction in life (a phenomenon some call the "low turning point"[52]). Peter Chadwick describes the despair that preceded his decision to begin forging a new identity:

I remember one day staring into a mirror on Ward 3 West at Charing Cross. My eyeballs were bulging, my skin was greasy and grainy, my hair like rats' tails ... I looked like everybody's image of a mental patient ... Reflecting on the pathetic sight that met my eyes I thought to myself, "Now I know that the days of the old mind *really are* dead. I, as I was, am really and truly *finished*. I start again, this time from the bottom, not with all my mother's self-sacrificial help but I make my *own* life, my own Self, and I do it *my* way this time." This was perhaps something that I'd always cryptically wanted. That day on the wards ... was nonetheless a final breaking of the umbilical cord with my mother and with the past and was a truly new beginning.[53]

The fact that some psychotic "breakdowns" eventually lead to positive change and personal growth challenges conventional notions of recovery. Such outcomes involve far more than abatement of debilitating symptoms – the hallmark of *clinical recovery* (also referred to as "remission"). In such instances it would perhaps be more fitting to speak of *psychospiritual recovery* with its connotations of regeneration, rebirth and renewal.

Conclusion

Psychosis has always attracted strong responses and given rise to extreme interpretations: considered by some as akin to a state of mystical illumination, but viewed by others as the epitome of human failure and psychological catastrophe. At their worst those who cling to the former belief demonstrate their ignorance of both phenomena. On the other hand, excessively pessimistic views fail to do justice to the richness and diversity of psychotic experience. Extremes of either kind are neither accurate nor helpful to those undergoing such crises and their social, emotional, and spiritual aftermath. Psychosis is a complex phenomenon that encompasses a broad spectrum of possibilities, positive and negative. Appreciating its constructive aspects, as well as those of a potentially detrimental nature, provides a sound basis for supporting healing and recovery.

Chapter Ten

Psychosis and Spirituality

If spirituality had not existed, people in psychosis would have invented it. The havoc of mental mechanisms experienced in psychosis seems to beg for spiritual or supernatural explanation.

Edward Podvoll[1]

Spiritual or seemingly spiritual experiences often occur in the course of spontaneous and drug-induced psychotic episodes. Such experiences are frequently a deeply moving, even transformative feature of psychoses of the self-healing type, spiritual emergencies, and psychedelic states. Spiritual phenomena of a more subtle kind are often present before, during, and after psychotic crises but may be overlooked due to their less dramatic form. Whether overt or not, spirituality plays a significant role in many psychoses and is often an important influence on subsequent adjustment, healing, and recovery.

These facts raise questions of great theoretical and practical importance. First and foremost, the occurrence of genuine spiritual phenomena during psychosis highlights the limitations of crude biomedical approaches – simplistic "chemical imbalance" hypotheses cannot account for them. On a practical level, putatively spiritual experiences present all concerned with complex challenges. While many psychotic phenomena seem to call for a supernatural explanation, such interpretations may *not* always be warranted. Determining whether these experiences are genuinely spiritual or merely illusory is often difficult, as is deciding how best to respond to them, illusory or not.

Healing the Soul

That spirituality is a quintessential aspect of human life is evidenced by the fact that all thinking people from time to time ponder the nature and meaning of their existence. While science has made tremendous progress elucidating the physical mechanisms underlying human life it cannot explain *why* we are here. Answers to questions pertaining to the great mysteries of life – Who am I? Why do I exist? What should I do with my life? What happens when I die? – must be sought at the deepest levels. In addition to metaphysical issues like these, individuals who undergo painful, life-changing ordeals often struggle with the inevitable question: Why did this happen to me? Facile explanations concerning genes and aberrant brain chemistry are unlikely to satisfy those who, during a crisis, felt themselves lifted into a world of celestial beauty or banished to a terrifying hellish realm.

Undergoing the profound upheaval of psychosis may rouse a previously dormant curiosity about spiritual and philosophical matters, especially if a person's former beliefs are unable to account for what they experienced and do not provide satisfactory guidance in the search for new bearings. Undergoing a severe emotional crisis shakes a person's identity and worldview to the core. While this can have problematic consequences such ordeals could serve as a kind of "wake-up call", as Jungian analyst and clinical professor of psychiatry Dr Jean Bolen explains:

> Illness is both soul-shaking and soul-evoking for the patient and for all others for whom the patient matters. We lose an innocence and we know vulnerability, we are no longer who we were before this event, and we will never be the same. We are in uncharted terrain, there is no turning back. Illness is a profound soul event … [that] makes us acutely aware of how precious life is and how precious a particular life is. Priorities shift. We may see the truth of what matters, who matters, and what we have been doing with our lives and have to decide what to do – now that we know. Significant relationships are tested and either come through strengthened or fail. Pain and fear bring us to our knees … Our spiritual and religious convictions or lack of them is called into question. Illness is an ordeal for both body and soul, and a time when healing of either or both can result.[2]

Some believe spiritual issues lie at the heart of certain kinds of mental disorder. In the Tibetan Buddhist tradition, for example, great emphasis is placed on the psychological consequences of spiritual dis-ease. As one authority states: "The general and basic cause of mental illness is thought to lie in leading a life that runs counter to one's deepest spiritual inclinations and insights and one's inherent disposition."[3] Traditional cultures recognise that spiritual harmony is one of the foundations of mental health and emotional wellbeing. Western cultures once acknowledged the role of spirituality in human life. It is an often overlooked fact that "psyche", the Ancient Greek word from which modern terms such as psychology and psychiatry are derived, refers to the human soul or spirit. In this context it is thought-provoking to realise that psychosis literally means "give soul or life to" and that psychiatry itself was originally understood to mean "healing of the soul".

It has been clearly demonstrated that religious and/or spiritual beliefs and practices can assist coping, healing and recovery.[4] A survey of a large number of studies published in the *American Journal of Psychiatry* and *Archives of General Psychiatry* found that the vast majority (92%) showed religious commitments had positive effects on mental health.[5] As well as being a source of strength, comfort, and guidance, spirituality can help reduce feelings of alienation, counteract the corrosive effects of stigmatisation, and function as a buffer against the impact of stressful events. Most importantly, it can help people maintain a sense of meaning and continuity in their lives – a boon during periods of uncertainty and loss of direction. Spirituality may play a vital role in the struggle to maintain a personally acceptable identity. Indeed, religious and/or spiritual beliefs are probably unique in their ability to foster a sense of personal worth, a feeling of being loved and valued despite one's problems and shortcomings, and a sense of connection to other people and life as a whole.[6]

"I Felt So Holy, But Now I'm Told It's A Disease"

People diagnosed with various kinds of mental illness frequently identify religious and/or spiritual beliefs and practices as important aids to coping and recovery. The findings of a recent survey of mental health patients are typical in that a large majority (80%) said their religious beliefs and activities helped them cope with symptoms and daily difficulties and nearly one third described such beliefs and practices as the most important things that kept them going.[7] Comparable findings have been reported by Australian researchers who also noted that many psychiatric patients feel their spiritual needs should be taken into account by those providing care and treatment:

Spiritual issues encompass what is most meaningful and central in human existence. In times of crisis, illness, and transition, spiritual issues are likely to come to the fore … spirituality was an important issue with the majority of patients. There was strong mention of the requirement of these patients' therapists to be aware of their spiritual beliefs and needs. A requirement was also expressed by patients for their spiritual needs to be taken into consideration when treatment was being planned. In other words, in a majority of these patients a spiritual intervention would not only be accepted but also desired. The outcome of this type of intervention on facilitating recovery and coping with psychological and physical problems is likely to be positive.[8]

Despite abundant evidence of its importance, on the whole mainstream psychiatry tends to ignore spirituality or dismiss it as irrelevant. This attitude is a product of several powerful influences. First and foremost, contemporary psychiatry is highly materialistic in that it sees *physical* factors (e.g. genes, neurotransmitters) as the principal cause of mental disorder and relies almost exclusively on *physical* methods of treatment (e.g. psychotropic medications). In this "scientific" paradigm spiritual phenomena are often considered too vague and subjective to be worthy of serious consideration. An additional influence is the fact that mental health clinicians rarely receive formal instruction on spirituality as part of their training. In the worst cases these combined influences could result in a tendency to pathologise spiritual beliefs and experiences, i.e. treating them as exotic mental symptoms which are a "part of the illness". More benign responses can involve simply overlooking spirituality (not asking about it), or treating it in a superficial manner, e.g. making a few cursory inquiries in order to tick the "Which religion are you?" box. Whether out of a sense of duty or as a way of passing the buck, the most that can often be expected is that a referral will be made to a minister of religion or pastoral counsellor.*

---

* This could be extremely beneficial if the training, experience, and personal orientation of the professional consulted adequately equip them to deal with the complex issues involved. However, partly due to lack of relevant training in assessing and responding to clients with mental health issues, many clergy do not feel comfortable dealing with such individuals. This is especially likely if a person is undergoing intense inner experiences. As Dr Grof has noted, "The Bible can be found in the drawers of many motels and hotels, and lip service is paid to God and religion in the speeches

 continued over page

Responding to psychosis in a positive and constructive way is difficult even when the presenting issues are relatively clear and straightforward. When complex religious and spiritual questions are involved – some of which might be personally and professionally challenging to clinicians and others concerned – the difficulties may be greatly increased. Furthermore, mental health professionals and other helpers (such as relatives and support workers) may fear that addressing spiritual issues could inadvertently reinforce unhealthy preoccupations and ungroundedness. Such concerns are especially pertinent in the case of individuals whose "reality testing" abilities are compromised. Faced with such complexity it can be tempting to consign these issues to the too-hard-basket. (It is not only clinicians and other helpers who may do this. People who undergo a psychotic upheaval often flee the experience, as evidenced by the "sealing-over" coping style described in *Chapter Eleven*. Indeed, individuals who may have been keenly interested in spirituality before experiencing psychosis sometimes develop a kind of "spiritual phobia" thereafter, actively avoiding all such matters for fear of stirring things up again.)

A host of influences have led to the present situation in which spirituality tends to be neglected, if it is not actively pathologised, in contemporary psychiatry. While partly a result of *legitimate* concerns, this attitude could result in "throwing out the baby with the bathwater" in some instances. If appropriate care is exercised it can often be extremely beneficial for mental health clinicians to acknowledge and address their clients' spiritual concerns. For example, in one study of individuals who had experienced acute psychosis over 30% reported an increase in religious/spiritual beliefs after diagnosis and 70% said such beliefs helped them cope better.[9] Interestingly – and in distinct contrast to what some might fear – the more religiously-inclined individuals in this study had *better* insight and were *more* compliant with treatment.

---

of many prominent politicians and other public figures. Yet, if a member of a typical congregation were to have a profound religious experience, its minister would very likely send him or her to a psychiatrist for medical treatment." [Grof, S. (1993) *Beyond the Brain*. Albany: State University of New York Press. p.334]

Jewels In The Psychotic Debris

Many astute observers of the human condition have noted a relationship between spiritual experience and certain kinds of mental disorder. Thus, the renowned Greek philosopher Socrates declared, "Our greatest blessings come to us by way of madness, provided the madness is given us by divine gift."[10] In modern times a number of the most perceptive psychologists and psychiatrists have insisted that spirituality must be granted a central role in mental health care. Anton Boisen, a true pioneer in this area, was quite adamant on this matter: "I feel that many forms of insanity are religious rather than medical problems and that they cannot be successfully treated until they are so recognised."[11] Indeed, Boisen went so far as to assert "Even the hospital patient who thinks himself as Christ may not be wholly mistaken".[12]

Psychiatrist Karl Jaspers pointed out that "Religious experience remains what it is, whether it occurs in saint or psychotic, or whether the person in whom it occurs is both at once."[13] Among contemporary mental health experts psychology professor David Lukoff is a leading proponent of the view that valid spiritual experiences sometimes occur in the course of acute psychosis. Professor Lukoff believes such episodes are best understood as "Psychotic Disorders with Mystical Features". He also contends that some disturbances diagnosed as acute psychosis are in fact spiritual experiences with psychosis-like aspects, phenomena he refers to as "Mystical Experiences with Psychotic Features".[14] While these notions have not been embraced by the mainstream mental health professions they are well-accepted in the burgeoning discipline of *transpersonal psychology*. General adoption of the transpersonal approach – particularly the notion that spirituality occupies a central role in any truly comprehensive view of the human mind and behaviour – would radically transform the way psychology and psychiatry are practiced.[15]

Until such time as this occurs those who have had apparently spiritual experiences while psychotic may take comfort from the views of Dr Edward Podvoll who insists "it is terribly important to become aware of the spiritual dimension of the psychotic ordeal."[16] A growing body of scientific evidence supports the validity of Dr Podvoll's advice. For example, research published in the *Journal for the Scientific Study of Religion* compared the experiences of psychiatric inpatients whose psychosis involved "religious delusions" with those of religious contemplatives (cloistered monks and nuns, meditation teachers). Interestingly, when various psychological tests were applied to the spiritual experiences of patients and contemplatives they were found to be very similar in form and content. This intriguing observation led these researchers to conclude that their findings "lend tentative support to the theoretical position that considers mystical experience in psychosis, and mystical experiences within various religious traditions, to be essentially the same."[17] Such findings appear to confirm Boisen's claim regarding "the hospital patient who thinks himself as Christ". (Significantly, this research also found a number of marked *differences* in the experiences and outlook of these two groups – a fact whose important implications are discussed later in this chapter.)

It is not difficult to find first-person accounts that accord with the preceding views. For example, during a prolonged psychotic episode (apparently provoked by mescaline), Mark Vonnegut had deeply moving spiritual insights:

> I thought about the things I had studied in religion, and about how much more of it seemed to make sense now. I had somehow touched what Jesus, Buddha, and others had been talking about. Formerly confusing phrases out of various scriptures came to me and each seemed perfectly beautifully clear. I became aware of a harmony and wholeness to life that had previously eluded me. Disconnectedness was very clearly illusory.[18]

The following experience, described in Morag Coate's auto-biographical memoir, *Beyond All Reason*, occurred while she was in an acute psychotic state:

> I got up from where I had been sitting ... Suddenly my whole being was filled with light and loveliness and with an upsurge of deeply moving feeling from within to meet and reciprocate the influence that flowed into me. I was in a state of the most vivid awareness and illumination. What can I say of it? A cloudless, cerulean blue sky of the mind, shot through with shafts of exquisite, warm, dazzling sunlight ... It seemed that some force or impulse from without were acting on me, looking into me; that I was in touch with a reality beyond my own; that I had made direct contact with the secret, ultimate source of life. What I had read of the accounts of others

acquired suddenly a new meaning. It flashed across my mind, "This is what the mystics mean by the direct experience of God."[19]

Several cases described earlier in this book also highlight the fact that profound spiritual experiences sometimes occur while people are in the throes of acute psychosis. In Dr Podvoll's view it is vital that these be acknowledged and affirmed: "Such experiences are of the utmost importance to people who have been in psychosis. In fact, they are the treasured possessions of the psychotic experience, jewels within the psychotic debris."[20] Sadly, the personal significance of such experiences is often ignored. As Sally Clay notes, such a derogatory attitude is certain to have negative consequences:

> A psychotic episode may contain within it the beginnings of a spiritual breakthrough. The spiritual qualities of extreme mental states are real and powerful, and they are part and parcel of the pain, confusion and dangerous quality of madness. To devalue or negate these spiritual aspects is to devalue or negate the person who experiences them, for these qualities are inseparable from the person. That is the true definition of stigma – a devaluation or negation that marks as shameful those qualities that are in a person's heart.[21]

Morag Coate's experience illustrates how invaluable the support of sensitive and open-minded helpers can be. Though she was previously advised to reject her experiences as meaningless symptoms of mental disorder, a turning point came when she finally found someone who followed Dr Podvoll's recommendations:

> It was a relief to be able to talk freely at last. Unlike the psychiatrists in the mental hospitals, Dr Upton was not a persistent questioner. Once the ice was broken he just let me talk, and it was his quality as a listener that led me on. He did directly influence me, but in a quiet and non-dominating way. He suggested to me that I had cast out too much when I rejected the whole content of my spiritual experiences. There might still be much that was valid in them. I was impressed by his comments, and by the way he listened, and his quickness to link up experiences of mine with those of other people. I no longer felt inwardly alone, and hope began to stir within me. My outside interests revived, I could listen to music with enjoyment, the world became a brighter place.[22]

The ineffable, other-worldly, "supernatural" phenomena reported by many people in acute psychotic states can be interpreted in a number of ways. While some accept them as valid spiritual experiences – "jewels in the psychotic debris" – to biomedical psychiatry they are evidence of the extent to which the psychotic mind has lost touch with reality. However, even phenomena which involve clearly illusory or severely distorted ideas and perceptions may sometimes originate in a true and noble spiritual impulse. This notion has a long history. Thus, the eighteenth century German philosopher Friedrich Hegel said: "In insanity the soul strives to restore itself to the perfect inner harmony out of existing contradiction."[23] Anton Boisen believed psychotic disturbances characterised by marked religious concern "are attempts at cure and reorganisation".[24] Contemporary authorities such as Edward Podvoll believe a heart-felt longing for spiritual transformation lies at the root of many acute psychotic episodes. These ideas underscore the importance of looking *beyond* overt symptoms to discern what a diagnosed person may have been endeavouring to achieve on a spiritual level.

Mystical Bedlam

Having discussed positive aspects of the spiritual dimensions of psychotic experience it is necessary to sound a note of caution. In-depth research convinced Anton Boisen that in acute psychotic crises "we are dealing with the operation of the most potent forces and the most delicate laws of the spiritual life".[25] Failure to understand and respect these could have a range of adverse consequences.

One way this might occur is if troubled individuals come to believe their problems are a consequence of things they have done or failed to do. This could lead to excruciating anxiety or guilt related to the conviction that they are being punished for their sins or have even been abandoned by God. That such beliefs may be relatively common is suggested by research which found almost one in four psychiatric patients felt sinful thoughts or acts may have contributed to their condition.[26] Nineteenth century Danish philosopher Søren Kierkegaard believed many mentally disturbed individuals are greatly tormented by such ideas: "The worst affliction of all is, and continues to be, that one does not know whether one's suffering is an illness of the mind or a sin."[27]

Delusional, hallucinatory, and other psychotic phenomena sometimes masquerade as genuine spiritual experiences. While their
erroneous nature might be obvious to others, people sometimes
become so engrossed in such experiences they lose the ability to
assess them correctly. The following statement is a rather extreme
illustration of this. Though the man concerned was convinced of the
spiritual profundity of his insights, to an impartial observer his highly
idiosyncratic ideas seem frankly bizarre:

> I have decided to reveal yet another secret! God is living on the
> 11 balls in the mist again. If a man takes a plank of wood and
> makes 12 holes and marks each hole, the eleventh with 11/0, then
> stands the board on the ground, looks through the twelfth hole,
> then looks up, thinks 12-24, while the woman – who must lie half
> to the left of the man – sees an apple, then it is possible that a child
> of God will be born. This has to be done in the woods, since you
> don't get the right contact with life indoors.[28]

If they are unable to exercise adequate "reality testing", individuals
under the sway of what they feel are valid spiritual ideas or experiences
might be led astray. Some could be exposed to serious danger or even
inflict harm on themselves or others. For example, at the height of
an acute psychotic episode Elizabeth Farr felt she was approaching
a state of spiritual enlightenment: "I walked around feeling as if I
was exposing the bareness of my soul before God". At one point
Farr (whose experiences were described in *Chapter Nine*) felt she was
being directed by the voices of supernatural beings to leap from a tall
building as a way of testing her spiritual commitment:

> The reason for my becoming so interested in religion, ESP, and
> the occult was that these were the closest things I could find that
> seemed to have any relation to what I was experiencing. I was
> susceptible to kooky ideas. I thought the voices came from other
> worlds ... I believed I was approaching an Enlightened state. The
> voices told me that in order to reach this Enlightened state I would
> have, at the appropriate moment, to jump from the seventh floor
> of a building and land on my head in a certain way. This would put
> me in a cosmic junction whereupon my spirit would be taken up
> from my body and transported to the parallel world where I would
> receive the ultimate Enlightenment.[29]

Fortunately, Elizabeth Farr was able to stop herself completing this test. Others are not so fortunate. Many have acted on delusional beliefs (e.g. "I must kill myself to prove I am immortal), or followed hallucinatory commands (e.g. a man believed God told him to castrate himself to atone for lustful thoughts), with tragic consequences.[30] Even if they do not result in physical harm, uncritical acceptance of seemingly spiritual imperatives could have undesirable effects of other kinds. As Jungian psychologist June Singer notes, social and emotional isolation is an all-too-common consequence of preoccupation with highly idiosyncratic "spiritual" notions:

> He may become obsessed with certain strange or eccentric ideas, probably ideas of apparently cosmic significance: he comes to feel that he is miraculously the possessor of a marvellous truth that no one has ever realised before. He may become an eccentric with prophetic leanings, but nothing ever comes of it because it all seems as real to him as it seems phoney to those who listen to him. As his friends turn cool toward him, he may then revert to a rather childish petulance and gradually cut himself off from contact with others, becoming a social isolate, a sad man with a mission in which nobody is interested.[31]

It is not unreasonable to ask: does this man have "spiritual" beliefs or do they have him? It is hardly surprising some people still accept the idea that certain types of mental disorder are a result of *possession* by supernatural forces. These situations readily devolve into a self-perpetuating cycle. Individuals who fall under the sway of dubious "spiritual" experiences may find it difficult to extricate themselves, especially if such experiences are helping meet their emotional needs or providing a temporary solution to complex personal problems. An individual with poor self-esteem might cling to the illusory belief they have a unique spiritual role or identity. As one young man explained, "My illness was a great ego-builder. Just think, God thought I was so special he was punishing me like this."

Even *genuine* spiritual phenomena could sometimes have untoward consequences. For example, aspects of Mark Vonnegut's experiences are highly reminiscent of the state of "cosmic consciousness" described by many bona fide mystics and saints throughout the ages.[32] However, while the experience was extraordinarily moving, Vonnegut soon found he was incapable of functioning in this state since

211

even simple tasks such as pruning trees became overwhelmingly complex:

> One saw cut would take forever. I was completely absorbed in the sawdust floating gently to the ground, the feel of the saw in my hands, the incredible patterns in the bark, the muscles in my arm pulling back and then pushing forward. Everything stretched infinitely in all directions ... I found myself being unable to stick with any one tree. I'd take a branch here, a couple there. It seemed I had been working for hours and hours but the sun hadn't moved at all. I began to wonder if I was hurting the trees and found myself apologising. Each tree began to take on a personality. I began to wonder if any of them liked me. I became completely absorbed in looking at each tree and began to notice that they were ever so slightly luminescent, shining with a soft inner light that played around the branches.[33]

As the intensity their experiences diminishes people are sometimes left with a deep feeling of loss and emptiness that could give rise to a distressing condition which has been referred to as "divine homesickness".[34] Elizabeth Keil (whose experiences were described in *Chapter Nine*), explains how she was overcome with profound sadness when her sense of spiritual wholeness and "cosmic oneness" eventually disappeared:

> Life, even with family and friends, was empty. I wondered if life was really worth all the effort it required of me. Weeks after dismissal from the hospital, at the point when I was completely in touch with everyday reality, I wept. I cried for all people because they could not see the perfection which existed. And, I cried for myself, because I had once *known* ... and *knew* no longer. Slowly, very slowly, a numbness overcame me ... I stumbled through the days like a robot.[35]

This state, characterised by a painful sense of inner desolation and spiritual aridity, is reminiscent of the "Dark Night of the Soul" described by the revered sixteenth century Catholic mystic, Saint John of the Cross.[36] If it is severe and prolonged such despair could lead to depression, possibly accompanied by suicidal ideation. Though individuals in this state may be diagnosed as suffering "post-psychotic depression", the fundamental cause of their malaise may in fact be unrequited spiritual longing.

Spiritual Discernment

While it is good to affirm the value of *authentic* spiritual phenomena it is important not to *over*-value them or succumb to the temptations of egocentricity and self-aggrandisement. Since even genuine experiences could foster beliefs or actions that are potentially harmful (psychologically if not physically), to safeguard against possible deception all apparently spiritual phenomena occurring in the context of psychosis should be subject to meticulous evaluation. As Professor James advised in his classic treatise, *The Varieties of Religious Experience*, "What comes must be sifted and tested, and run the gauntlet of confrontation with the total content of experience, just like what comes from the outer world of sense."[37]

Some supposedly "spiritual" notions are clearly irrational or even patently bizarre (e.g. the "secret" involving a plank of wood in the preceding section). Differentiating genuine and illusory spiritual phenomena in such cases is a fairly straightforward matter. However, when a person's experiences or beliefs are less extreme or unusual the task can become far more difficult. Furthermore, it is often not a simple issue of either/or. In acute psychosis genuine spiritual experiences may be mixed up with hallucinatory phenomena and delusional ideas. Anton Boisen described his own psychotic crisis as "an experience which was at once mental disorder of the most profound and unmistakable variety and also of unquestionable religious value".[38] While Morag Coate's psychosis involved a blissful "direct experience of God", she was also subject to paranoid ideas: "I was myself a camera. The views of people that I obtained through my own eyes were being recorded elsewhere to make some kind of three-dimensional film." Such admixtures are consistent with Professor Lukoff's suggestions regarding possible overlap of mystical and psychotic phenomena.

It is just as unwise and potentially misleading to claim *all* acute psychotic episodes are psychospiritual crises as it is to deny that *any* are. The latter belief is common among adherents of biological psychiatry who subscribe to the view that all psychotic disorders are solely the unfortunate result of a malfunction in the diagnosed person's brain. Many mental health experts reject this overly simplistic approach to the complex phenomenon of psychosis, particularly because of its insensitivity to the lived experience of those in crisis. However, in their zeal to promote holistic, spiritually-sensitive views some well-meaning proponents of "alternative" approaches are inclined to overlook the fact that psychosis encompasses a broad range of experiences, *not all of which entail spiritual phenomena or spontaneous self-healing processes.*[*] So intent are some on emphasising the "cosmic" or mystical import of psychosis they turn a blind eye to the real suffering, disorganisation, and disability that occur in the wake of many episodes. (Conveniently for those intent on glorifying psychosis such untoward outcomes can be blamed on what they see as inept or insensitive psychiatric treatment rather than being attributed to the inherently negative effects of certain kinds of mental disturbance.)

While all religions encourage adherents to remain open and receptive to spiritual influences they also emphasise the importance of exercising informed judgement in such matters. In the Christian tradition St Paul exhorts the faithful: "Test everything; hold fast what is good."[39] In a similar vein St John urges caution regarding experiences involving "spirits": "Beloved, do not believe every spirit, but test the spirits to see whether they are of God; for many false prophets have gone out into the world."[40] Apparently spiritual phenomena such as experiencing blissful or ecstatic states, seeing sublime visions, hearing other-worldly voices, or feeling one has a superhuman identity or role, could be a blessing if genuine. However, falling prey to false or illusory pseudospiritual experiences could lead to serious problems. A great deal rests on correct assessment. While conventional psychiatry is inclined to pathologise spirituality, there are dangers, too, in spiritualising pathology.

The fact that there are no objective, universally-accepted criteria for assessing the validity of spiritual phenomena ensures this area is fraught with difficulty. If a person says God speaks to them, there is no way of *proving* whether or not this might actually be true. Such uncertainty means judgements are often made on the basis of personal

---

[*] Readers interested in considering these matters in greater depth are referred to the work of transpersonal psychologist Ken Wilber whose concept of the "pre/trans fallacy" – i.e. failure to differentiate *pre*personal and *trans*personal mental states – is highly relevant to the issues in this chapter. See Wilber, K. (1996) *Eye to Eye: The Quest for the New Paradigm.* Boston: Shambala. An erudite discussion of the use of this concept to clarify features schizophrenia and mystical experience have in common, and their crucial differences, can be found in Wilber,K. (1980) *The Atman Project: A Transpersonal View of Human Development.* Wheaton, Illinois: Theosophical Publishing House.

beliefs and predilections, thus leaving them open to the possibility of bias and distortion. A confirmed atheist is certain to be more sceptical about spirituality than an ardent believer. However, since spiritual or quasi-spiritual phenomena are a crucial aspect of many acute psychotic episodes, it is best to avoid potentially misleading judgements and seek a more impartial evaluation. Fortunately, guidelines which have stood the test of time and proven relevant in a broad range of circumstances have been devised for this purpose.

Before proceeding it should be noted that differentiating genuine and erroneous spiritual phenomena is not the only relevant task. Sometimes, even *genuine* experiences might have untoward consequences. For instance, certain experiences may be so powerful and intense they overwhelm the person concerned, provoking irrational behaviour and a temporary impairment of judgement (and possibly giving rise to a "spiritual emergency" of the kind described in *Chapter Six*). All reputable authorities agree the only reliable way to assess the validity of nominally spiritual phenomena is to examine their effects: "You shall know them by their fruits". Anton Boisen made a similar observation:

> There is no line of demarcation between valid religious experiences and the abnormal conditions and phenomena which to the [psychiatrist] are evidences of insanity. The distinguishing thing, as I see it, is not the presence or absence of the abnormal and the erroneous and the morbid, but the direction or tendency of the change which may be taking place.[41]

The criteria outlined below provide a practical means of assessing the effects of a person's beliefs and experiences on their life as a whole and other people. If these prove negative it is reasonable to assume the phenomena in question are either not truly spiritual or that they have been misinterpreted or acted upon incorrectly.* Sufficient time should be allowed for the initial impact of a crisis to subside since episodes which eventually prove spiritually enriching or transformative are sometimes marked by agitation, preoccupation, and inflation during

---

* If delusional beliefs or hallucinatory experiences have primarily *positive* effects it could be asked whether it matters that such phenomena are, strictly-speaking, illusory. After all, some people believe *all* religious beliefs are a form of self-deception, and more than one "expert" has suggested that Jesus Christ probably suffered from paranoid schizophrenia characterised by grandiose messianic delusions!

the early phases. Only when there has been adequate opportunity for stabilisation and integration will the enduring effects, positive or negative, of a psychotic crisis become evident.

Peace versus Agitation

Authentic spiritual experiences and beliefs: Contribute to enhancement of mental peace, serenity, and an abiding state of emotional equanimity. St Paul declared: "The fruit of the Spirit is love, joy, peace, patience, kindness, goodness, gentleness, self-control".[42]

Erroneous spiritual experiences and beliefs: Tend to foster impulsiveness, impatience, seriousness, inflexibility and lack of reflection. May contribute to superficial improvement in mental and emotional stability by masking anxiety and inner uncertainty, but are likely to exacerbate fear, guilt, anger, and despair in the long-term.

Growth versus Stagnation

Authentic spiritual experiences and beliefs: Are life-enhancing. Nourish the spirit, inspire and guide in a positive way, help people love and accept themselves and others, foster inner strength and personal responsibility, facilitate acceptance of reality and an ability to deal with complexity and uncertainty, enhance enjoyment and appreciation of life.

Erroneous spiritual experiences and beliefs: Preoccupation with erroneous ideas fosters misguided or inflexible behaviour which impairs adaptation and inhibits personal growth. In extreme cases may condemn a person to a limited, unproductive, socially impoverished way of life ("sad man on a mission").

Humility versus Inflation

Authentic spiritual experiences and beliefs: Promote humility and an attitude of reverence for life in all its myriad forms. Foster selflessness ("Others have greater needs than me") and willing acceptance of limitations and shortcomings. Accommodate a sense of humour that helps counteract pride or tendencies to take oneself too seriously.

Erroneous spiritual experiences and beliefs: May foster an attitude characterised by pride, arrogance, and an inflated or grossly exaggerated sense of self-importance that culminates in development of grandiose delusional beliefs (e.g. "I am the Chosen One").

Balance versus Preoccupation

Authentic spiritual experiences and beliefs: Are kept in perspective and understood to be but one facet of life. Are consistent with beliefs held before the psychotic crisis occurred and capable of being integrated into a harmonious, life-affirming personal belief system.

Erroneous spiritual experiences and beliefs: Lack of appropriate balance and perspective may result in a tendency to overemphasise irrational notions or become preoccupied with trivial issues. Phenomena with the power to dominate and entrance the mind often possess an addictive quality and may readily become the predominant focus of a person's life.

Free Will versus Compulsion

Authentic spiritual experiences and beliefs: Do not impair free will. Person may surrender to certain legitimate beliefs or experiences but is able to exercises choice and demonstrate mature self-control. Good "reality testing" is maintained, enabling person to question and critically evaluate his or her beliefs and experiences.

Erroneous spiritual experiences and beliefs: May be so compelling and mesmerizing that choice, free will, and self-control are compromised. Certain phenomena (e.g. voices) may involve specific orders or demand unquestioning obedience. In extreme cases person may become enslaved by phenomena that obsess and possess them to such an extent they are unwilling or unable to question or challenge them.[*]

Legitimacy versus Eccentricity

Authentic spiritual experiences and beliefs: While varying in specific form and content from one person to another nonetheless meet legitimacy criteria established by recognised authorities, e.g. religious

---

[*] In traditional shamanic cultures the ability to enter and exit the spirit world *at will* is considered one of the distinguishing characteristics of a genuine shaman. Anthropologist Michael Harner reports that in one of the South American Indian tribes he studied there was a man who wandered the forest day and night talking to spirits. "I asked if this man was a shaman. 'No,' they said, 'he's crazy.' Was he crazy because he was seeing things? No, because they had seen them too. He was crazy because he was out of control – he couldn't turn it off." [Lukoff, D. (1990) Divine Madness: Shamanistic Initiatory Crisis and Psychosis. *Shaman's Drum*, Winter 1990-1991, p.27].

tradition, respected teachers, sacred texts. Novel ideas, insights or beliefs are consistent with those of others with a comparable religious and/or spiritual philosophy and world view.

Erroneous spiritual experiences and beliefs: Are often highly idiosyncratic, eccentric, or bizarre and diverge substantially from generally accepted standards. Some ideas may be patently irrational, self-contradictory or incomprehensibly "autistic", i.e. person concerned understands them but nobody else can.

Inclusiveness versus Isolation

Authentic spiritual experiences and beliefs: Build bridges between people by fostering an awareness of the fundamental unity of life and sense of trust in the universe. Enhance the capacity for love and intimacy in relationships which may grow into genuine compassion for the whole of humanity and all living beings.

Erroneous spiritual experiences and beliefs: Fanatical ideas ("I alone possess the truth") create barriers that shut a person off from others in increasing isolation, seclusiveness, and self-absorption. May devolve into a narcissistically constricted "all about me" attitude that results in ever-diminishing sensitivity to the feelings and needs of others.

Anyone experiencing phenomena of a seemingly spiritual nature is advised to give careful consideration to the following:

Spiritual guidance

Most authorities agree it is not advisable for anyone to rely solely on their own judgement when assessing the validity of spiritual experiences and beliefs – particularly when they are of an unusual or highly idiosyncratic kind. The assistance of an appropriately qualified and experienced spiritual guide and/or adviser should be sought in such cases. As well as providing containment and facilitating groundedness, a trusted spiritual guide can support accurate reality testing by countering the distorting effect of personal blind spots or biases. Due to the complexity of the issues involved the person performing this function should possess sophisticated spiritual understanding *and* sound knowledge of the basic principles of mental health.

Psychological explanation

Many ostensibly spiritual phenomena have a *psychological* rather than metaphysical basis. The "fevered" imagination of an individual in the throes of acute psychosis is capable of generating an extraordinarily rich variety of compelling ideas and vivid mental imagery. Psychological needs sometimes cause the resulting "waking dream" to take a specifically "spiritual" form. For example, an unconsciously-driven need to compensate for feelings of personal inadequacy and insecurity might result in development of a so-called "messiah complex". Experiences involving "supernatural" entities such as spirits, demons, or ghosts are often the result of split-off and projected aspects of unconscious mental contents:

> The psychological interpretation of the so-called "demons" and "ghosts" is that on some levels they are the embodied forms we give to our negative projections, those dark forces in ourselves which are too awful to admit into consciousness and which are then projected outward and turned against ourselves. In terms of Western psychology, these could be explained as ego-alien unconscious material and impulses that are projected as destructive forces that are perceived as an outer form which then possess us (audio-visual hallucinations, etc). Those are our own ghosts, so to speak ... Ghosts are also the imprints of mental habits and thought patterns whose unconscious hold is so strong that they are constantly projected, unawares, onto the world ... From the inner point of view, these "demons" can also be explained as the negative archetypes of the collective unconscious, archetypes which overtake us from within.[43]

Containment and grounding

Many of the difficulties encountered by individuals in acute psychotic states are due to the fact that their feelings, beliefs, and experiences tend to be incompatible with those of other people and the world of everyday reality. The differences are often so great that a "clash of realities" occurs. Timely exercise of self-control and self-restraint can reduce the risk of untoward consequences. Given the potential for enchantment and ego inflation associated with emergence of powerful spiritual energies, psychiatrist Stanislav Grof offers this sage advice: "It is essential to refrain from acting out while under their spell and not to make any important decisions until we again have both feet on the ground."[44] This can be easier if the person concerned is able to recognise that, while it may *seem* as if profound events are occurring "out there" in the surrounding environment, the images, ideas, and feelings preoccupying them are actually subjective, *inner* experiences.

Walking on Water Wasn't Built in a Day

Psychedelic drugs sometimes facilitate the occurrence of profound spiritual experiences. However, as famed Beat Generation author Jack Kerouac said after first taking psilocybin ("magic mushrooms"): "Walking on water wasn't built in a day."[45] *There is a tremendous difference between having spiritual experiences and leading a spiritual life.* Actions speak louder than words. In this context it is instructive to consider some additional findings of the previously described research which found that the spiritual experiences of a group of psychiatric inpatients were very similar to those of religious contemplatives. This research also noted "a significant difference between psychotics and contemplatives on dimensions of personality structure and maturity".[46] While the contemplatives' lives were devoted to selfless service based on compassionate awareness of the needs of others, these patients were more narcissistic and self-centred, with limited empathic understanding and a high level of "ego-grasping" personality traits (excessive control, resistance, rigidity, striving). Sally Clay tells how clinging to her sublime experiences had exactly the opposite effect to what she intended: "I was determined to hold onto my spiritual visions at any cost, even, as it turned out, at the cost of losing my humanity."[47] Having spiritual experiences is not in itself sufficient to improve a person's life. If not properly integrated and accompanied by a mature level of personal responsibility, such experiences could even prove more of a hindrance than a help.

The Most Powerful Medicine for Recovery from Psychosis

While there is no question authentic spiritual phenomena sometimes occur in the course of acute psychotic episodes, merely having such experiences is no guarantee they will foster adaptation, growth, and healing. Certain phenomena may be so powerful they overwhelm the rational mind, giving rise to misguided ideas and maladaptive behaviour. Furthermore, people could respond to *genuine* experiences in ways that ultimately prove detrimental to recovery. Such responses are not uncommon. As Dr Podvoll observed in people diagnosed with bipolar disorder, "It is a typical and painful paradox of mania that, while seeking to transcend an individual ego, one lapses into bullying egocentricity".[48]

Many who have profound spiritual experiences struggle to apply in their everyday lives the insights gained. Even Anton Boisen had difficulty living in the spirit of the truths revealed during his psychotic episodes:

> Throughout those entire periods it was my best self that was dominant, something strong and deep and tender and intense, which was, I still believe, more than just myself. My great difficulty in the period of "normality" is to remain true to the vision which came to me then. I must recognise that in this present life of active participation in the world of men I am very far from having maintained the mystical identification which I felt so keenly during the disturbance.[49]

One of the great ironies of psychotic crises is that even those which entail *genuine* spiritual phenomena could exacerbate a person's difficulties if they are not responded to with wisdom and humility.

What is required to ensure a beneficial outcome? There are sound practical reasons all spiritual and/or religious traditions stress the importance of developing compassionate concern for the welfare of others. Adhering to this principle is an extremely effective way of guarding against any temptation to misconstrue spiritual experiences or use them for personal gain. In Dr Podvoll's view this precept, one of the cornerstones of Buddhism, has profound implications for healing and recovery:

> In the Buddhist tradition, dissolving ego-centricity is the basis of anything that can be called "spiritual" ... The materialism of ego – its territoriality, possessiveness, need for confirmation, attachment to self, protection of self, and eventual aggrandisement of self – is the greatest threat to both the patient's recovery and a harmonious community. Relaxing one's personal territory and being able to open up to the experience of others is a fruition of true community ... spirituality that recognises and relates to a world of experience beyond the confines of ego is the bottom-line individual and collective discipline ... With a gradual shedding of the restricting blinders of ego comes greater appreciation of the sensory world and

the possibility of recognising sacredness and dignity in ordinary life. This, I have found, is *the* most powerful medicine for recovery from psychosis, and a major inspiration to shift one's allegiance to sanity.[50]

Applying bona fide discernment criteria (as outlined above) and being constantly mindful of the feelings and needs of others are the best way of ensuring inner experiences find their rightful place in the service of a truly spiritual life.

Chapter Eleven

An Environment of Sanity

The process of recovery in general, and from psychosis in particular,
depends on creating an atmosphere of simplicity, warmth, and dignity.
Edward Podvoll[1]

The clinical term "psychosis" encompasses a diverse range of extreme mental states and conditions which, while involving overtly similar behaviours, vary greatly in form, cause, and personal significance. Many of the problems that befall affected individuals and their helpers are a direct result of the widespread failure to appreciate these critical differences and respond to them in adequate and appropriate ways. Although individuals who display characteristic psychotic symptoms (hallucinations, delusions, loss of contact with reality) could be having radically different inner experiences and grappling with personal crises of a very different kind, once diagnosed with a psychotic "illness" they tend to be treated in a strikingly uniform manner, with most receiving psychotropic medications which they may be advised to take for long periods, possibly indefinitely. Such medications are likely to constitute the only significant treatment for many.

This chapter and the next outline ways of responding to psychotic crises and their aftermath that will foster healing and recovery while reducing the risk of iatrogenic harm. Drawing on the accumulated wisdom and expertise of many people – individuals with first-hand experience of psychosis as well as mental health clinicians and others – these practical strategies constitute an *holistic approach* which treats body, mind, and soul as a unified whole. This approach aims to alleviate emotional distress while helping to restore psychological, social, spiritual, and biological balance.

Ancient Commonsense Wisdom

A central premise of this book is that individuals who have experienced psychosis are not fundamentally different to other human beings.

In keeping with this idea it is assumed the kinds of things *most* people find helpful during times of difficulty are also likely to benefit those affected by psychosis. Rather than involving complex techniques which can only be administered by specialists with years of training, the strategies outlined below are largely based on practical common sense. Although some might baulk at this notion, a lifetime of experience convinced Professor Ciompi of the value of such measures:

> The therapeutic principles ... are very straight forward. Essentially, they correspond to an ancient commonsense wisdom: More than anything else, the "insane" are confused, anxious, hypersensitive, and vulnerable people; therefore, anything contributing to a relaxed, simple, clearly defined environment will have a beneficial effect on the intricate pattern of their thoughts and emotions. Such an approach makes sense not only to the medical specialists but also – and this is far more important in everyday life – to the nursing staff as well as to family members, employers, and lay helpers. Together with the professionals they become able to lay, on these grounds, solid therapeutic foundations without which even the most sophisticated medical treatments will remain suspended in a vacuum, so to speak.[2]

Responding Positively To Psychosis

The variability and inherent complexity of psychotic phenomena ensure that any synopsis of therapeutic strategies is bound to be incomplete. Adding to the difficulty of providing general advice is the fact that the needs of individuals experiencing spiritual emergencies or psychotic crises of the self-healing type are significantly different to those of persons whose symptoms are manifestations of a psychotic breakdown, psychological irruption, or coping reaction. Furthermore, the needs and circumstances of people experiencing their first or second acute psychotic episode ("early psychosis") differ markedly from those of individuals enmeshed in the severe and prolonged psychosocial dysfunction which is the hallmark of "chronic mental illness". Nevertheless, widespread adoption of the following recommendations would improve the outlook for people experiencing psychosis for the first time as well as reducing the number who spiral downward to "chronic" status.

Some of the strategies discussed below are *generic* in the sense of being beneficial to all who experience psychosis, whether it is benign or otherwise. A healing environment is such a generic factor. *Specific* strategies, by contrast, while not applicable to everyone may nonetheless be of benefit to some, e.g. use of "anti-psychotic" and other psychotropic medications. The following topics are discussed in this chapter:

• Therapeutic asylum
• Guidance and support
• Holistic assessment
• Healing environments

Topics discussed in the next chapter include:

• Self-help and self-responsibility
• Self-treatment: cultivating sanity
• Using medication wisely

Therapeutic Asylum

People in an acute psychotic state are often hyper-vigilant, highly aroused, and excitable. Individuals who are irritable and suspicious may become more so, and might even become hostile or aggressive, if they feel they are being mistreated or coerced. Even those who are having intrinsically pleasurable experiences (e.g. elation, grandiosity, "cosmic" insights) are often prone to becoming agitated and over-stimulated as a result of their burgeoning hypersensitivity. In any event, distress and confusion engendered by the inevitable "clash of realities" is likely to provoke anxiety, defensiveness, and a tendency to misinterpret the environment. An overwhelming onslaught of conflicting inner and outer stimuli could set in train an emotional chain-reaction that fuels a self-perpetuating cycle of disconnection from consensual reality ("spinning out").

It has long been known that quiet, calm and orderly surroundings have a beneficial effect on disturbed minds. Early mental hospitals were referred to as "asylums" precisely because the best of them offered inmates *asylum* in the sense of a sanctuary and place of refuge and safety. As sensitive observers have frequently noted, "The psyche, as much as the body, needs a safe place in which to recover or be healed."[3]

225

Professor Luc Ciompi's research demonstrated that individuals in the throes of psychotic crises can benefit greatly from calm, low-stimulus environments in which they feel safe and protected:

> In acute phases, when they are confused, hypersensitive, unable to cope with anything unfamiliar or to process complex information, and likely to misinterpret events in a delusional manner, what is needed above all is a quiet, relaxed, and natural atmosphere, a relatively small space in which they can feel protected. Hectic goings-on should be avoided, and the people dealing with them should be few in number, calm, reliable, understanding, and, above all, healthy themselves. Patients whose affects are supposedly blunted, but whose reactions are still quite vehement under the surface, need a similar milieu.[4]

Simple, relaxed, orderly surroundings can do more than just help distressed, highly agitated individuals feel calmer. As Dr Podvoll observed, the feeling of inner tranquillity that such environments induce may help bring some acute psychotic episodes to a natural resolution relatively quickly:

> The early situation of psychosis is usually very fragile and flickers back and forth between clarity and confusion. The amount of this flickering is often conditioned by who one is with and how one is being treated. When the environment is a safe one, with healthy friendships and patience, the psychosis may resolve itself in short order. On the other hand, when a psychosis that might naturally last only several hours or days is over-reacted to by others in an attempt to suppress it as quickly as possible (as with over-medicating or other subjugating techniques), the disoriented one often fights against the effects of what he feels is an intrusion and a punishing abuse of his already-fragile mind. Such situations commonly lead to months or years of aggravated struggle with oneself and with psychiatric and legal authorities (while the psychosis worsens).[5]

A number of carefully conducted research studies have lent strong support to the claim that some acute psychotic episodes will abate spontaneously in optimally supportive environments. One of the most significant of these, the *Soteria Project*, ran from 1971 to 1983 in San Jose, California and involved a small (6 bed) community-based residence that provided a home-like sanctuary for young people experiencing acute psychosis of recent onset.[*] Its clinical director, psychiatrist Loren Mosher, was Chief of the Centre for Studies of Schizophrenia at the US National Institute of Mental Health and editor-in-chief of the *Schizophrenia Bulletin*, a highly-regarded international psychiatric journal. A key aspect of Soteria's philosophy was that acute psychosis was considered a "crisis in development" rather than an incurable mental illness. In keeping with this philosophy, Soteria residents received support and guidance from a team of specially selected staff (none of whom were mental health clinicians) who endeavoured to engender a simple, home-like, safe, warm, supportive, unhurried, tolerant, non-intrusive social environment.[6]

Soteria residents were not routinely given medication during their first six weeks in the programme. If they did not appear to be improving after this time they received a trial period of neuroleptic treatment on a case-by-case basis. Dr Mosher has reported that during the first five years of Soteria's existence there were fewer than a dozen occasions when it was deemed necessary to administer medication during the first six weeks.[7] For research purposes a comparison was made between the Soteria residents and a comparable group of young people who received treatment in a conventional psychiatric facility (thus acting as a control group). One of the most significant findings was that, during the first six weeks, the two groups experienced similar improvement in their psychotic symptoms:

> To our surprise, six weeks after admission our patients and control patients are basically indistinguishable in terms of symptoms, even though one hundred percent of the control patients have had therapeutic courses of neuroleptics and no Soteria subjects had. We did not expect symptoms to be alleviated by six weeks of interpersonal intervention. We thought it would take more like six months.[8]

---

[*] Retrospective analysis has shown that Soteria residents during this period would have been diagnosed with schizophreniform disorder (58%) or schizophrenia (42%) according to *DSM-IV* criteria. Approximately one third had previously experienced an episode of acute psychosis. Bola, J. and Mosher,L. (2003) Treatment of Acute Psychosis Without Neuroleptics: Two-Year Outcomes From the Soteria Project. *Journal of Nervous and Mental Disease*, Vol.191, 219-229.

No formal therapy was conducted at Soteria. Rather, the emphasis was on creating a supportive community in which the total environment helped instil positive expectations and provided an opportunity to develop greater self-understanding:

> Soteria's atmosphere was imbued with the expectation that recovery from psychosis was to be expected ... Perhaps the most important therapeutic ingredient in Soteria emerged from the quality of relationships that formed, in part, because of the additional treatment time allowed. Within staff-resident relationships, an integrative context was created to promote understanding and the discovery of meaning within the subjective experience of psychosis. Residents were encouraged to acknowledge precipitating events and emotions and to discuss and eventually place them into perspective within the continuity of their life and social network.[9]

Soteria residents spent an average of five months in the programme while those receiving conventional treatment remained in hospital about one month. Two years after leaving their programmes the two groups were compared on various criteria. The former Soteria participants tended to be working at a significantly higher occupational level and were more often living independently or with peers than those treated in hospital.[10]

Research conducted by Professor Ciompi and his colleagues reached very similar conclusions to those of the Soteria Project. A core feature of Ciompi's programme was the provision of a small (6-8 beds) home-like environment in which residents were helped to grow through the "severe developmental crisis" of acute psychosis. Particular emphasis was given to ensuring new residents were protected from frightening or noxious stimuli while at their most vulnerable:

> Each patient is assigned his own carer who stays constantly with him during the initial and most acute phase. He is cared for in the "soft room", which is a large and pleasant one on the ground floor. There are only cushions and mattresses in this room so as to avoid any sort of danger or over-stimulation. The main purpose of this phase is to reduce anxiety and tension by providing the patient with constant human support and guidance by calming him down, or by implementing relaxation techniques such as massage, holding hands, short walks, or other physical activities. Next comes

the activating phase, characterised by gradually getting back in touch with reality – first by negotiating simple household and gardening chores within the sheltered environment of the therapeutic setting, and later doing the shopping and going for walks near the house.[11]

In contrast to Soteria, Professor Ciompi's community provided formal therapies including psychotherapy and sociotherapy. "Milieu therapy" – i.e. using environmental influences, particularly the social surroundings, to foster positive change – was strongly emphasised. Thus, characteristics such as orderliness, structure, and predictability induced calmness and tranquillity, while relationships characterised by warmth, sensitivity, and acceptance facilitated development of trust and feelings of personal security.

Anti-psychotic medication was not routinely administered in Ciompi's therapeutic community. Rather, drugs were used only if a situation arose involving serious danger to a resident or others, if no improvement occurred within the first 3 to 4 weeks of admission, or if a resident seemed on the verge of an impending relapse that could not be prevented by other means. The majority of people remained in the programme between one and four months. Data from 51 residents was analysed on completion of the research.[*] Among this group, 20 had received no neuroleptic drugs whatever while in the programme while the remaining 31 received neuroleptic treatment approximately 2/3 of the time. Average daily medication dosages for the drug-treated residents were estimated to be around 1/3 of the usual European dosage and between 1/5-1/10 of the usual American dosage.

In a report published in the *British Journal of Psychiatry* these researchers stated that, in settings which provide adequate and continuous emotional support combined with sociotherapy and psychotherapy, a low-dose or drug-free approach is a feasible alternative to standard treatment for many people experiencing acute psychosis. Professor Ciompi described one of the most important findings as follows:

---

[*] Of the 56 individuals participating in this research, 39 were assigned a diagnosis of schizophrenia and 14 were diagnosed with schizophreniform disorder according to *DSM-III-R* criteria. Diagnoses of the remaining three participants were reported as "uncertain".

In contrast to the usually tense and bewildering admission wards, a therapeutic setting as relaxing, secure, and supportive as possible would be indicated, especially for highly agitated and frightened psychotic patients ... In the warm, open, supportive and relaxed emotional atmosphere of a small and stimulus-protected open house ... highly psychotic patients quite often improve or even recover within days or weeks, with no or only minimal neuroleptic medication.[12]

Mosher and Ciompi based their findings on research primarily involving people experiencing their first or second psychotic episode and diagnosed with schizophreniform disorder or schizophrenia. In 2008 the *Schizophrenia Bulletin* published a review which concluded: "the Soteria paradigm yields equal (and in certain specific areas, better) results in the treatment of schizophrenia when compared with conventional, medication-based approaches."[13] If persons with so-called "schizophrenia spectrum disorders" benefit from calm, low-stimulus, supportive environments there is no doubt such environments would have salutary effects in cases involving psychoses of an inherently more benign nature. As noted earlier, psychedelic crises will usually resolve naturally if subjects receive warm, non-judgemental support in a tranquil setting. Those undergoing self-healing psychoses or spiritual emergencies are also more likely to successfully navigate such crises if they are supported in safe, emotionally nurturing surroundings.*

Guidance and Support

Many people assume that formal qualifications in a mental health discipline and extensive clinical experience are mandatory for anyone wishing to assist individuals struggling with psychosis. While such qualifications have their value, the nature of psychosis is such that very simple measures are sometimes extremely beneficial. Dr Podvoll explains:

> It is definitely possible to be of great use to someone in psychosis without knowing the almost unbearable details of the apparatus of their minds. Even children and elderly people – scarcely suspecting the complexity of the psychotic experience – through kind and

---

* For up-to-date information about the Soteria approach see www.soterianetwork.org.

intimate relationships, have been known to give comfort to people lost in psychosis.[14]

Other people can have a powerful effect on someone experiencing or recovering from psychosis. Whether this proves helpful or harmful largely depends on their attitudes, beliefs, and personal characteristics. Sadly, it is common for hypersensitive, emotionally vulnerable individuals to encounter people who are thoughtless and uncaring (oftentimes inadvertently so). Certain types of people have a disturbing effect on psychotic individuals due to peculiarities in their manner and behaviour. Even in nominally therapeutic settings, people in the throes of a psychotic upheaval or its emotional aftermath may be exposed to harsh, insensitive or controlling attitudes (therapeutic aggression). Though their intentions may be good, would-be helpers sometimes act in ways that unwittingly have a deleterious effect. As Dr Perry explains, fear of mentally disturbed individuals often provokes a reflex withdrawal which, even if subtle, could have devastating consequences:

> What is absolutely crucial to the individual who is beginning to "space out" is the emotional response of the persons in his surroundings. If they are appalled, bewildered, and afraid, and have the feeling they are separated by a yawning chasm from this individual who has drifted into another world that is no longer recognisable as part of human experience, then the individual in the plight feels himself isolated and alone. Panic seizes him when he realizes he has dropped out of the world of human communication ... there is another more deadly withdrawal that occurs. The persons in the surroundings withdraw from him and his strange state. Even if they are trying to be kind and tolerant, they may at a subtle level seem demeaning, and may at least convey a hardly perceptible recoil; that to the individual in his very heightened state of discernment is very perceptible indeed. It makes a gigantic impact on him, and tends to aggravate his own withdrawal from their response.[15]

Ideally, individuals experiencing an acute psychotic crisis would be supported by a community of helpers who are neither fearful nor judgemental and who look upon what is occurring as personally meaningful rather than as a totally negative event to be diagnosed and suppressed as quickly as possible. As Carl Jung noted, even *one* open and emotionally receptive person may be enough to save the individual in crisis from the terror of feeling totally alone:

> One should not underrate the disastrous shock which patients undergo when they find themselves assailed by the intrusion of strange contents, which they are unable to integrate. The mere fact that they have such ideas isolates them from their fellow-beings and exposes them to an irresistible panic, which often marks the outbreak of the manifest psychosis. If, on the other hand, they meet with an adequate understanding ... they do not fall into a panic, because they are still understood by a human being and thus preserved from the disastrous shock of complete isolation.[16]

Individuals in an acute psychotic "altered state" sometimes demonstrate an almost preternatural sensitivity to their surroundings, particularly the interpersonal environment and the "vibes", good or bad, they sense emanating from other people. If they are admitted to a hospital ward, such people sometimes display an uncanny ability to see through outer appearances and are often able to astutely assess the prevailing atmosphere – including the attitudes, motives, and subtle patterns of deference among the staff.

Sensitive, compassionate, open-minded helpers can make an immensely valuable contribution to creating a healing environment, whether in a psychiatric ward, therapeutic community, or diagnosed person's own home. Dr Mosher feels the Soteria community's effectiveness was the result of both its calm, low-stimulus environment and the benign influence of a small complement of specially-selected support personnel. These staff were selected, not on the basis of formal qualifications, but because they possessed desirable personal characteristics such as being tolerant, motivated, enthusiastic, positive, flexible and psychologically strong.[17] Rather than engaging in formal therapies, Soteria staff felt their most important role was to provide the often highly distressed residents with a calm, reassuring presence. Simply "being with" acutely disturbed individuals was considered more beneficial than anything staff might be involved in "doing to" them in the guise of formal therapy:

> All the troubled residents of Soteria are mentally in a very different place than the staff members are, but the staff try to do everything they can to be in that place with them. They try to share the patients'

psychological space – without reinforcing it but also without trying to force them to give it up. Staff members try to protect the patients, be with them, be real, be honest, be simple (meaning not delivering complicated interpretive statements), and to take seriously the fact that this person is in a painful, traumatic life crisis [which] has a deep, powerful effect ... The staff members take the psychosis seriously, try to pay attention, deal with it, hope that the person can get through it and not come out of it as a psychological cripple.[18]

Listening attentively and accepting without judgement whatever a person may be thinking, feeling and experiencing establishes a supportive context that provides "asylum" and containment. Without such support, anxiety-provoking experiences might intensify to such a point they trigger a self-perpetuating cycle of emotional turmoil.

The need for empathic support and understanding becomes especially great during the protracted recuperative phase which often occurs in the wake of a psychotic episode. Recovering individuals frequently feel extremely uncertain or even lost during this period, and some remain mentally fragile and emotionally vulnerable for a considerable time. It is vital that helpers show great patience and are able to accept that progress may initially be agonisingly slow for all concerned. Paradoxically, not pushing or trying to hurry recovery facilitates natural healing. Although active involvement is often vital, Professor Ciompi believes at times it is important for helpers "to be able to do nothing at all, to sit with them in silence ... [to] keep still and listen."[19]

Helpers can play a key role in supporting the development of positive attitudes and expectations. One way of doing this is to encourage the diagnosed person to remain open to the possibility their experiences, strange and painful as they may have been, reflect the occurrence, not of a "psychotic illness" but a personal crisis which holds the potential for growth and healing. One of the traditional functions of a healer is to act as a carrier of hope for those who are temporarily unable to feel hopeful. In Professor Bleuler's opinion, relating constantly and actively to the diagnosed person's "healthy" aspects is one of the most therapeutically beneficial strategies of all.[20]

Psychiatry has a long-standing practice of scrupulously segregating those involved in providing treatment from those receiving it. This radical separation into "us" (staff) and "them" (patients) is based on the spurious assumption that patients have all the problems while staff are exemplars of "normality" and mental health. In reality, the two groups have far more in common than is generally acknowledged. (The fact that sanity and madness lie on a continuum was discussed in *Chapter Two*.) Truly effective helpers, lay and professional, acknowledge their own problems and endeavour to deal with them in a constructive way. This does *not* mean helpers need to be "perfect" before they can assist others, nor should a diagnosed person's family and friends aspire to becoming amateur therapists. However, if they are not actively engaged in cultivating their *own* mental health and sanity, helpers are less likely to be able to provide the calm, grounded, simple human presence so beneficial to those recovering from psychosis. The surest way to learn what recovery really entails is for helpers to acknowledge their own woundedness and make a personal commitment to living the spirit of recovery in their own lives.

Holistic Assessment

So sharply does the approach outlined above contrast with the conventional psychiatric practice of administering antipsychotic medications at the earliest opportunity to people experiencing acute psychosis that certain clarifications are in order. Most importantly, it would be unwise to assume *every* individual experiencing psychosis would necessarily do better if, instead of receiving standard medical treatment, they simply went to some quiet place to await spontaneous healing. Many have chosen this course only to experience unpleasant, possibly harmful, consequences.

It is vital to appreciate that, while *some* acute psychotic episodes are inherently transitory, others are not. Psychotic crises predominantly reflecting the operation of innate self-healing mechanisms tend to be fairly brief and will usually reach a natural conclusion if the autonomous process at work is allowed to proceed unimpeded. By contrast, mental disturbances which are manifestations of a psychological breakdown or coping strategy (Boisen's "drifting" and "concealment" reactions) may result in prolonged difficulties and persistent symptoms (positive and negative). While they do not necessarily culminate in permanent disability, such disturbances call for different responses to those warranted for psychospiritual crises. To ensure people receive the most appropriate assistance it is vital they are carefully assessed to ascertain the true nature of their psychotic experiences and the predominant issues with which they are grappling.

Conventional psychiatric assessment is based on a procedure known as a *mental status examination* during which the interviewing clinician is alert to various signs and symptoms that provide clues regarding the subject's psychological state. In unskilled or insensitive hands this can easily devolve into a crude "symptom hunting" exercise. In any event, such assessment invariably results in a *DSM* diagnosis. These descriptive labels, now a clinical and bureaucratic formality and a necessary prelude to medical treatment, convey little about the subjective and inner dimensions of psychotic experience. In this context Anton Boisen's sage advice is worth repeating:

> The descriptive groupings are not without significance but we would probably be better off if our psychiatric staffs would stop giving so much attention to a meaningless classification and more attention to the attempt to understand the real meaning of the experiences with which they are dealing.[21]

Holistic assessment demands far more than psychiatric knowledge and familiarity with conventional diagnostic categories. It involves a sincere attempt to understand the person being assessed in his or her entirety – body, mind, and soul – within the context of their life as a whole. It requires an ability to look *beyond* symptoms and behaviours in an attempt to appreciate the inner meaning and significance of the person's experiences, past and present. Given the fluctuating, highly individual, inherently unpredictable nature of acute psychosis, this type of assessment is necessarily an *ongoing process* rather than a "one off" clinical procedure.

Assessment should occur in a simple, tranquil, low-stimulus setting – ideally an "asylum" environment which instils natural feelings of safety and security. Interviewers who foster trust and confidence in the person being assessed (and other informants) will inevitably gain a more accurate impression of what is and has been occurring.

Whether assessment occurs in a sanctuary-like environment or clinical setting it is highly desirable that there be a *medication-free observation period* of at least several days. There are two sound reasons for this. Firstly, once powerful psychoactive medications are administered people undergoing assessment are no longer in a "natural" state and it could be difficult to discern their true feelings, thoughts, and experiences (this is especially so in regard to the extremely subtle and evanescent realm of inner experience). Furthermore, the possibility that some acute psychotic episodes will come to a natural end is negated by failing to withhold medication for a time. Unfortunately, it is not always feasible to adhere to these recommendations. There may be little choice but to administer medication if the person concerned is experiencing extreme distress, is "acting out" in a dangerous manner, or engages in serious self-harming behaviour. In such cases the minimum effective dose should be used and efforts made to find the least restrictive means possible of reducing the risk of harm to self or others.

Comprehensive holistic assessment includes the following:

- Physical health
- Substance use
- Psychosocial stressors
- Type of psychotic disturbance
- "Acute" or "chronic" status
- "Insight" and "reality testing"
- Predominant needs and concerns
- Personal coping style/attitude to psychosis
- Inner life and "history of sanity"

Physical health
Some psychotic disturbances are a result of physical illness or injury which impairs brain functioning. Mental disorders with a predominantly physical causation are often marked by confusion, memory impairment, disorientation (affected person is unsure of the time, date, where they are), and prominent hallucinations of a *non-auditory* nature (e.g. seeing or smelling things, unusual physical sensations). Everyone experiencing psychosis should have a thorough medical examination as soon as practicable to exclude the possibility they might have an "organic" mental disorder.

Substance use
Since chemical substances of various kinds can provoke psychosis it is important to assess a person's recent history of illicit drug use, if any. This should include the type of drugs taken, frequency of use (e.g. rarely, occasionally, regularly), and level of consumption (e.g. light, moderate, heavy).

While expert assessment is warranted if illicit drug use has been more than minor, it is possible for lay helpers to formulate a rough hypothesis about the part such use may have played in provoking a psychotic episode. As explained in *Chapter Seven*, prolonged heavy consumption of potent stimulants like cocaine and amphetamines can cause severe disturbances in the activity of key neurotransmitters. In such cases, psychosis could be the direct result of a substance-induced chemical imbalance in the user's brain. By contrast, if an episode occurs in the context of very light or occasional consumption of marijuana or psychedelics it is more likely a crisis was imminent and drugs have served as a catalyst or trigger. For individuals trapped in a "no exit" situation illicit drugs might be "the straw that breaks the camel's back". Experiences that are so unsettling they constitute a spiritual emergency sometimes occur in the context of drug experimentation. Such crises could be provoked by a *single* exposure to a potent psychedelic, especially if taken by emotionally unstable individuals in an uncontrolled setting.

People *currently* abusing drugs and/or alcohol present a special challenge as such behaviour can cloud the picture and make accurate assessment problematic. Consequently, it is highly desirable for people to abstain from substance use for a reasonable period prior to assessment to minimise the difficulty of differentiating drug effects from spontaneous psychological and/or spiritual phenomena.

Psychosocial stressors

Although psychosis sometimes seems to "strike out of the blue" it is usually the case that developmental influences have contributed to a person's "psychosis proneness" and that the episode itself has been triggered by specific circumstances or events. While the nature of potential psychosocial "triggers" varies greatly their common feature is that they are felt to be highly stressful.[22] Some stressors are easily identified, e.g. unexpected change or loss, financial pressure. However, triggers sometimes involve a situation or event whose significance might not be obvious to others but which is experienced as highly distressing due to its peculiar meaning to the affected person. Such *idiosyncratic stressors* frequently involve events which represent a threat to a vulnerable individual's fragile self-image or deliver a blow to their already tenuous self-esteem. Even apparently trivial incidents (such as an insensitive comment or overheard remark) could have a shattering impact.

It is now widely accepted that the risk of relapse for persons with an established history of schizophrenia increases significantly when they are exposed to stress exceeding a critical threshold level.[23] It has been found that, in the three weeks preceding onset of a psychotic episode, many people have experienced an excess of stress-inducing changes or crises ("life events").[24] Research has repeatedly demonstrated that persons diagnosed with schizophrenia can be strongly affected by the emotional climate in their family. The three components of so-called "expressed emotion" (or EE) are *criticism* (negative comments about what the diagnosed person does, thinks, or feels), *hostility* (criticisms and rejection), and *emotional over-involvement* (over-protectiveness, intrusiveness, emotional display, excessive praise, self-sacrifice, preoccupation). Some studies have found that in the two years following hospital discharge, 66% of those living in families with high levels of EE experienced relapse compared to 27% in low EE families, and that relapse rates increase with number of hours per week spent in direct contact with high EE relatives. Measures which help to reduce high EE levels (e.g. psychoeducational programmes) can result in a significantly lower incidence of relapse.[25]

Identifying psychosocial stressors which may have triggered a psychotic episode is important for several reasons. If sources of critical stress are not identified there is little chance of reducing or avoiding them, resulting in a high risk of relapse and reliance on the "stress-buffering" effect of neuroleptic drugs. If steps are taken to identify and deal with potential triggers (inner and outer), it may be possible to reduce both relapse risk and need for medication. The feasibility of this approach has been demonstrated in families: when high EE levels are reduced and support increased, relapse rates are lower even for people receiving less medication.[26]

Individuals exposed to stress that exceeds their relapse threshold do not generally become psychotic all of a sudden. Rather, onset of an episode typically occurs in a series of stages which unfold in a characteristic sequence over a period lasting from several days to a few weeks or longer.[27] At the beginning of this process people often become aware of changes in their feelings, thinking, perceptions, and behaviour – so-called "prodromal symptoms" – that indicate relapse could be imminent. Such changes can serve as personal *warning signals* indicating a need to take steps to avert a possible full-blown psychotic episode (see *Chapter Fourteen*).

Type of psychotic disturbance

Psychotic disorders discussed in this book are categorised into various types, not on the basis of symptoms as in the conventional psychiatric approach, but according to deeper characteristics such as the reason the crisis occurred and the purpose various symptoms might be serving in the affected person's life (the "method in the madness"). A number of *psychological crises* that might culminate in acute psychosis were discussed in *Chapter Five*, while psychoses reflecting the occurrence of profound *psychospiritual crises* were discussed in *Chapter Six*.

Guidelines for differentiating various types of psychosis were outlined in *Chapter Nine*. The task could still prove difficult, even for those with considerable knowledge and experience. Consequently, it is vital to remain as open as possible and to attend closely to what the affected person is saying and doing – as well as to what might be communicated in things they *don't* say or do. It can be helpful to hold in mind the question, "Could this person's unusual behaviour be serving some important purpose, however obscure?"

A *mixture* of the different types sometimes occurs. For example, Anton Boisen had frankly "paranoid" experiences in the course of what proved to be a spiritually enriching self-healing process. Since there can be dramatic changes from hour to hour during some florid psychotic episodes, assessment must focus on identifying themes and attitudes that have been predominant over a sustained period (days, weeks or longer).

"Acute" or "chronic" status

To determine what type of therapeutic approach is most appropriate for a given individual it is necessary to gain a sense of their current state of psychological and social adjustment (sometimes referred to, rather crudely, as their "level of functioning"). In making such an assessment it must be remembered there is a vast difference between the needs of people experiencing their first or second psychotic episode and those who have reached "chronic" status after repeated hospitalisations and lengthy periods of treatment. Those in the former group typically have predominantly "positive" symptoms (hallucinations, delusions) and a reasonable level of motivation and social competence, while those in the latter tend to be afflicted with "negative" symptoms (lack of motivation, poverty of thought and speech, social and emotional withdrawal), the hallmarks of severe psychiatric disability.

Individuals with lengthy psychiatric histories characterised by extended periods of institutionalisation, isolation, and poor social functioning often lack the motivation and ability to participate in formal therapies. Furthermore, those who are prone to feelings of persecution ("paranoia") tend to have difficulty making use of the opportunities offered by open therapeutic communities such as Soteria due to their inability to trust and co-operate with fellow residents and support staff. Consequently, they are more likely to benefit from highly structured, rehabilitation-focused programmes that focus on boosting confidence and self-esteem and teaching practical social and living skills. Professor Ciompi explains these contrasting approaches as follows:

> Efforts to create different therapeutic settings for various stages [have] only just begun, but we can already recognise a certain contrast between the two types. In the former, which we might call "maternal", acutely anxious patients are calmed and soothed in an indulgent but protective atmosphere; in the latter, more "paternal" type, limits are set and demands imposed in a kind but respectful way, so as to stimulate chronic patients and gradually draw them out of their shell.[28]

"Insight" and "reality testing"

As a psychotic crisis subsides people often realise the thoughts, feelings, and experiences that totally preoccupied them during the episode were actually dream-like phenomena that occurred on a purely subjective level. Those who develop such understanding and who are able to see their ordeal as an *inner* process are described in clinical terminology as having "insight". By contrast, some people display a limited ability to recognise the subjective nature of their often highly idiosyncratic ideas, feelings, and experiences. Such a "lack of insight", when combined with a marked tendency to disown and project inner experiences and feelings onto the environment and other people, can result in what clinicians refer to as "impaired reality testing".

Psychoses originating in "concealment" reactions often result in psychological disconnection and isolative behaviour. An underlying lack of basic trust may be reflected in "paranoia" and suspiciousness (e.g. perceiving others as potential enemies) and overt or covert hostility. Such persons often have difficulty developing two-way relationships with others and may adamantly deny their need for help.

Possessing a reasonable degree of "insight" and an ability to correctly "test reality" allows reflection on the personal meaning and significance of psychotic experiences that is difficult or impossible for those who lack such capacities.

Predominant needs and concerns
Individuals who experience psychosis have often grappled with a variety of long-standing personal difficulties which contributed to their "psychosis proneness". Common problems include low self-esteem, poor self-image, lack of self-confidence, fraught interpersonal relations, and troubled social adjustment. While psychotic crises of the self-healing type may contribute to constructive resolution of such issues, the effects of stigmatisation, loss of hope, and other iatrogenic influences could cause them to become even worse.

Identifying needs and issues for which people may require support or guidance is a key focus of holistic assessment. Individuals vary greatly in this regard – even if they have the same psychiatric diagnosis. While those who have undergone a self-healing crisis or spiritual emergency do not necessarily lack confidence or the ability to fulfil domestic and occupational roles (for which reason they may be described as "high functioning"), they might have trouble understanding and integrating the experience into their post-psychotic life. At the other extreme, some people could require ongoing assistance with basic needs and activities such as self-care, domestic chores, and socialising.

Spiritual issues and concerns occupy a central role in many people's lives. Though they may appear totally meaningless to insensitive eyes, genuine spiritual phenomena can occur in the course of some acute psychotic episodes. However, since illusory experiences sometimes masquerade as legitimate spiritual phenomena, astute discernment is vital (see *Chapter Ten*).

Personal coping style and attitude to psychosis
People respond to and cope with disturbing experiences in a variety of characteristic ways. Those who have recently experienced a psychotic episode often utilise one or other of two distinct coping styles termed "integration" and "sealing-over" respectively.[29] Curiosity is one of the cardinal distinguishing features of the two styles: those who *integrate*

tend to feel curious about their experiences and try to understand and learn from them, while people who *seal-over* are inclined to actively avoid speaking about what happened and will often try to put it out of their minds as much as possible. The principal characteristics of the two coping styles are as follows:[30]

Individuals with an *integrating* coping style:
• Are aware of a connection between thoughts and feelings experienced during psychosis and emotional conflicts before and after the episode
• Experience psychosis as personal rather than totally foreign or imposed by some unknown influence or agency
• Are curious about their psychotic experiences and emotionally invested in trying to understand them
• See psychosis as a source of new information about themselves and endeavour to use this to modify their beliefs and behaviour
• Are able to see positive as well as negative aspects to psychosis and like some of the unusual feelings and ideas experienced during the episode
• Feel psychotic experience has had a significant impact on their life
• Actively enlist help of others in an ongoing effort to deal with psychosis and life issues generally

Individuals with a *sealing-over* coping style:
• Isolate thoughts and feelings experienced during psychosis from emotional conflicts present before and after the episode
• See psychosis as an encapsulated, circumscribed event totally alien to and distinct from their usual mental life and view themselves as having fallen victim to a medical and/or biological illness
• Lack curiosity about their psychotic experiences and are not emotionally invested in trying to understand them
• Do not see psychosis as a source of new information about themselves and seek to return to their previous identity, opinions and behaviour
• Are unable to see any positive aspects to psychosis and are repelled by feelings and ideas experienced during the episode
• Deny the importance or impact of the psychosis on their life
• Tend not to enlist help of others in dealing with issues related to psychosis and general life problems

These characteristics are broad generalisations that describe opposite ends of a continuum. In reality, a *mixture* of the two coping styles is often evident. Furthermore, people might selectively integrate certain aspects of a psychotic episode but seal-over others.

The sealing-over coping style is exemplified in these remarks by a person speaking about her most recent psychotic episode:

> I'd like to kind of place this experience in the back of my mind. It was a gross experience in a sense … But I don't think about it very often … very infrequently, in fact. The only time that I think about it in daily life is if someone is talking about what I did that fall. Then, that's the only time it really pops up … To me it's unnecessary to dwell on it. There are so many other things I have to figure out in my daily life … why regurgitate and regurgitate over and over in your head? It doesn't accomplish anything.[31]

Whether overtly or covertly, those who seal-over often convey a clear message to others: "I don't want to talk about it". By contrast, the approach adopted by Jeanette Keil epitomises an integrating coping style. After being diagnosed with acute schizophrenia, Keil (whose experiences were discussed in *Chapter Nine*) worked hard to find meaning in her psychotic ordeal:

> As I endeavoured to comprehend what happened I realised schizophrenia is not like chickenpox. One does not suffer a schizophrenic episode, then recover and return to the same life. The psychotic experience is not easily forgotten. It must be dealt with in whatever way possible … I tried to make my way through available literature on the subject. Working towards comprehension of my schizophrenic episode was the only thing that made day to day living bearable for me … two years after the initial occurrence I started to write a journal. Writing about my experiences gave me the confidence to begin trusting my own thoughts. Ultimately, the journal helped me come to grips with my illness by allowing me to develop thoughts which I had been unable to express verbally. With increased confidence I began to trust my own understanding of the experience. I began to feel that even if all my thoughts about schizophrenia did not fall within the bounds of traditional psychiatric models, they might still be of some personal value.[32]

Seeing continuity between thoughts and feelings which arose during psychosis and personal problems that existed before the episode is one of the hallmarks of an integrating coping style. In recognising such continuity, people may begin to appreciate how aspects of the psychotic crisis were related to their long-standing difficulties and concerns.

As well as a personal coping style people develop a specific *attitude* toward their psychotic experiences. Broadly speaking this could be positive, e.g. "Psychosis helped me grow in certain ways", or negative, e.g. "It is hard for me to think of anything good about what happened". (While such attitudes are largely a result of conscious choice, personal coping style tends to be shaped more by automatic and unconscious psychological defence mechanisms.[33])

As explained later in this chapter, the attitude people adopt toward their psychotic experiences, together with their personal coping style, can affect their recovery prospects.

Inner life and "history of sanity"

Conventional psychiatric assessment focuses on identifying symptoms for the purpose of assigning a clinical diagnosis. An holistic approach, by contrast, is founded on the belief that no matter how troubled or dysfunctional a person might be, they always amount to far more than a conglomeration of symptoms, deficits, and handicaps. Sensitive attention to the whole person invariably reveals healthy, "normal" characteristics and abilities, as well as a history of personal achievements and successes.

This statement holds true for all who have experienced psychosis – including those diagnosed with schizophrenia, commonly seen as the most destructive psychotic disorder. A lifetime working alongside individuals with this diagnosis convinced Professor Manfred Bleuler that "behind the psychotic manifestations there are an intact personality, intact intellectual abilities, and very human and warm feelings."[34] Indeed, hidden behind the psychotic symptoms a *normal* inner life continues to exist in every such person: "The fact that a normal life is running its course parallel to and behind the schizophrenic life is undoubtedly one of psychiatry's important and assured realisations. Kind-natured care personnel of schizophrenics have probably always known this."[35] Bleuler explained this notion as follows:

The obvious symptomatology is but one level of the schizophrenic's personality. A healthy life exists buried beneath this confusion. Somewhere deep within himself [he] is in touch with reality despite his hallucinations. He has common sense in spite of his delusions and confused thinking. He hides a warm and human heart behind his sometimes shocking affective behaviour.[36]

Professor Bleuler believed such observations are true even of those most severely disabled – so-called "chronic schizophrenics" – a view which contrasts sharply to that of many clinicians who believe schizophrenia, in its most severe form, can subvert the entire personality, causing its irreversible destruction. Bleuler was certain there always exists a "rich and human inner life" concealed by the psychotic façade:

> Of great relevance seems to me the clinical observation that even in these chronic patients who have never improved with respect to hospital status, skilful examination reveals hidden behind the psychosis an intact inner life ... the ability to reason and to think logically is never lost, but continues along with the illogical and chaotic inner life. And even more, I found it fascinating to discover and to evoke very normal, very fine emotions, signs of an intact and warm emotional life in chronic schizophrenics.[37]

If these claims are true of severely disabled individuals they are certain to apply to those less adversely affected by psychosis and its aftermath.

Sadly, in the lives of many people the most prominent landmarks seem to be the crises, breakdowns, and hospitalisations (often documented in excruciating detail in their medical files). When people have a long history of pain and suffering it can be easy – for them and others – to lose sight of the positive aspects of their lives. However, no matter how extreme a person's difficulties may have been, intertwined with stories of frustration, failure and loss there are invariably instances in which they experienced success in certain endeavours (however small), and felt a sense of personal pride, satisfaction, and dignity. Dr Podvoll refers to this as the *history of sanity* which always exists alongside a history of mental disorder.[38]

The more obvious aspects of this history are readily uncovered, e.g. scholastic or occupational accomplishments, natural talents and abilities, admirable personal qualities, successful relationships. However, many significant aspects are subtle or fleeting and thus easily overlooked. Examples include simple acts of kindness or generosity toward others, expressions of gratitude, spiritual sensitivity, feelings of appreciation for the natural world of plants and animals, and heartfelt concern for the environment.

Ignoring this positive history can inadvertently reinforce feelings of worthlessness and inadequacy, while recognising it affirms a person's inherent goodness, human dignity, and fundamental sanity.

A Healing Environment

Sadly, it has become difficult to find places that provide genuine asylum to people in the throes of acute psychosis and its emotional aftermath. Mainstream hospitals and clinics no longer even attempt to provide the warm, home-like environments crucial to the success of initiatives such as Soteria and Ciompi's therapeutic community. Fortunately, innovative programmes in various parts of the world have furnished further evidence regarding the viability of such approaches and clarified the environmental characteristics that facilitate natural healing and recovery.*

Without substantial financial and human resources it is no longer possible to set up ideal healing environments incorporating residential facilities for clients and support staff. However, since a great deal has been learnt about the qualities and characteristics which constitute the essential ingredients of such environments, less elaborate alternatives are still feasible. Armed with knowledge of these, motivated individuals or groups can make a tangible contribution to improving the circumstances of anyone struggling with psychosis. Even if they are only able to integrate *some* of these into an individual's living situation, caring relatives and friends, lay and professional helpers, or teams of volunteers, can help create an environment that alleviates

---

* Important exemplars include therapeutic household communities founded by Dr Edward Podvoll (see next chapter) and various experimental Scandinavian programmes – see, for example, Lehtinen,V. et al. (2000) Two-Year Outcome in First-Episode Psychosis Treated According to an Integrated Model. Is Immediate Neuroleptisation Always Needed? *European Psychiatry*, Vol.15, Issue 5, 312-320; Cullberg, J. et al. (2002) One Year Outcome in First Episode Psychosis Patients in the Swedish Parachute Project. *Acta Psychiatrica Scandinavica*, 106: 276-285.

distress, makes deterioration less likely, and fosters growth and development.

When they first begin to recover, individuals who have endured a severe mental disturbance face a host of challenges which highlight the importance of the right kinds of support being available – as well as suggesting how easily things can go wrong in their absence. The earliest stages of recovery entail a gradual "coming out": with each tentative step a person's vista expands a little as they slowly emerge from an isolated and enclosed "dream world" and begin reconnecting with everyday reality. Dr Podvoll's description of the initial phases of this precarious journey highlights its potential pitfalls:

> Moments of recovery often occur in much the same way. They may be tentative, quickly withdrawn, hesitant, practicing motions, as though by trial and error … Even when one is well on the way to recovery … the "dislocating wound" of psychosis, the wound that leaves one estranged from conventional psychological moorings, may continue to exert its influence. The residuals from all that one has been through manifest themselves in a peculiar hypersensitivity as soon as one tries to re-orient to the outside world … In the immediate "coming out" stage, one's world seems incredibly fragile; one may feel broken, ragged, or simply worn out ... At the beginning of recovery one feels an edginess, like a pull in two directions at once – into the world of human drama and into a dream world. At times both are equally accessible, and it is not always clear which way is forward and which way backward. This situation can last a surprisingly long time. Even after months of appearing free from delusions or "interferences", someone may still experience interruptions of consciousness that hold one in fascination and obsession. A word or words can set this off – particularly harsh, judgemental words ... This is why many people who are recovering from psychosis appear to be so tentative. They fear they will become carried away too easily and react too quickly, especially to anger and the urge to withdraw.[39]

Though their florid symptoms might have abated, people often remain emotionally and mentally fragile for a considerable time after a psychotic episode. The importance of stable and tranquil surroundings cannot be overstated, especially during the earliest stages of recovery. Extensive evidence demonstrates that the essential characteristics of healing environments include the following:

- An atmosphere of dignity and respect
- Non-judgemental acceptance
- Respect for individuality
- Therapeutic containment
- Positive attitudes and expectations
- Structured activity and routines
- Confiding relationships

An atmosphere of dignity and respect

Since steady and predictable surroundings have a stabilising effect on mind and emotions they constitute the foundations of a recovery-promoting environment. The physical setting plays a vital, though often undervalued, role. Clean, orderly, aesthetically-pleasing spaces have a calming, soothing, and emotionally-uplifting effect (if only subliminally at first), in sharp contrast to the jarring impact of chaotic environments punctured by loud music and other noise, people coming and going at all hours, incessant smoking and substance abuse. Healthy, life-affirming environments provide a foundation for healing and recovery and a context in which other beneficial influences can take effect.

Healing environments are characterised by *hospitality* – i.e. friendly and generous reception of residents and visitors (historically, hospitals were so named because they embodied the ideal of offering hospitality to the sick and needy). The simple experience of being received with kindness, warmth, and emotional generosity invariably has salutary effects. Regarding a recovering individual not as a "patient" but as a fellow human-being who happens to be struggling will bolster their confidence and self-belief. The therapeutic power of such influences should not be underestimated. As Dr Mosher explains, they were at the heart of Soteria's philosophy:

> I thought that sincere human involvement and understanding were critical to healing interactions … The idea was to treat people as people, as human beings, with dignity and respect.[40]

Though many would doubtless agree with these simple sentiments, they are all too easily overlooked in the frenetic bustle of modern clinical settings.

Non-judgemental acceptance

Many people report that one of the most difficult and frustrating aspects of experiencing psychosis and subsequent treatment was feeling they were not taken seriously or properly listened to by those around them. Sadly, this complaint often extends to those who were supposed to be helping. The message conveyed by such indifference is that the person's experiences and ideas are meaningless, of no value, best eradicated as quickly as possible. Finding no-one who will listen condemns a troubled individual to deeper isolation.

A tangible way of contributing to a healing atmosphere is to listen with respectful interest to a person's ideas and concerns – including those that may be hard to understand or empathise with. This does *not* necessarily entail accepting everything at face value or colluding with outlandish notions. Nevertheless, open-minded listening can help alleviate feelings of loneliness and isolation which, if not always obvious, are invariably present. A heart-felt experience of connecting with another human being could be a turning point for some. As Dr Perry testifies, the simple act of listening empathically, with genuine interest and concern, sometimes has a profound effect:

> When I was first entering upon medicine on the way toward psychiatry, my cousin's wife told me about a psychosis she had had and about the ideas, feelings, and delusional beliefs that had filled her mind. She wound up her account with one emphatic admonition: "What makes the crucial difference to a patient is to be able to talk all about it to someone who will really listen." She clearly pointed to this as the thing that had allowed her to get over her psychosis. I never forgot that tip, and have always put it into practice. Many others since have told me of their recovering from psychosis when they found an understanding listener.[41]

This advice is bound to be challenging at times, perhaps especially when people in the throes of psychosis speak in a chaotic manner or express seemingly nonsensical ideas. Those who are excessively intellectual often find it difficult to attend to such utterances without judgement. Nevertheless, Dr Perry believes it is legitimate to assume *everything* people say or are preoccupied with is rich in personal meaning, obscure as it may be, that those who listen with mind and heart open are sometimes able to discern:

This significance often eludes us at first, but sooner or later we come to recognise that there is an emotional truth lurking behind the somewhat inscrutable play of image and symbol. In fact, following the line of thought in an individual in this psychic state, or "space", is quite like trying to grasp the metaphorical meaning in the lines of an obscure poem. The less one tries to transliterate it into rational talk, and the more one flows along with it, the more it speaks its own meaning.[42]

Even if it is not possible to understand or even follow what someone is saying, it is still possible to reduce their sense of isolation by allowing them to feel they have the ear of a sympathetic listener.

Respect for individuality
Everyone who experiences psychosis has a uniquely individual and distinctive inner life, pattern of symptoms, repertoire of past and present experiences, and idiosyncratic array of psychological characteristics and biological propensities. These crucial variations are not always adequately acknowledged in modern clinical settings where there is a tendency to treat people in a similar, routinised manner (an oversight that sometimes devolves into a production-line approach).

A practical way of honouring individuality is to treat people's experiences with an attitude of respectful curiosity. This does not necessarily entail in-depth scrutiny of their psychotic symptoms (though it sometimes may) but simply remaining open and receptive so people feel free to speak about whatever they wish. Anton Boisen's own experience of institutional invalidation led him to strongly emphasise this point:

> In the hospital to which I was sent as a patient little attention was paid to my ideas. It was assumed that such disorders were rooted in some as yet undiscovered organic [biological] factor and that the ideas were secondary or accidental. Such a view has been fairly common in the psychiatric world. The great advances have come however with the recognition of the tremendous significance to the patient of his ideas and emotions. They are to him reality, grim, terrifying, torturing, mocking, fascinating, and if we are to arrive at any true understanding of our patient and of the world in which he lives we must know what is on his mind.[43]

Everyone experiencing psychosis responds to it in a highly individual way. While some are curious and wish to understand and learn from their experiences (an integrating coping style) others may try to forget about them (sealing-over). Mainstream psychiatry selectively encourages the latter response. A more respectful attitude involves accepting each person's natural inclinations in this regard. By endeavouring to accommodate *both* coping styles the Soteria community embodied such an attitude. Dr Mosher points out that while only 60% of residents chose to "face" their psychotic experiences, individual choice was always respected:

> Some people who come to Soteria want nothing to do with their madness; they spend all their time running as fast as they can away from it, and that is all right. But if they feel that they in some way want to go through that process without anybody trying to abort it or force it into some pigeon hole or divert it, then we allow them to try to do this.[44]

Such an approach leaves room for the possibility a person's preferred coping style and attitude toward psychosis might change over time.

Therapeutic containment
The chief goal of conventional psychiatric treatment is to eradicate a person's symptoms and prevent them recurring. "Anti-psychotic" and "mood-stabilising" drugs are the most common means of achieving these aims. Such measures may be helpful, at least in the short-term, e.g. for individuals tormented by distressing delusional beliefs or malevolent hallucinations that cannot be alleviated by other means. However, medications are often used excessively in a determined effort to banish such symptoms completely ("therapeutic aggression").

Suppressive measures may seem entirely appropriate to those who view psychosis as a strictly medical affliction. However, this diagnosis encompasses a variety of different kinds of phenomena, some of which (spiritual emergencies, self-healing psychoses) entail potentially transformative inner processes which may be stifled or thwarted by insensitive handling. Furthermore, psychoses of the coping strategy type are rooted in psychological conflicts that tend to be entirely overlooked by techniques that focus solely on eradicating symptoms. From an holistic perspective it is preferable to address underlying *causes* of a condition rather than simply suppressing its symptomatic manifestations. Stanislav Grof's pioneering research into psychedelic and other altered states of consciousness (*Chapter Eight*) led him to propose the following maxim for those whose aim is not just to treat but to heal: "An important task of therapy is to lead to a situation where symptoms *need not appear*, not to a situation where they *cannot appear*."[45]

Containment refers to use of various measures aimed at ensuring the physical and psychological safety of a person experiencing psychotic symptoms and the protection of other people and the surrounding environment. Such measures might include confining a person to a specific location or vicinity, curtailing behaviour that threatens harm to self or others or which could result in property damage, and restricting socially unacceptable or grossly inappropriate behaviour. Setting of boundaries and limits must, of course, be done as gently and respectfully as possible. Contrary to what some are inclined to believe, this kind of limit-setting can be very reassuring, especially to those experiencing poor impulse control or severe identity disturbances (which could involve temporary fragmentation or even complete loss of ego boundaries).

Therapeutic containment entails the provision of adequate emotional support while encouraging people to give full expression to their feelings, thoughts, and experiences in a safe and constructive way. Suitable modalities include art (drawing, painting, sculpting), writing (journal, poetry), music, singing, dancing, and creative movement. These activities might also be used to complement or amplify verbal expression (talking). As Carl Jung recognised, activities such as these help people distance themselves from disturbing inner experiences:

> Even with ordinary therapeutic measures you can get the patient's mind at a sufficiently safe distance from the unconscious, for instance by inducing him to draw or paint a picture of his psychic situation. (Painting is rather more effective, since by means of the colours his feelings are drawn into the picture too.) In this way the apparently incomprehensible and unmanageable chaos of his total situation is visualised and objectified; it can be observed at a distance by his conscious mind … The effect of this method is evidently due to the fact that the original chaotic and frightening impression is replaced by the picture which, as it were, covers it up … and whenever the patient is reminded of his original experience

by its menacing emotional effects, the picture he has made of it interposes itself between him and the experience and keeps his terror at bay.[46]

Small amounts of medication – sufficient to "take the edge off" anxiety-provoking or overwhelming experiences without stopping them entirely – might sometimes be used in conjunction with expressive measures. However, in contrast to a strictly suppressive approach, containment allows a person's experiences – including symptoms – to continue, thereby leaving open the possibility of exploring and examining them, as those with an integrating coping style may wish to do.

Positive attitudes and expectations

Individuals who have experienced a psychotic episode are generally encouraged to accept they have a "psychotic illness" caused by a disturbance in their brain and that medications will help rectify the "chemical imbalance" allegedly responsible for their disorder. People are often told they have an incurable affliction ("like diabetes") and are likely to require life-long medical treatment. Though such notions are well-meant, many people find them distressing, if not depressing. While it is imperative to beware of romanticising psychosis with patently fanciful notions (e.g. that *every* episode involves a mystical inner journey or elevated "altered state of consciousness"), unnecessarily pessimistic views should also be scrupulously avoided.

Many people find it reassuring to consider the similarity of acute psychosis to the normal experience of dreaming. The fact that all human beings have vivid "hallucinatory" experiences and compelling "delusional" ideas in dreams has been noted by many astute observers of the human mind. Jung was the first modern psychiatric researcher to point out that an acutely psychotic individual is like a person dreaming while awake.

Emphasising the meaning and significance of the profound life crisis of psychosis provides a counterbalance to conventional views. Acknowledging that psychosis can have positive as well as negative aspects – as the cases discussed earlier demonstrate – can help avoid the burden of hopelessness evoked by "broken brain" ideology. Maryanne Handel's views epitomise a balanced attitude toward psychotic experience. After enduring a long struggle with frightening symptoms that included persecutory delusions and nightmarish hallucinations, she eventually came to feel it had been a "meaningful disturbance" which resulted in significant personal growth (*Chapter Six*). Looking back on how the psychotic ordeal affected her life she said:

> The whole experience means something. It's not just a meaningless chaos that's come to persecute you or to hurt you for no reason. It does mean something. Knowing that was valuable to me. What I experienced was like this inner journey full of temptations and so on. And you are able to come out of it, but come out of it changed on the inside and different. I wanted to have this feeling that I could change through it and that I would be allowed to become normal again. Knowing that was very important to me because it was like a promise that I could. And it gave me hope that I would come out of it. That hope sort of led me on.[47]

Rather than viewing it as an entirely negative condition permanently embedded in a person's genetic and biochemical makeup, testimonials such as this highlight a dynamic understanding of acute psychosis as a dramatic life-changing crisis. Encouraging people to view psychosis as a crisis they *experienced* rather than an illness they have *got* can help free them from despair and galvanise their desire to deal with the issues raised in a more positive and hopeful way.

Helping people to develop a more constructive interpretation of their situation and experiences establishes a foundation for practical action. A variety of other measures can help restore self-confidence and foster hope. Acknowledging a person's achievements and positive attributes ("history of sanity") can help heal the damage inflicted by isolation and stigmatisation. Affirming the existence of an intact inner life which continues in spite of psychosis, as Professor Manfred Bleuler and others have observed, can enhance a person's sense of self-worth and foster confidence in diagnosed individuals and helpers alike.

The atmosphere of the Soteria community was imbued with the belief that people can grow through the upheaval of psychosis. Indeed, residents were actively encouraged to *expect* they would recover. Far from being a superficial ploy to make people feel better, such positive expectations can act as self-fulfilling prophecies which actually increase the likelihood of recovery, as Professor Ciompi's research has shown.[48]

The human body is naturally endowed with an astonishing variety of mechanisms to combat illness, repair injury, and restore normal physical functioning. Those struggling with severe mental disturbance may find it reassuring to realise that the human *mind* also possesses a repertoire of remarkable self-healing abilities. Although this phenomenon is not recognised in orthodox medicine, it is a central premise of Jungian psychology. Carl Jung was among the first to realise *the psyche is a self-regulating system* with an innate ability to rebalance and reorder itself in the service of the journey toward psychological and spiritual wholeness. Anton Boisen viewed these natural mental self-healing abilities as reflections of the "healing power of nature":

> This interpretation means that *in the ailments of the mind no less than in those of the body we can see the manifestation of the healing power of nature so familiar to the physician.* Nature itself in ways far beyond our comprehension is constantly seeking to heal and to save. All that the best physician can do is to help nature in removing the obstacles to the free flow of life-giving forces. Nor does nature wait for the physician to act. This is perhaps even more true in the mental realm than it is in the physical ... nature itself is the chief actor in most of the cures that are actually affected.[49]

Recognising the existence of natural inner healing processes fosters hopefulness. It is vital, however, to guard against unrealistic or distorted beliefs – such as that people can just sit back and passively await spontaneous recovery. In this context *excessively* positive attitudes and expectations are just as undesirable as excessively negative ones. This has been confirmed by studies of individuals diagnosed with schizophrenia which found that the less negative people are about their future, the better their prognosis is likely to be. Interestingly, having a strongly positive attitude toward the future is less important in this regard than *not* having a negative one:

> Romantic idealisation of the psychotic episode is just as much a distortion as unrealistic despair ... patients with good outcome were not enamoured of their illness or psychotic experience. At the same time, however, they did not reject it as irrelevant or devalue it as unimportant. They dealt with it as a real event with vital implications in their lives. One might say their attitude was neither positive nor negative, but *realistic* ... a relationship between attitude and outcome is present. Specifically, the less negative patients were about their future, the better their outcome. Conversely, a

very positive attitude about the future was not associated with good outcome. Thus, the absence of a negative attitude appears critical.[50]

It is common for people to go through periods of uncertainty (possibly prolonged) and many "ups and downs" before they develop a settled attitude towards their psychotic experiences and future. Helpers with an open-minded, life-affirming outlook can provide invaluable support and encouragement during this time.

Structured activity and routines

At the height of an acute psychotic episode, when a diagnosed individual's experiences and symptoms are intense and their behaviour is at its most chaotic and unpredictable, they may effectively be "in a world of their own" for a time. The paramount need during this phase is for a low-stimulus "asylum" environment that provides an appropriate degree of limit-setting and containment. The immediate aftermath of such an episode may entail a period of post-psychotic retreat. Since this is often a crucial phase of the healing process, premature attempts to "push" people out of it could prove harmful. However, concerned helpers sometimes err on the side of caution and adopt an excessively gentle approach that could inadvertently contribute to prolonging idleness and fostering dependency.

Environments that foster healing and recovery are not an unbroken succession of lazy Sunday afternoons. It is unwise for anybody to spend too long passively awaiting the return of energy and motivation. Even if it is extremely basic to begin with, a simple daily routine of practical activity helps counteract tendencies toward aimless drifting, boredom, and physical and mental sluggishness (tendencies exacerbated by over-use of medication). Simple exercise routines (walking, jogging, swimming, bicycle riding, dancing, yoga) and household chores (shopping, cleaning, cooking, gardening) help integrate body and mind and foster a sense of stability and groundedness ("being in your body") – a boon to those with a tendency to "space out" or drift into the psychotic "dream world".

Carl Jung's experiences while grappling with powerful archetypal images during the tumultuous period he called his "confrontation with the unconscious" brought home the importance of maintaining stable relations with other people and fulfilling everyday duties and responsibilities. Such practical obligations helped him remain grounded and were an essential counterbalance to the tendency to become lost in the "other" world:

> Particularly at this time ... I needed a point of support in "this world", and I may say my family and my professional work were that to me. It was most essential for me to have a normal life in the real world as a counterpoise to that strange inner world. My family and profession remained the base to which I could always return, assuring me that I was an actually existing, ordinary person. The unconscious contents could have driven me out of my wits. But my family, and the knowledge: I have a medical diploma from a Swiss university, I must help my patients, I have a wife and five children, I live at 228 Seestrasse in Küsnacht – these were actualities which made demands upon me and proved to me again and again that I really existed, that I was not a blank page whirling about in the winds of the spirit ... I aimed, after all, at *this* world and *this* life. No matter how deeply absorbed or how blown about I was, I always knew that everything I was experiencing was ultimately directed at this real life of mine. I meant to meet its obligations and fulfil its meanings ... Thus my family and my profession always remained a joyful reality and a guarantee that I also had a normal existence.[51]

Having something tangible to do each day (domestic chores, housework, exercise) and regular commitments (rehabilitation programmes, therapy sessions, voluntary work) provide points of focus and help impose a sense of structure and direction. Daily routines can also provide a reassuring sense of order and predictability during unsettled periods. Making a sincere effort to honour all obligations and commitments (e.g. appointments) is a major challenge for some and an opportunity to practice self-discipline and self-control. Simple activities such as tidying one's room, attending to personal hygiene and grooming, and wearing clean clothes help instil a sense of wellbeing and will eventually contribute to improved self-confidence.

Getting started is often the hardest part. Sometimes people might need to literally *force* themselves into action, at least until they have overcome their initial resistance and developed a stable routine. Emma Pierce's struggle illustrates the benefits of a determined effort to overcome lethargy and inertia:

It came as a great surprise to me to find that my lethargy, over a long period of time, had actually robbed me of physical ability. I can now appreciate the total sanity of those people who face crisis by keeping up the ordinary tasks in a religious routine … It goes a long way to keeping the mind on an even keel … No matter how dopey, lethargic, depressed I felt, if I really wanted to I could physically move my arms and legs and make them perform as I so ordered. This forced me to face the fact that the messy house was messy because, essentially, I didn't feel like cleaning it up … In time I was forced to recognise that when I commanded my limbs into action against lethargy, the lethargy left and after a period of time, I felt better. Certainly a large part of feeling better, even happier, was the sense of achievement, both with what I had done, be it in making a bed or sweeping a floor, and overcoming lethargy.[52]

As their motivation and energy improve it is essential that people begin accepting greater responsibility for their life and recovery. While this may be an extremely daunting prospect for some – especially those whose confidence has been shattered – it is a crucial element in the process of rebuilding self-esteem and self-reliance.

From time to time it is good for people in recovery to be exposed to new situations and responsibilities. Deliberately putting themselves into situations which force them out of their "comfort zone" may help people discover untapped strengths and abilities. Sudden confrontation with stressful situations, or unexpected changes in environment and routine, sometimes mobilise hidden potentials, even in severely disabled individuals.[*]

Confiding relationships
Some people who experience psychosis have had long-standing problems (often related to poor self-image and lack of confidence) that have contributed to difficulty in interpersonal relationships.

---

[*] This fact led Professor Manfred Bleuler to prize the remedial value, for those diagnosed with "chronic schizophrenia", of sensitively timed confrontation with new situations, routines, and responsibilities. As he noted, "sudden confrontation with a new and surprising social situation demanding action: giving the patient unexpected responsibilities, early discharge from the hospital, sudden changes of hospital, and so on" may function as a kind of shock treatment that "shakes the patient out of his autism". Bleuler, M. (1970) Some Results of Research In Schizophrenia. *Behavioral Science*, Vol.15, 211-219.

Even if they did not previously have such problems, undergoing a psychotic crisis can have a devastating impact. Stigmatisation could so erode a person's confidence they come to feel they lack any human worth. These problems are compounded by erosion of former social connections. With their confidence shattered and feeling irrevocably cut off from others, some people retreat into a shell of aloofness and emotional shut-down.

Given safe, supportive surroundings some people may have sufficient reserves of confidence and ego-strength to emerge from their cocoon-like existence more or less on their own. However, some are so traumatised by their ordeals, or have such deep-seated interpersonal difficulties, they may require assistance of a specific kind to help them with the onerous task of re-connecting with the world around them. This may take the form of another person whose calm, reassuring presence furnishes a bridge back to everyday life. A young woman who had completely cut herself off from others explains how reassuring it was to find someone she felt might accept and understand her:

> Meeting you made me feel like a traveller who's been lost in a land where no one speaks his language. Worst of all, the traveller doesn't even know where he should be going. He feels completely lost and helpless and alone. Then, suddenly, he meets a stranger who can speak English. Even if the stranger doesn't know the way to go, it feels so much better to be able to share the problem with someone, to have him understand how badly you feel. If you're not alone, you don't feel hopeless any more. Somehow it gives you life and a willingness to fight again.[53]

Individuals who have become estranged from the world are sometimes able to start the process of reconnecting with others through the development of a trusting relationship with another human being. In the first instance this might be a counsellor or therapist, but since theoretical knowledge and clinical skills are less critical to this endeavour (at least in the beginning) than are personal qualities like patience, gentleness, and non-judgemental acceptance, a relationship of this kind could just as well involve a relative, caring friend, or compassionate lay helper. To the extent it provides a sense of safety and refuge, such a relationship can itself function as a kind of asylum.

As well as helping to alleviate fear and loneliness, a healing relationship provides a space in which a wounded individual can practice interacting with another human being in relative safety and so begin the task of rebuilding their fragile identity and confidence. For some, the greatest challenge in this undertaking involves learning to trust and open up to another person. Difficult as this may be, it could result in personal transformation, as the following account illustrates. This woman explains how learning to trust her therapist allowed her to feel she was a real person, not an "outsider" looking in on the world:

> I had drawn so far inside myself and so far away from the world, I had to be shown not only that the world was safe but also that I belonged to it, that I was in fact a person ... But none of this can happen without the all-important but ever so elusive element of trust ... It was not so difficult to trust my therapist with words, with information [but to] "let him in" would have felt like such a violation and a betrayal to myself and to the world that had kept me safe from other people for so long ... Part of me wanted to trust him totally, but an equally tenacious part of my mind said no and I did not know why. The fight went back and forth ... [until eventually] I experienced a feeling I did not remember ever having before – it was a total and unselfish caring for another human being. Finally I was able to trust my therapist enough to make myself vulnerable and to care ... I know that I have the capacity to care, but overcoming what seems to be an inborn terror often seems as difficult as scaling a granite wall without ropes.[54]

Such testimonials lend support to Jung's contention that "a schizophrenic ceases to be a schizophrenic when he meets someone by whom he feels understood".[55] For some, a trusting relationship with another person could be a crucial stepping stone toward greater involvement with the world as a whole.

Conclusion

Anyone wishing to understand what a healing environment entails might find it helpful to ask themselves the following questions: What kind of place would I like to spend time in if I was going through a severe emotional ordeal? What sort of people would I like around me? While in this place, what sorts of things might help me feel better? What would assist my recovery? In assessing an existing therapeutic environment (such as a hospital ward, community-based clinic, or rehabilitation programme) one might ask: How does being in this place make me feel? What are its good points? What seems to be lacking? How could it be improved?

Chapter Twelve

Healing and Recovery

Everyone has the capacity to recover from psychosis.

Edward Podvoll[1]

Anton Boisen was among the first to recognise that psychotic crises can take a variety of forms, some of which are best understood as problem-solving experiences. He also noted that the most severe crises tend to "make or break", such that a person may come through an episode "in better shape than he had been for years", or else suffer a major (though not necessarily irreversible) setback. Boisen spent many years investigating why some who experience psychosis recover completely and go on to lead satisfying and fulfilling lives, while others become stuck or even go downhill, with some becoming mired in prolonged disability. He concluded that the outcome is strongly influenced by *psychosocial* factors, among which the following are especially important:[2]

- The amount and quality of social support people receive
- The honesty and sincerity with which they face their difficulties
- The balance of assets and liabilities in their character and life situation

Contemporary evidence supports Boisen's conclusions. Since he conducted his research long before the advent of modern psychiatric medications, Boisen was not in a position to assess their influence on recovery. However, many people find such drugs helpful, despite their adverse effects. While medication and other physical therapies heavily overshadow psychosocial measures in mainstream psychiatric treatment, there is no reason the factors Boisen identified are any less relevant now than they were in his day. A holistic approach emphasises these influences, combining them with judicious use of medication if it proves helpful. Topics covered in this chapter include:

- Self-help and self-responsibility
- Self-treatment: cultivating sanity
- Using medication wisely

Self-Help and Self-Responsibility

Within the purview of mainstream psychiatry people diagnosed with psychotic disorders have tended to be seen as essentially passive "victims" of their condition who are capable of little more than "compliance" with recommended treatment. Recent years have brought belated recognition that these infantilising perceptions are quite erroneous and that – like every other human being – such persons are highly active agents in their own lives.[3] This agency manifests in a multitude of ways. For instance, people are constantly making decisions regarding what to make of their experiences, whether or not to accept treatment (including medication), and the kind of involvement they want with mental health services and other supports. Furthermore, many people employ a variety of coping strategies which range from simple manoeuvres (e.g. social withdrawal) to more elaborate measures (e.g. cognitive behavioural techniques) in an effort to alleviate anxiety-provoking experiences such as distressing thoughts or hostile voices.[4]

A period of profound disorientation often occurs in the wake of a person's first psychotic episode and the "clash of realities" that accompanies it. The ordeal invariably raises many questions: Why did this happen? Was any of it true? Could it happen again? As soon as the crisis has passed many people endeavour to put it behind them so they can get on with their lives (sealing-over). Some may be able to do this but, if a second or third crisis occurs, painful facts must be faced. Many who find themselves in this situation cling to the hope some simple remedy – such as an all-purpose pill – will solve their problems. However, even if a helpful medication regime is available, psychosis and its psychosocial aftermath entail many aspects not amenable to such treatment, e.g. damaged self-esteem, stigmatisation, loss of direction and purpose. Some may try to avoid discomfort by living in denial and hoping a miracle cure will be found. Others take the path of least resistance and allow themselves to drift aimlessly through life.

In Alcoholics Anonymous (AA) and other 12-step programmes, those who do not acknowledge their problems and accept responsibility for them are said to be "in denial". Recovery demands a willingness to face reality. People must eventually acknowledge and start coming to terms with the fact that something happened which led to them receiving a psychiatric diagnosis. Some people accept that they have a mental illness and willingly comply with recommended psychiatric treatment. However, relinquishing denial does *not* necessarily mean having to accept a strictly medical view of psychosis. Such explanations might suit some people but be unacceptable to others. The non-medical constructions of psychotic experience outlined in this book are bound to be more intuitively acceptable to many. Whatever view is finally adopted, it must be compatible with a person's own experiences, beliefs, and values.*

Of all the things that can help improve mental health and wellbeing, a person's own efforts are among the most important. In a recent survey in which people were asked what most helped their recovery, various kinds of self-help were identified as extremely important.[5] Beneficial influences nominated by the greatest proportion were:

- Determination to get better (82%)
- Understanding the illness (81%)
- Taking responsibility for helping themselves (68%)
- Finding their own ways to manage the illness (64%)

Like many others, Esso Leete reached a turning point when she decided to take control of her life and begin the work of recovery:

Sadly, for years I had expected someone else to "fix" me. However, I finally realised, after many clinical disappointments, that this task fell to me alone and that no one else could really make me better. I approached this task very seriously, conscientiously working to get my life back together. For the first time, I then felt ready to take responsibility for myself, including management of my illness, and I feel it was at this point that my recovery really began.[6]

The following are among the many practical ways people can play an active role in their healing and recovery:

Self-understanding and self-education
Learning about the nature and causes of psychosis can help people better understand their own experiences and behaviour. Under-

---

* Various compromise positions involving "partial" or "conditional" acceptance are possible. For example, some people may refuse a psychiatric label but willingly accept offers of support and even take medications if they prove helpful. Others may accept a psychiatric diagnosis initially but eventually reject it in favour of their own interpretation of their experiences.

standing the various inner and outer influences that can help or hinder healing and recovery fosters a sense of control and opens up a range of possibilities for constructive action.

Developing a realistically hopeful attitude
Positive attitudes and expectations have a beneficial effect on natural healing processes. Eliminating negative attitudes and pessimistic expectations which can act as self-fulfilling prophecies is especially important. Some may find it helpful to think of the psychosis as an intense personal crisis which happened to them rather than as an illness they have got.

Cultivating self-esteem
The stigma and negativity associated with mental illness can harm a diagnosed person's self-image and self-esteem. Consequently, taking active steps to counter these influences, and making an effort to develop and maintain a personally acceptable identity and sense of self-worth are crucial tasks. Acknowledging one's inherent human worth and "history of sanity" can be very helpful, especially to those lacking external sources of validation.

Adopting a healthy lifestyle
A well-balanced nutritious diet, regular exercise, and adequate rest and sleep help sustain mental and physical health as well as promoting vitality and sense of personal wellbeing. These measures also strengthen the natural restorative mechanisms of body and mind that play a vital role in healing and recovery.

Avoiding substance abuse
In addition to having detrimental effects on physical and mental health, abuse of illicit substances and/or excessive consumption of social drugs such as caffeine and alcohol can exacerbate psychotic symptoms or even trigger relapse. Consequently, social drugs should be used in moderation and potentially "pro-psychotic" street drugs avoided entirely.

Using medication wisely
Those who require psychotropic medication, either temporarily or for extended periods, must assume responsibility for ensuring they use it

wisely. Making an effort to learn about the therapeutic and side effects of medications fosters a sense of control and encourages realistic expectations about what these drugs can and cannot be expected to do. Wise use entails using medications as one tool among many to promote healing and recovery (see "Using Medication Wisely" below.)

Learning practical strategies for managing symptoms
Many people discover ways of preventing or alleviating symptoms and other difficulties through a combination of experience and trial-and-error. People can add to what they learn in this way by making an effort to expand their repertoire of coping skills, e.g. through careful self-observation and a process of experimentation based on strategies and techniques learnt from others, books, self-help manuals, and training courses.

Learning to manage stress
Excessive stress can cause established symptoms to become more severe and could trigger a psychotic episode ("relapse") in susceptible individuals. Effective stress management is thus a fundamental component in every person's repertoire of coping strategies and survival skills.

Monitoring prodromal symptoms
Prodromal symptom monitoring entails learning to recognise characteristic changes which indicate a person has exceeded their stress tolerance and might be at risk of experiencing relapse. Individuals who are able to accurately identify these subtle inner changes can use them as personal "warning signals" which indicate the need to take steps to reduce stress and increase supports before a crisis point is reached. This is an essential skill for anyone whose treatment involves using medication on an intermittent basis.

Utilising counselling or psychotherapy
"Talking therapy" provides a context in which to identify and address personal problems and concerns. The ongoing support and guidance of a trusted therapist or counsellor can be an invaluable aid while working on issues such as lack of confidence, low self-esteem, and loss of direction and purpose.

Acknowledging and nurturing spirituality

Even if it is not always recognised as such, spirituality is an important facet of human life. Though profound spiritual experiences sometimes arise in the context of acute psychosis, such phenomena are rarely dealt with in an appropriate or adequate manner. Nevertheless, the comfort, strength, guidance, and meaning provided by spiritual beliefs and practices can be a boon during the often fraught journey of healing.

Seeking and accepting help

Experiencing psychosis and its aftermath is hard. Even if effective therapies are available, affected individuals must contend with a multitude of challenges. While some people are reluctant to accept their need for help, many eventually come to value the support and assistance that caring and compassionate helpers can provide. There is much wisdom in the GROW aphorism, "You alone can do it, but you can't do it alone".

Richard Weingarten's story epitomises the attitude of self-responsibility alluded to above. Over time he discovered there were many things he could do to nurture his mental health and emotional wellbeing:

> My health really began to improve in 1986 when I saw that my therapists were limited in what they could do for me, and I began to do things for myself … I tended to blame everything on my "illness". As it turned out, I had many problems that were caused or made problematic by the lack of meaningful activities and a strong social network, or just being out of tune with my environment. Perhaps the biggest danger was seeing myself as a "sick person" … I began to make real progress when I took control of my life and began doing things that utilised my strengths and abilities, and received some recognition … when I began to take on real challenges and saw that I could meet them successfully, I felt more hopeful about myself and my future. It was about this time also that I began to see myself as a therapist and devised coping mechanisms to deal with my problems and situations that were causing me difficulty … I try hard to keep the amount of stress I encounter to a minimum. I get the exercise I need, eat the right foods, get the right amount of sleep and rest – very important – and generate

the amount and kinds of activities I need that allow me to keep my life interesting and moving forward.[7]

Recovery depends on cultivating a positive attitude and being prepared to do the necessary work. As Dr Podvoll explains, "It requires a shift of allegiance to 'living well', to cultivating one's own health and sanity."[8]

Self-Treatment: Cultivating Sanity

Despite the fact that psychosis is a *mental* condition, conventional Western approaches to mental health rarely provide guidance regarding care of the mind. However, this usually neglected aspect of self-help is so important it warrants special consideration.

Though most people who experience psychosis eventually recover, little is known about how this actually occurs. Formal psychiatric assessment relies on relatively crude measures such as symptom severity to gauge "clinical progress".[9] This leaves unanswered many vital questions. In particular, it reveals nothing about *subjective* aspects of recovery, such as what people experience and feel as they emerge from their "waking dream", and how the mind gradually re-orients to everyday reality.

Dr Edward Podvoll's pioneering research provides a glimpse into this ordinarily hidden realm. Tracking the recovery process in minute detail allowed him to identify the critical mental events that occur as people gradually emerge from a psychotic altered state. One of his principal contributions to understanding the mind in recovery is his realisation that moments of sanity – "islands of clarity" as he calls them – occur continually, even while people are in the throes of a psychotic episode. In his view, they are manifestations of the disturbed individual's inherent sanity:

> Spontaneous flashes of clarity occur all the time during psychosis. They are generally experienced as moments of freshness of mind, or relaxation from intensified mind. These flashes represent a fundamental intelligence of the "intrinsic health" that exists beneath the psychotic delusions.[10]

Similar observations have been made by some of the most eminent figures in the history of psychiatry. For example, German psychiatrist

Karl Jaspers noted in his seminal treatise on psychopathology that "momentary insight" is a common occurrence even in the midst of a florid psychosis:

> In acute psychoses there are transient states of far-reaching insight. The patient returns from his fantastic experiences for a moment ... Sometimes at the beginning of a process we find considerable insight, the correction of delusions, the proper assessment of voices, etc., which one might well consider as recovery ... but insight of this sort is quite transient. We can occasionally observe how it comes and goes within a few hours or days. Sometimes clear consciousness will arise in the very middle of the schizophrenic experiences. The patients will say afterwards, "For a moment I was again aware that I was disturbed", or "Suddenly I was quite aware that the whole thing was nonsense" ... the momentary insight which emerges is more far-reaching than the content of most of the verbal utterances suggest.[11]

Because "islands of clarity" are so brief – especially when they first appear – they often go unnoticed. The few clinicians who are aware of this phenomenon tend to see it as simply another bizarre anomaly of the severely disturbed mind. However, Dr Podvoll's research convinced him these natural mental events constitute the very *seeds of recovery*. In his opinion, full recovery from psychosis depends on recognising, acknowledging, and protecting these spontaneous interruptions of the waking dream state.

This conclusion is consistent with a notion central to Eastern spiritual traditions, Buddhist psychology in particular, which hold that the human mind possesses a quality of *inherent sanity* – an incorruptible state that continues to exist behind the periods of mental and emotional unrest which inevitably occur from time to time. (A notion reminiscent of Professor Manfred Bleuler's observation that an "intact inner life" always exists behind the psychotic façade, even in the most severely deteriorated "chronic" individuals.) While Western approaches use methods such as stress management techniques to *induce* mental and physical relaxation, practitioners of meditation believe calming the mind uncovers an *already existing* state of tranquillity and inner peace.

In addition to using externally-imposed measures to promote mental wellbeing it is possible to work directly with spontaneous moments of natural recovery as they arise. The first requirement in using this approach is an ability to recognise "islands of clarity" which can take various forms, such as the following:

Doubts: may arise at any time, even in the midst of a florid psychosis, causing a person to ask, "Am I only dreaming?" The most convincing delusion or vivid hallucination might be temporarily punctured by moments of doubt and uncertainty: "Is this true?", "Are these voices real?", "Could such strange things really be happening?" The first hint of doubt is sometimes heralded by a niggling feeling "something is wrong".*

Sudden insights: Karl Jaspers noted that there can be moments when, in a flash, people see through their dream-like experiences: "Suddenly I was quite aware the whole thing was nonsense". At such times people sometimes feel they understand what has gone wrong and can see quite clearly what they need to do to get well again.

Awakenings: people may have experiences of "coming to", as if they had suddenly woken from a dream. Such moments are characterised by a sense of renewed mental clarity and alertness and heightened awareness of the surrounding environment ("coming to one's senses"). Joanne Greenberg describes a moment when she "suddenly had a revelation or a mystical conjunction of some kind, and became aware of being alive. I was aware that I was alive and wanted to live. I really took off pretty much after that."[12]

"Clicking in": a vivid sensation of reconnecting with one's self, body, and the physical environment. Sometimes described as a feeling of "stepping back into oneself" attended by a sense of being solidly grounded in reality once more.

Dr Podvoll has observed that recognising and affirming "islands of clarity" facilitates their occurrence and encourages them to accumulate

---

* Doubt is sometimes personified in hallucinatory voices. Jung noted that people sometimes hear "correcting voices" which talk about their symptoms: "It is remarkable that not a few patients who delight in neologisms and bizarre delusional ideas … are often corrected by their voices. One of my patients, for example, was twitted by the voices about her delusions of grandeur, or the voices commanded her to tell the doctor who was examining her delusions 'not to bother himself with these things.'" Jung, C.G. (1974) *The Psychology of Dementia Praecox*. Princeton: Princeton University Press. p.90.

and merge into sequences that eventually spread into many areas of a person's life:

> There is a moment in the midst of madness when things suddenly begin to make sense again. One feels that one has come back into oneself. One has become the "operator" … It is an island of clarity where one is suddenly freed from the fixed mind of delusion. Some people describe this as a feeling, almost a physical sensation, of "clicking in". Frequently this moment carries with it an uncanny confidence that the worst is over and that one will become well again. Sometimes the moment is fleeting, sometimes it endures. But however brief, moments of recovery from psychosis are universal experiences – yet everyone who suffers with psychosis experiences them and reacts to them in different ways … They are fragile moments, and they need to be acknowledged and respected. This simple act will greatly facilitate anyone's recovery from psychosis.[13]

Although moments of recovery occur continuously ("In retrospect, one is always surprised that islands of clarity have been happening all along, and much earlier than one had recognised at the time"), when psychotic experiences are intense they may quickly be swamped by mental phenomena which distract and enthral the mind. Sometimes they are *deliberately* abandoned, as when a person wakes momentarily and is horrified to realise he or she has been immersed in an illusory world. The "seduction of madness" represents a great temptation for some. As one person said, "There were times when I was aware, in a sense, that I was acting on a delusion. One part of me seemed to say, 'Keep your mouth shut, you know this is a delusion and it will pass.' But the other side of me wanted the delusion, preferred to have things this way."[14] A great deal hinges on the choices people make, as Dr Podvoll emphasises: "The difference between guarding and abandoning one's intelligence and sanity during a psychosis has very great consequences, yet only a hair's breadth separates them."[15]

There are simple practical ways to foster the occurrence and recognition of islands of clarity. Anything which promotes synchronisation of mind and body tends to promote their appearance. Activities which engage the senses and enable a person to practice being fully focused in the present moment are especially beneficial. When performed with full attention, "grounding" activities like

271

domestic chores (shopping, cleaning, cooking) and exercise (walking, swimming, jogging, bicycle riding) help integrate mind and body into a harmonious state which will facilitate recovery.

As people become more connected to the world around them, practices which help to calm and rest the mind can be extremely beneficial. At an appropriate time, meditation and similar "mind training" techniques are invaluable recovery tools:

> Caring for one's mind in general involves the ability to continually bring back the attention of a wandering mind and to focus concentration ... The formal practice of meditation is also referred to as "resting the mind". This sense of rest means quieting down the mind ... When practiced correctly, this kind of resting also inevitably leads to a relaxation of the body ... At the point when someone reaches a fairly stable state of recovery, he needs to begin to *take responsibility for taming his mind*. Some kind of "mind training" is required, because only that can allow one to break the weak links in the psychotic chain reaction ... It is the tendency to attach to and identify with thoughts and emotions that is at the root of the psychotic chain reaction, and it is the one most directly cut through by the practice of mindfulness meditation, and perhaps other traditional mind trainings as well ... From this point of view it is important that at a certain time in recovery from psychosis one engages in some discipline(s) that allows one to slow down the speed of mind and weaken powerful internal habits of attachment and subsequent trance.[16]

While engrossed in intense psychotic experiences (and possibly for a considerable time afterwards) people may have difficulty recognising islands of clarity as they occur. For this reason, the presence of others who are able to affirm these precious moments can be of great assistance.[*]

---

[*] Dr Podvoll and his colleagues have developed a comprehensive home-based treatment approach based on the principles outlined above. This is elaborated in his book *Recovering Sanity: A Compassionate Approach to Understanding and Treating Psychosis* (Shambhala, 2003) and implemented in a therapeutic community of individual treatment households located in the USA and Canada (www.windhorseassociates.com).

Using Medication Wisely

Many people feel modern psychotherapeutic medications are a godsend. Neuroleptics, commonly known as "anti-psychotic" drugs, certainly provide some people with welcome relief from tormenting symptoms such as anxiety-provoking thoughts (e.g. "persecutory delusions") and hostile "voices", while mood-stabilising drugs, on their own or in tandem with neuroleptics, can help limit the disruption of extreme mood swings. The prophylactic actions of both classes of medication are now widely relied on to reduce the likelihood of people experiencing further psychotic episodes: so-called "relapse prevention".

While such treatment is sometimes beneficial, widespread misuse has resulted in the role of these drugs becoming one of the most hotly debated topics in contemporary mental health care. Psychiatric medications are sometimes prescribed inappropriately and are often given in excessive doses or continued longer than necessary, practices that only exacerbate their deleterious effects. There are many legitimate grounds for concern about the way these drugs are often now used. In an unusually candid statement the president of American Psychiatric Association recently acknowledged the "widespread concern of the over-medicalization of mental disorders and the over-use of medications" before belatedly admitting "many patients are being prescribed the wrong drugs or drugs they don't need. These charges are true … a 'pill and an appointment' has dominated treatment."[17]

Since neuroleptic drugs were first introduced to psychiatry in the early 1950s their usefulness has been bedevilled by their numerous physical, mental, and social side effects. Introduction of clozapine in the early 1990s promised a new era of the so-called "second generation" or "atypical" neuroleptics. As well as clozapine this broad class now includes risperidone, olanzapine, quetiapine, amisulpride, aripiprazole, ziprasidone and others. An injectable preparation of risperidone (Risperdal Consta) recently became the first atypical to be used as a long-acting "depot" medication.

Despite what many still believe, with the possible exception of clozapine atypical neuroleptics as a group are *not* more effective than the older medications.[18] Independent research (i.e. not sponsored by the pharmaceutical industry) comparing efficacy and side effect profiles of the two groups has revealed that heavily publicised claims regarding

the unparalleled superiority of the newer drugs are erroneous.[19]* In
January 2009 a scathing editorial in the prestigious medical journal,
The Lancet, included these remarks:

> Antipsychotic drugs differ in their potencies and have a wide range
> of adverse-effect profiles, with nothing that clearly distinguishes the
> two major groups ... the second-generation drugs have no special
> atypical characteristics that separate them from the typical, or first-
> generation, antipsychotics. As a group they are no more efficacious,
> do not improve specific symptoms, have no clearly different side-
> effect profiles than the first-generation antipsychotics, and are less
> cost effective. The spurious invention of the atypicals can now
> be regarded as invention only, cleverly manipulated by the drug
> industry for marketing purposes and only now being exposed.[20]

The above comments notwithstanding, if neuroleptic and other
psychotropic drugs are used with wisdom and skill – never simply as
a way of "managing" people – they can sometimes be a valuable aid in
the work of healing and recovery.

An asylum of the kind described in *Chapter Eleven* is the ideal
environment in which to care for people in the throes of psychosis. As
the research of Loren Mosher, Luc Ciompi and others demonstrated,
psychotic crises often reach a natural conclusion if such conditions
are provided. While this is especially likely with inherently transient
episodes (spiritual emergencies, self-healing psychoses), it may also be
true of other types of acute psychosis. Since psychotic crises are often
triggered by excessive stress, calm, supportive, low-stimulus settings
are sometimes sufficient to disrupt the emotional chain-reaction that
can cause hypersensitive individuals to "spin out". Since stress often
exacerbates existing symptoms, such settings can have a natural "anti-
psychotic" effect.

---

* Cambridge University psychiatrist Dr Peter Jones, leader of the first major
independent study comparing the two groups of drugs, believes that for nearly two
decades the psychiatric profession was "beguiled" into thinking the atypical medications
were vastly superior. How could such a massive deception have occurred?
  Part of the answer can be found in a 2003 publication entitled *Is Psychiatry For
Sale?* by British psychiatrist Joanna Moncrieff, in which Dr Fuller Torrey states: "Dr
Moncrieff's question has already been answered in the United States, where it is clear
that psychiatry has already been sold. The buyer was Big Pharma. The sale price has
not been disclosed, but rumour has it that the pharmaceutical industry got a bargain."
[Cited in Bentall, R. (2009) *Doctoring The Mind*. London: Allen Lane. p.202]

Because asylums of this kind are not readily available it is often necessary to resort to other ways of helping people re-establish emotional equilibrium and regain self-control. Anti-psychotic medications are arguably the simplest and quickest means of doing this. In this context it is noteworthy that even in Soteria and Professor Ciompi's community, some acutely psychotic individuals did *not* respond satisfactorily to the tranquil ambiance in the first six weeks and were subsequently given medication. (It is worth bearing in mind that a non-medical understanding of psychosis does not necessarily imply strictly non-medical treatment in every instance.)

In *Chapter Three* it was suggested constitutional hypersensitivity is often a major contributor to psychosis proneness. This helps to explain why neuroleptics are sometimes beneficial. One of the principal effects of these drugs, Professor Manfred Bleuler notes, is to induce a state of calmness by dampening the intensity of the brain's responses to inner (psychodynamic) and outer (environmental) stimuli:

> Neuroleptics act by changing the activity or the sensitivity of definite neurological systems. The therapeutic consequence consists mainly in *calming agitation* and *diminishing the sensitivity to stimulation* both by psychodynamic experience and by experience from the outer world.[21]

Neuroleptics reduce the activity of specific receptors in the brain, especially those involving the neurotransmitter dopamine (so-called D2 receptors). Psychopharmacologist Dr David Healy, an international authority on therapeutic use of psychotropic medication, explains what occurs when a neuroleptic drug attaches itself ("binds") to such receptors:

> What binding to D2 receptors does is to produce a feeling of indifference, a sense of being shielded from stress, a "who cares" feeling that many people under stress find immensely useful. Neuroleptics are also called "major tranquillisers" for this reason. But the tranquillisation they produce is not like the wave of calm relaxation that Librium, Valium, and alcohol bring about ... It is much more a case of finding oneself not getting worked up than finding oneself tranquillised down ... they produce a feeling of detachment – of being less bothered by what had formerly been bothering ... more able to focus on tasks that need doing, less in a

daydream, not distracted by internal dialogues, strange thoughts, or intrusive imagery.[22]

The practical value of the neuroleptics lies in their ability to shield psychologically vulnerable individuals from stress by muting the impact of inner and outer experience on their exquisitely sensitive nervous systems. This stress-buffering action has two beneficial consequences: *therapeutic effects* such as calming those who are anxious and bewildered and alleviating distressing symptoms like hostile voices and frightening delusional beliefs; a *prophylactic effect* due to the drugs' ability to help hypersensitive individuals not get too "worked up", decreasing their likelihood of experiencing another episode, i.e. they reduce "relapse" risk. Dr Podvoll summarises possible beneficial effects of these drugs thus:

> By this time, it is well known that medications are not a "cure" for psychosis, that they do not specifically affect voices, visions, or delusions. Primarily, they have been given to control behaviour. But at times, they do lower the "amplitude" of outrageous sensory phenomena, or they lower the excitement and panic caused when the senses are in disarray ... They may give a patient an opportunity to live with some relatively quiet moments, when the sensory phenomena are not so imperious, and when one can turn away from the hallucinatory demands to live in "two places at once". There may be some precious spare time to relax, to begin to approximate reality, and to gain some semblance of dignity by not appearing to others as continuously distracted and forgetful.[23]

Observing the following ten simple principles can help optimise potential benefits of psychotropic medications while reducing the risk of adverse effects.

(1) A holistic approach
Far from being a consequence of a "chemical imbalance" in the brain, the crisis of acute psychosis is a result of a multitude of biological, psychological, social and spiritual factors interacting in highly individual sequences and combinations. Since a complex interplay of factors is involved, the person concerned is invariably affected in numerous ways. To be optimally beneficial, treatment must address the full range of their experiences, needs, and difficulties. Such a

holistic approach allows for the judicious use of medication if it proves helpful, while recognising that it does not work in isolation from all the other influences that affect a person's life.

Medication can never be an adequate substitute for treating the whole person since people only do as well as their *total* circumstances allow. In this context it is instructive to reflect on modern approaches to management of hypertension (high blood pressure). It is known that even with a medical condition like this, drugs are not always necessary. Many people can control their blood pressure by using lifestyle measures such as losing weight, reducing alcohol and salt intake, quitting smoking, exercise and stress-management. Some people may need anti-hypertensive medication temporarily – until lifestyle measures take effect – or for longer periods. The latter group includes those who are unable or unwilling to reduce their blood pressure without drugs.

The key components of a healing environment were outlined in *Chapter Eleven.* Even if they do not remove the need for medication entirely, such conditions may reduce the amounts required. With adequate support medication may even become unnecessary for some people. Those with persistent symptoms might be able to reduce their need for long-term "maintenance" treatment, and increase the effectiveness of the medication they receive, by adopting a healthy lifestyle which incorporates effective stress-management.

(2) Medication-free assessment

The fact that acute psychosis can involve a number of quite different kinds of experience challenges the wisdom of administering drugs as the first response to *everyone* undergoing such crises. Spiritual emergencies, self-healing psychoses, and crises provoked by short-term use of illicit substances tend to be transient, with the episode coming to an end as the inner process reaches completion or the drug effects wear off. In such cases, tranquillising medications could impair natural healing mechanisms or even cause people to be "frozen" in psychosis. Studies by reputable researchers leave little doubt some people experiencing acute psychosis fare better – or at least no worse – in the long-term if they do not receive neuroleptic treatment.[24]

Whenever feasible – and in the absence of physical or psychological risk to those concerned – people experiencing acute psychosis should have the benefit of a medication-free assessment period. During this time an effort should be made to ascertain the type of psychosis occurring (using guidelines in *Chapter Nine*), and whether medication is really necessary.

(3) Individualised treatment
Though they may have received similar diagnoses, people experiencing psychosis remain unique individuals, each with their own set of past and present life experiences, distinctive symptoms, and highly idiosyncratic array of psychological and biochemical sensitivities. In view of these variations it is vital that treatment be individualised.

Subjective responses to neuroleptic medication provide an indicator as to the likely success of such treatment. The way a person feels when first given these drugs sometimes predicts whether or not they will be beneficial in the long-term. Some people experience an unpleasant reaction – a so-called "dysphoric response" – that leaves them feeling tired, drowsy, goofy, lazy, dull, fuzzy, zombified, drugged, slowed down, and "like a hangover without a headache".[25] Some may have difficulty describing their state apart from saying something doesn't feel quite right in their brain. By contrast, those experiencing a positive response report feeling calmer, more relaxed, less worried, and less fearful.[26]

From the beginning dysphoric responders may complain that medication is making them worse. This feeling is often persistent, i.e. it tends *not* to diminish, even when people have had time to "get used to" the medication. Clinical research suggests that individuals whose initial reaction is negative tend to respond poorly to ongoing treatment and could even deteriorate on such therapy.[27] In view of this, dysphoric responders should either not be treated with neuroleptic medication or, if it is considered essential, only be given very small doses and their responses closely monitored.

(4) Non-drug coping strategies
Some people do not gain appreciable benefit from neuroleptic treatment. Such individuals are now likely to be described as "treatment resistant". In a determined effort to overcome such resistance some clinicians administer ever-increasing doses, try one medication after another hoping to find one that will "work", or experiment with combinations of different drugs ("polypharmacy"). However, if it is clear a person is not benefiting it may be wisest to forgo neuroleptic treatment altogether, as Professor Richard Bentall suggests:

Although most modern recipients of psychiatric care find that neuroleptics to some extent control their symptoms, it is doubtful whether any are *cured* by this kind of treatment, and a substantial minority obtain no benefit whatsoever. Despite extensive research, no one has found a way of predicting in advance which patients will respond to neuroleptic treatment. However, there is very good evidence that patients who fail to benefit from one type of neuroleptic will fail to respond to any other. These persistent "neuroleptic non-responders" would almost certainly do better if given no neuroleptic treatment whatsoever, yet drug-free strategies for managing symptoms are almost never considered.[28]

When treating people with persistent symptoms like hallucinations and delusions psychiatrists have long assumed there was no alternative to "anti-psychotic" medications. However, it is now known that *non-pharmacological strategies* are sometimes extremely effective in alleviating, possibly even preventing, these and other distressing phenomena. Cognitive behaviour techniques (CBT) can assuage some intrusive or threatening "voices" and delusional beliefs.[29] Early research suggests trans-cranial magnetic stimulation (TMS) may be beneficial for some people.[30]

One of the most important developments of recent times has been the recognition that, by utilising a process of trial-and-error, many people gradually acquire a repertoire of practical strategies and techniques they use to prevent, minimise, or cope with psychotic symptoms and other troubling experiences.[31] For example, some people are able to stop or lessen disturbing "voices" using simple strategies such as relaxation, distraction, selective listening, and auditory counter-simulation via stereo headphones or earplugs.[32] Though notoriously resistant to medical treatment, "negative" symptoms like loss of motivation and lack of emotional expressiveness ("blunt affect") may be amenable to psychosocial techniques.[33] Self-help manuals based on the cumulative experience of diagnosed persons are certain to become an important resource for disseminating non-drug coping strategies. Effective use of such strategies could reduce the amount of medication people need and might, in some cases, eliminate it entirely.

(5) Minimal effective dose

If medication is deemed necessary it is vital it be used with great care and skill. Potential benefits of psychotropic drugs are soon outweighed by their detrimental effects if used inappropriately or excessively. As well as having physical side effects, indiscriminate use could have adverse mental effects that hinder recovery. For instance, neuroleptic-induced "psychic indifference" could result in loss of drive and spontaneity and reduced sensitivity to *normal* feelings, thoughts, and sensations.

It used to be standard clinical practice for people in a floridly psychotic state to be immediately given copious amounts of medication in an effort to eradicate their symptoms as rapidly as possible. However, the simplistic notion "more is better" does not apply to neuroleptics. Skilful treatment is guided by the motto, "start low, go slow, stay low". In other words, if medication is required it should be given in very small amounts initially and the treated person's responses closely monitored. If it is necessary to increase the dose this should be done in small steps, with the maximum dosage remaining as low as possible consistent with the aims of effective treatment.

Young people experiencing their first acute episode may be especially sensitive to psychotropic medications and only need very small doses to elicit a substantial response. Extremely low dosages are sometimes sufficient for "neuroleptic naïve" individuals who have not previously had such drugs.[34] It is now recognised that even those diagnosed with "chronic" schizophrenia can often be successfully stabilised on far lower doses than were once thought necessary.[35]

(6) Early medication-reduction trial

Although many who experience a psychotic crisis will have no more episodes, people are often advised to continue taking medication for some time as a precautionary measure. Many clinicians recommend that people take anti-psychotic medication for a year or two after an episode and only reduce it thereafter if they are completely symptom free. While this conservative approach results in a lower incidence of relapse it comes at the cost of exposing many people to prolonged drug treatment they probably do not need.

There is currently no simple way to distinguish individuals who have had a one-off experience from those who may be prone to further episodes. The only practical method of determining whether a person requires ongoing medication is to observe what happens if they stop it. Some authorities recommend that, a few weeks after their symptoms abate, those experiencing psychosis for the first time should slowly reduce their medication and, if feasible, stop it completely.[36] It is vital such an experiment be conducted in a mature and responsible manner. In view of possible risks, individuals prone to violent, aggressive, or serious self-harming behaviour should be excluded from such a trial unless their safety and that of others can be assured.

With the exception of those who have only had very small amounts of medication a short time, *neuroleptic dosages should always be reduced slowly.* As well as decreasing the likelihood of withdrawal reactions, research has established that relapse is much more likely following rapid dose reduction than it is when the dosage is reduced gradually. For people diagnosed with schizophrenia, relapse rates are three times higher when treatment is stopped abruptly as compared to reducing it slowly.[37]

Because of the highly individual nature of the situation there are no hard and fast rules regarding the rate at which neuroleptic medication can be safely reduced. Dr Podvoll recommends reducing medication in ten consecutive steps, each amounting to 10% of the initial dosage. After each reduction the treated person should remain on the new dose until they feel ready to take the next step.[38] If problems occur at any stage the dose should be kept steady, or even increased a little, until everybody involved feels confident to proceed. It is vital to have patience, take as long as necessary for each step (there could be months between one reduction and the next), and be prepared for even slower reductions toward the end of this process.

(7) Relapse or re-emergence?

If symptoms return during a medication-reduction trial most psychiatric clinicians advise returning to the original dosage and remaining on it for some time before contemplating another such trial. If symptoms should recur during a second trial, long-term treatment is likely to be recommended, i.e. at least several years and possibly indefinitely. This view is based on the assumption that symptom recurrence indicates the presence of a persistent psychotic "illness" which can only be kept under control with continuous medication (the role of neuroleptics is often likened to that of insulin in treating diabetes for this reason). Though this assumption may be valid in some cases, a different interpretation of this state of affairs may be warranted.

In some instances what occurs when anti-psychotic medication is stopped is that a potentially healing or transformative inner process that has not yet reached completion is released from suppressive control. This is especially likely in respect to psychoses of the self-healing type and spiritual emergencies, in which case it would be more appropriate to view the psychosis-like phenomena as manifestations of a "re-emergence" than as signs of clinical "relapse". In such cases, reinstating medication – accompanied by the message that the person concerned has an incurable "psychotic illness" – could exacerbate their distress and contribute to life-long suffering and disability.

(8) Maintenance treatment

In discussing the role of medication it is necessary to distinguish between those who have only had one or two acute psychotic episodes (so-called "early psychosis") and those with lengthy psychiatric histories characterised by multiple hospital admissions, i.e. "chronic mental illness".

If they receive adequate support, some belonging to the former group will recover naturally without medical treatment. Others may find medication helpful in the short-term but be able to manage without it once the crisis has been satisfactorily resolved. Some in this group may continue having disturbing or disruptive experiences that make it difficult for them to function satisfactorily. In some instances these experiences may be so intense or deeply entrenched they cannot readily be dealt with by non-pharmacological means. Furthermore, individuals who develop "paranoid" symptoms as a result of their tendency to externalise inner conflicts may be unable to trust others sufficiently to avail themselves of effective help and support. For such individuals medication might provide a necessary means of containment, as Dr Grof explains:

> Systematic use of the mechanism of projection – disowning one's inner experiences and attributing them to influences coming from other people and from external circumstances – is a severe obstacle to the kind of psychological approach we described here. People suffering from severe paranoid states, hostile acoustic hallucinations ("voices"), and delusions of persecution consistently engage in projection of such unconscious contents and act under their influence. They cannot be reached with the new strategies, even if some aspects of their experiences seem to belong to the category of spiritual emergency. Unless it is possible by systematic

psychotherapeutic work to create a situation in which they have adequate insight into the nature of the process and a significant degree of trust, such people may require suppressive medication.[39]

Some individuals might need neuroleptic or other psychotropic medications on an ongoing basis to ensure their mental and emotional stability. Among those receiving such treatment ("neuroleptic maintenance") are some who may be able to use medication on an intermittent rather than continuous basis, i.e. taking it only at specific times such as if they are feeling excessively stressed or have developed "prodromal symptoms" which could be early warning signs of impending relapse.[40]

Long-term treatment does *not* necessarily mean it must be maintained indefinitely. Human beings grow and change over time and some people who might once have needed medication may reach a point when it is no longer necessary.[41] Some experts believe even those diagnosed with "chronic schizophrenia" should periodically have their medications gradually reduced on a trial basis in order to assess their ongoing need for such treatment. A study published in the *American Journal of Psychiatry* suggested up to 50% of people might be capable of managing without long-term medication:

> The question arises of what proportion of chronic schizophrenic outpatients may not need to be on anti-psychotics, either because they would do well without medication or because they would not do well on drugs for reasons including failure to find optimal drug or dose level, non-compliance, or toxicity. Judging by this review, the proportion of such patients may be as high as 50% … *The major principle we wish to stress is that every chronic schizophrenia outpatient maintained on anti-psychotic medication should have the benefit of an adequate trial without drugs* … Our review of drug discontinuance studies in outpatient schizophrenics maintained on anti-psychotics suggested that perhaps as many as 50% of such patients might not be worse off if their medications were withdrawn. In view of the long-term complications of anti-psychotic drug therapy – primarily tardive dyskinesia – an attempt should be made to determine the feasibility of drug discontinuance in every patient.[42]

Common sense dictates such a trial should generally not be undertaken unless the psychological and social circumstances of those concerned provide reasonable grounds for anticipating a successful outcome.

(9) Use of benzodiazepines
It is increasingly common for people diagnosed with psychosis to be given medications belonging to the *benzodiazepine* family (these drugs, also known as "minor tranquilisers", were discussed in *Chapter Seven*). Some people find benzodiazepines extremely helpful, and it may even be possible to use them instead of "heavier" neuroleptics in some cases. Indications relevant to psychosis include:

a) Stress, anxiety, insomnia
Benzodiazepines are effective anxiolytic (anxiety-reducing) medications which are often used to alleviate persistent symptoms of anxiety, tension, panic, and post-traumatic stress disorder (PTSD). These drugs can also help reduce the distress, agitation, and anxiety that commonly occur during acute psychotic episodes. Timely administration of a drug such as diazepam (Valium) when a person is developing warning signs ("prodromal symptoms") that suggest a psychotic episode may be imminent might help prevent a full-blown relapse from occurring.[43] Agitated and emotionally overwrought individuals often have difficulty sleeping and can get caught in a self-perpetuating cycle of anxiety and distress. Short-term use of hypnotic (sleep-inducing) benzodiazepines can help break this destructive cycle.

b) Psychotic agitation
When administered during an acute psychotic episode these drugs can dramatically reduce a disturbed individual's level of arousal thereby alleviating anxiety, agitation, excitement, hyperactivity and emotional distress. Severely agitated, aggressive, or hostile individuals are sometimes given the potent, short-acting benzodiazepine midazolam by intramuscular injection. This rapidly induces profound sedation with subsequent amnesia for the period during which the drug was acting.

c) Positive and negative symptoms
In addition to alleviating anxiety, tension, and agitation, benzodiazepines may also help to ameliorate "positive" psychotic symptoms such as hallucinations, delusions, and thought disorder in some people.[44]

The anti-psychotic effect of benzodiazepines may be related to their ability to block release of dopamine in the brain.[45] While "negative" symptoms like loss of motivation, reduced emotional responsiveness, and withdrawal often respond little, if at all, to neuroleptic treatment, benzodiazepines might ameliorate them.[46] Persons in a stuporous catatonic state are sometimes dramatically released from this extreme emotional "shut-down" when administered diazepam or similar benzodiazepine.[47] The effectiveness (albeit temporary) of anxiolytic therapy is illustrated in the following anecdote concerning a young woman in an acute catatonic state:

> Apparently overwhelmed by auditory hallucinations and environ-mental stimuli competing for her attention, she stands in one spot all day, immobilised. She is unable to answer simple questions, each hesitant phrase trailing off unfinished. She appears frightened, highly aroused and her pupils are widely dilated. Within one hour of taking a moderate dose (5 to 10 milligrams) of diazepam (Valium) she has completely returned to her normal self – capable, outgoing and calm. After a few hours the effect of the drug wears off and the patient is again extremely psychotic. Taking the drug regularly, the patient's psychosis is well controlled but, after a week, tolerance to the anti-psychotic effect of the drug develops and higher doses are required to achieve the same benefit. The effectiveness of the benzodiazepines in this case and in other psychotics may be due to a reduction in the patient's level of arousal.[48]

Everyone taking benzodiazepines should be aware of the following facts. These drugs are fast-acting, effective anxiolytics with relatively few side effects compared to neuroleptics. Significantly, they do not cause neurological disturbances such as akathisia, dyskinesia, and akinesia. Possible side effects include sedation (sleepiness), lethargy, and cognitive disturbances (impairment of memory and learning, confusion, ataxia). Abrupt cessation of benzodiazepines may pro-voke a withdrawal syndrome characterised by anxiety ("rebound anxiety"), irritability, faintness, sleep disturbance, bizarre dreams, and exacerbation of psychotic symptoms. A *tolerance* to the drugs' therapeutic action develops fairly rapidly so that ever-larger doses may be needed to achieve the desired effect. Prolonged use could lead to psychological *dependence* in certain individuals. In view of these risks caution is warranted. Benzodiazepines should be used sparingly and prolonged routine use avoided. To minimise risk it is advisable to use the lowest effective dose on an "as needed" basis rather than in a set daily routine. Such restrictions allow for short-term use (a few days up to a few weeks) to promote sleep and reduce anxiety and agitation.

(10) Risk minimisation strategies

Neuroleptic medications have potentially debilitating side effects including neurological disorders (extrapyramidal symptoms) such as dystonia, akathisia, and tardive dyskinesia. While these might be somewhat less prevalent with so-called "atypical" neuroleptics, this group of medications is *more* likely than the older drugs to cause metabolic and endocrine disorders such as weight gain/obesity, abnormally elevated blood lipids, and disturbances of glucose metabolism, including type 2 diabetes. Although the mechanisms underlying such adverse effects are not well understood, a range of simple practical measures can reduce the risk of these and other medication-related complications.

a) Minimise cumulative exposure
The first principle of risk reduction entails minimising cumulative exposure to neuroleptic and other drugs by using the lowest possible doses consistent with effective treatment and reducing or stopping the medication as soon as it is safe to do so. Using neuroleptics on an intermittent "as needed" basis could be a feasible alternative to continuous treatment for some people. It may sometimes be possible to use drugs belonging to the benzodiazepine family (see above) rather than the more side-effect-prone neuroleptics.

b) Lifestyle measures
Lifestyle measures that can reduce the risk of neuroleptic-induced metabolic, endocrine, cardiovascular, and other disorders include the following:

- Weight control (obesity is a major risk factor for diabetes and heart disease)
- A nutritious, well-balanced diet (low in sugar and saturated fat, high fibre)
- Adequate exercise (minimum of 30 minutes per day of vigorous activity)
- No smoking (whether actively or passively inhaled)

- Limited consumption of "social" drugs (i.e. reduce caffeine and alcohol)
- Avoidance of illicit substances (especially pro-psychotic "street" drugs)
- Stress management (e.g. exercise, guided imagery, progressive relaxation)
- Nutritional supplementation (including antioxidants and omega-3 fatty acids)

Benefits of the above measures include strengthening and detoxifying the body, boosting the immune system, enhancing vitality, reducing anxiety, and alleviating depression.

c) Nutritional supplements

The health-promoting and health-protecting properties of a wide variety of nutrients have been scientifically proven. Two specific groups of nutrients may be particularly beneficial for people receiving psychiatric treatment.

Antioxidants

"Free radicals" are toxic compounds produced within the body as a natural by-product of metabolic processes involving oxygen. These compounds can damage cellular membranes and internal structures (including DNA) thus impairing their ability to function optimally. Cell damage induced by free radicals plays a major role in the aging process and many medical conditions.[49] Stress stimulates the production of adrenal hormones (adrenaline, noradrenaline) which generate large numbers of free radicals when metabolised. As well as those produced within the body there are many external sources of free radicals such as toxic chemicals (e.g. pesticides, herbicides), environmental pollutants (e.g. motor vehicle exhaust fumes, heavy metals), radiation (including solar radiation and medical X-rays), food preservatives, alcohol, tobacco smoke, and pharmaceutical drugs.

Some neurological side effects may be related to cellular damage caused by free radicals produced by the metabolic break-down of dopamine and other neurotransmitters. Prolonged administration of psychiatric drugs can result in continuous exposure to large quantities of free radicals that damage synaptic terminals in the brain. Tardive dyskinesia (TD) and other neurological side effects could be among the consequences of such damage.[50]

The human body produces substances called "antioxidants" that protect it against free radical damage. These natural antioxidants can be augmented by others obtained from dietary sources. Antioxidant-rich nutrients act as *neuroprotective* agents which can help to reduce free radical damage.[51] To the extent that they are able to heal existing damage it is possible these nutrients could also act as *neurorestorative* agents.

In addition to protecting the brain, antioxidants act throughout the entire body to counteract harmful effects of free radicals which contribute to numerous medical disorders and conditions.[52] Potential benefits include:

- Protection against the damaging effects of drugs and other toxic chemicals
- Strengthening the body's immune system and natural healing mechanisms
- Reducing heart disease risk by increasing HDL ("good") cholesterol levels
- Improving insulin action in people with non-insulin-dependent diabetes

Key nutrient antioxidants include vitamins E (alpha tocopherol), C (ascorbic acid), and A, B group vitamins, betacarotene, bioflavanoids, and manganese, copper, zinc, and selenium. Rich dietary sources of antioxidants include fresh fruits and vegetables, garlic, legumes, whole grains, nuts (almonds, sunflower seeds), some spices (ginger, turmeric), herbs such as ginkgo (*Gingko biloba*), milk thistle (*Silybum marianum*), St John's Wort (*Hypericum perforatum*), and green tea (*Camellia sinensis*).

Antioxidant intake can be enhanced by increasing consumption of foods, herbs and spices listed above. Further protection can be obtained through nutritional supplements, especially vitamin C (1000mg per day) and vitamin E (800IU per day).

Omega-3 essential fatty acids

These vital nutrients are now known to have a wide range of beneficial effects on physical and mental health. Scientific studies have demonstrated that omega-3 essential fatty acids can help prevent or ameliorate medical conditions to which people treated with atypical neuroleptics may be especially susceptible. These nutrients have cardio-protective effects that can reduce the risk of coronary artery disease, heart attack and stroke. By decreasing insulin resistance they can help to prevent type 2 diabetes. They also inhibit blood-vessel damage, the principal cause of many long-term complications of diabetes.

Seafood is by far the richest dietary source of omega-3 fatty acids. Oily cold-water fish (Atlantic salmon, ocean trout, tuna, sardines, mackerel, herring) contain the largest amounts of the omega-3 fats EPA and DHA which play a key role in maintaining optimal structure and functioning of the human brain. Fish-oil capsules are a convenient, readily available, inexpensive source of these nutrients.

Psychiatrist Dr Andrew Stoll, an internationally recognised authority in this area, recommends 1 to 2 grams (1000-2000 milligrams) of total omega-3 fatty acids (EPA plus DHA) per day to support optimal general health and wellbeing and contribute to enhanced mood and cognitive functioning.[53]

As a general recommendation everyone being treated with psychiatric medications would be well advised to adopt the health-promoting lifestyle measures listed above. Since some people's diets may be deficient in key nutrients it would be prudent to also take nutritional supplements as an additional protective measure, especially omega-3 essential fatty acids and antioxidants (vitamins C and E in particular).

As well as having beneficial effects on physical health, recent research suggests antioxidant and omega-3 supplementation might help improve therapeutic outcomes for people receiving neuroleptic treatment for schizophrenia.[54] Such regimes may also have *preventive* effects as suggested by recent ground-breaking research which found omega-3 supplementation (1.5 grams per day) during the prodromal phase resulted in significantly reduced likelihood of psychosis among adolescents considered at extremely high risk of developing a psychotic disorder.[55]

If they are used wisely, psychiatric medications are undoubtedly helpful to some people who have experienced psychosis. Neuroleptics sometimes alleviate persistent debilitating symptoms, and people who might otherwise feel in constant danger of being overwhelmed could experience a welcome sense of inner calmness and mental stability on neuroleptic and/or mood-stabilising medications. Professor Ciompi's views are in accord with those advocated in this book:

As for medication, and the neuroleptics in particular, the view developed here does not question their potential usefulness, either in acute conditions or as preventive measures against relapses. Their ability to reduce sensitivity to stress and the vehemence of emotions, and thus to act as an effective "brake" in cases of psychotic "runaway", suggests that their main function is as general buffers. Although this function may certainly be advantageous in some situations, it may be superfluous or even harmful in others ... Medication represents a potentially useful tool that is best employed when a patient's total social and personal situation is taken into account. The results from the Soteria Project indicate that drug therapy can become unnecessary even for acute schizophrenics if other conditions for therapy are particularly favourable.[56]

Sadly, heavy-handed use of psychotropic drugs is common. Many problems are a direct result of psychiatry's long-standing failure to distinguish benign psychotic episodes from those of a more insidious nature. Though the value of psychosocial therapies has been clearly demonstrated, drugs are frequently used not as an aid to such measures, but as a substitute for them. The beguiling promise of a "quick fix" for complex psychological and emotional problems all too often overshadows the hallowed medical precept *primum non nocere* – first, do no harm.

It is impossible to know what Anton Boisen would have thought about the current emphasis on psychiatric medications. However, he did warn that the physical treatments applied to schizophrenia in his day "may produce peace of mind, but they are not likely to contribute to the constructive solution of the problem with which the schizophrenic patient is grappling so desperately."[57]

Note: See *Healing Schizophrenia: Using Medication Wisely* by John Watkins (Melbourne: Michelle Anderson, 2006) for detailed information on using medication in the context of a holistic approach to schizophrenia and other psychotic disorders and guidelines for safely reducing and/or stopping neuroleptic treatment.

The Travail of Recovery

A major theme of this book is that full recovery from psychosis is possible. This chapter emphasised *islands of clarity* as these natural mental phenomena constitute the very seeds of recovery. However, the fact that recovery is an ever-present possibility does not mean it is easy or automatic. Seeds require appropriate conditions and constant nurturing if they are to bear fruit. An *environment of sanity* (as described in the preceding chapter) provides ideal conditions for nurturing recovery. Beyond this, a great deal depends on a person's own willingness and determination. The nineteenth century French physician Jean-Martin Charcot maintained that "There is a particular moment between health and sickness when everything depends on the patient."[58] The arduous journey of recovery is comprised of many such moments.

As well coming to terms with the impact of their psychotic experiences, people must often struggle with damaged self-esteem, stigmatisation, loss of hope and a host of other wounds. Meeting these daunting challenges calls for courage and tenacity, as Dr Podvoll emphasises:

> In its own way, the journey to recovery is just as dramatic and hectic as the descent into madness itself. Just as madness forces a confrontation with oneself, so does recovery. Moreover, recovery is not a temporary process, a fire through which to be burnished and then forever healed; it is an ongoing achievement in which one may have to face essential realities about oneself over and over again. But anyone recovering needs to learn how to return to normal life on earth and needs especially to know the obstacles one faces ... We should make no mistake about this point: In the end, no matter how much help is provided, full recovery from psychosis requires valiant personal action and a lifelong commitment to health.[59]

Dr Podvoll's research led him to conclude that true healing entails mastering the *psychology of recovery*. This is so, he feels, because as helpful as the kindness and support of others may be, psychosis originates in subtle mental processes only affected individuals themselves can influence:

> As much as such comfort and respite is a blessing to someone in the pain of psychosis, it is not sufficient to counteract the powerful tendency of psychosis to reproduce and recycle itself. Until the person in psychosis can recognise for himself the roots of the wild and exaggerated mental events that intrigue and come to dominate

him, he will be subject to continuing cycles of seduction, confusion, and despair … Ultimately, recovery depends on how much a person in psychosis is both willing and capable of relating precisely to the details of his mind, on his own, alone with his experience. Only this kind of precise observation can reveal the cause and effect of the mental events from which that person suffers.[60]

A lifetime of research led Professor Ciompi to feel that many effective therapeutic measures correspond to *ancient commonsense wisdom*. Many people come to appreciate the value of simplifying their lives and striving for balance. Emma Pierce epitomises the notion of making a commitment to living well and actively cultivating health and sanity:

My getting well focused on changing my thinking, changing my actions, and as a result my relationship with myself and the world around me changed. My getting well focused on developing as a good ordinary human being; not expecting miracles, taking life as it came; not wasting my time wishing for what could never be or fearing what might be. My getting well focused on being in control of myself, of deciding who I was, where I was going, what I wanted to do with my life. My getting well focused on the care and concern for those around me; on forgetting about placing myself at the centre of my universe. My getting well focused on taking care and control of my body; on eating a decent diet without being neurotic about having or not having this or that food. Exercise needed to be regular and natural. I didn't need the body of Marilyn Monroe, but I didn't want to look like Dracula either. My getting well focused on accepting who I was, right there and then, right here and now, at any given point in my life … My getting well focused on keeping a balance in every sphere of myself and my life.[61]

Conventional psychiatric treatment is often deemed a success if a person has been "stabilised" and their psychosis has gone into "remission". But even when this outcome is welcomed by all concerned many challenges still remain. Yet, when the work of recovery is embraced wholeheartedly, real healing may begin.

Epilogue

Unshrinking Psychosis

There is a crack in everything.
That's how the light gets in.

Leonard Cohen

As this book neared completion I found myself reflecting, not without some discomfort, on how much of my life has been consumed by matters most people would rather not think about. Can I really say why I have grappled so long with these issues in spite of their often maddening complexity? The question evokes a surge of feelings and springs a trapdoor to memory-filled chambers in the private museum of my mind. The hall of memory is lined with distorting mirrors, but some things I can clearly recall.

The Diggings

A claustrophobic emotional atmosphere pervaded my childhood home and an ever-present threat of sudden unanticipated violence hung over my early years like a concrete sky. This stultifying ambience constellated a secret inner world, at once a sanctuary of inviolable innocence and repository of vengeful fantasies. My parents – caring ghostly mother and intelligent, emotionally leaden father – faltered often as they juggled more lives than their battered hands could hold. Their frequent mishaps frayed the delicate tapestry of my soul. Thankfully, their goodness and decency also left impressions that remain with me.

Growing up in the social and spiritual wasteland of Melbourne's western suburbs in the 1950s was a recipe for alienation and despair. I knew something vital was missing from my life and often felt I didn't belong but, as none of my peers seemed to share these concerns, feared my inability to fit in meant that something was seriously wrong with me. I learnt to hide my discomfort and gradually fashioned a persona sufficiently acceptable to get me through school and the empty rituals of youthful social life that substituted for rites of passage in the stunted world in which I found myself an often bewildered participant. The brittle fortress of my severely introverted personality concealed a vulnerable heart. Numerous invisible injuries sustained along the way ensured I reached adolescence deeply wounded: reticent, hypersensitive, emotionally shut-in – yet with a burgeoning inner life well hidden from view. (Unusual behaviour on both sides of my family going back several generations makes me wonder what role hereditary factors, or perhaps some less tangible ancestral legacy, might have played in my emotional evolution.)

Happy Daze On The Hippy Trail

The Age of Aquarius arrived at exactly the right time for me. Becoming a hippy in my early 20s came very naturally as I was temperamentally drawn to a lifestyle centred on soul-searching, rebellion, non-conformism, and pursuit of answers to "cosmic" mysteries and meaning-of-life questions. Clad in tie-dyed rags and sandalwood beads, I wandered this path for many years following my nose. Only much later did I begin to appreciate the extent to which my prolonged hippy phase – with its emphasis on Eastern philosophies, altered states of consciousness, free love, and spirituality – had been impelled by powerful unconscious forces: a noble yearning for truth and authenticity on the one hand, fear of life and dread of being fully present in the world on the other.

Drugs, an essential component of every self-respecting hippy's repertoire, proved a major turning point in my life and were the catalyst of many subsequent developments. As well as magically cleansing the doors of perception ("If the doors of perception were cleansed, everything will appear to man as it is, infinite", said William Blake), they served as potent rocket fuel for a fledgling space cadet intent on fleeing the terrible gravity of the material world and looming responsibilities of adulthood. Psychotropic drugs – especially psychedelics such as LSD and psilocybin – revealed directly, at times very forcefully, the radiance and intricacy of the human mind. However, contrary to romantic hippy lore it soon became clear they had a darker side.

Psychedelic drugs granted me vivid glimpses of heaven *and* hell (a phenomenon I was later to understand when I stumbled across the writings of Aldous Huxley and other pioneer explorers of inner space). By affording me access to awe-inspiring inner realms they demonstrated the reality of mental states other than ordinary waking consciousness. These mind-expanding substances unveiled a world of possibilities – including my own horrifying potential for madness. I shudder now when I think how cavalier dabbling with powerful mind-altering substances by someone as ungrounded and prone to "spacing out" as I then was could so easily have resulted in me plunging into a howling spiritual abyss or getting lost in some endless paranoid nightmare, not temporarily as happened often enough, but permanently. I don't know what saved me but am only grateful it did. Though spared this dire fate in youth I know there are within me still psychotic propensities that (god forbid) might one day prevail given the right circumstances. I do not doubt that my arduous life-long effort to explain madness has been partly motivated by an unconscious compulsion to forge an impregnable intellectual armour that might somehow protect me from this dreaded prospect.

Crazy Remedies

Like so many things that happened in my early years I just seemed to wander into nursing. During my hippy days a number of friends had spun out and then crash-landed in various psychiatric hospitals. When visiting them I was often introduced to other patients they had befriended – generally similar young folk whose faltering attempts to navigate reality had also gone awry. Though I didn't then know what the term meant, I invariably found those diagnosed with schizophrenia the most intriguing – doubtless because I recognised them as sensitive kindred souls. On one of these visits somebody happened to mention that the hospital staff actually got paid to sit around all day talking to these fascinating characters. My application was soon accepted.

I am grateful I trained under the old apprenticeship scheme because it emphasised hands-on learning. Whatever else might be said about them, old-style mental hospitals in the 1970s provided an incomparable education. Within a short time I had been exposed to the full gamut of experiences these "bins" (as the staff tended to call them) had to offer, from bathing and feeding elderly dementia patients to wrestling floridly psychotic men in the often violent locked admission wards. I was a diligent student and soon mastered the basic concepts and adopted the secret jargon. This brought rewards. For a while I enjoyed being acknowledged as someone who "knew his stuff", but within me the nagging feeling grew inexorably that it was all a sham. When doing the one thing I felt really mattered – talking to patients and trying to understand their experiences so I could offer more than a superficial response or temporary solution, I felt completely impotent. If my colleagues felt the same way they never showed it. Once again I wondered if it was just me – perhaps I wasn't cut out for this kind of work? I kept these doubts to myself and continued to act the part but knew I would not be able to go on pretending or ignoring the feeling that we were truly "the blind leading the blind".

Few of my colleagues seemed bothered by the glaringly obvious limitations of our understanding of issues we were routinely called upon to deal with. Most seemed to think problems could be solved without appreciating their real nature. In private many admitted all we were doing was applying "emotional band-aids", but most seemed content to go on doing so. Regarding his early clinical training Carl Jung said, "The main art the students of psychiatry had to learn in those days was how not to listen to their patients."[1] The usual approach was astoundingly superficial: "Patients were labelled, rubber-stamped with a diagnosis, and, for the most part, that settled the matter. The psychology of the mental patient played no role whatsoever."[2] He could have been talking about us. Eventually I could no longer tolerate the status quo, which then primarily involved mind-numbing doses of potent but often ineffective medications and multiple courses of memory-erasing ECT ("shock treatment") – to which regime the more kindly-disposed sometimes added a dollop of superficial reassurance. The gentle caress of a fallen angel's Rescue Remedy was no match for chlorpromazine's hammer blows. Though I often felt lost and alone, my yearning for answers to heart-felt questions would not abate. Little did I then realise what an intriguing journey my restless seeking would take me on.

Beyond The Brain

Once I had mastered the art of evading the autistic gaze of institutionalised charge nurses I took to absconding from the wards and going alone to the (usually deserted) mental health library where

I began what was at first an almost entirely random search. An intriguing pattern soon emerged – the items I found most interesting were not reports on the latest scientific research but musty old books and yellowing journals that generally hadn't been borrowed or even opened for years. I still recall the mixture of excitement and relief I experienced as I began finding bits of information which, even if they didn't fully answer my questions, at least assured me I was on the right track and pointed a way forward. Jung was the first reputable authority I came across who spoke of things I had long suspected but which my learned colleagues never even mentioned. Reflecting on his earliest days as a trainee psychiatrist Jung said:

> Within my first months at the Clinic I realised that the thing I lacked was a *real psychopathology*, a science which showed what was happening in the mind during a psychosis. I could never be satisfied with the idea that all the patients produced, especially the schizophrenics, was nonsense and chaotic gibberish. On the contrary, I soon convinced myself that their productions meant something which could be understood, if only one were able to find out what it was ... Psychiatry has entirely neglected the study of the psychotic mind, in spite of the fact that an investigation of this kind is not only important from a merely scientific and theoretical point of view, but also from the standpoint of practical therapy.[3]

These words spoke to my heart, and as I read them I knew I was no longer alone. Real psychology at last! How astounding to find others travelled this path over a century ago. Emboldened by these discoveries I eagerly sought Jung's writings on psychosis and allied subjects. *The Psychology of Dementia Praecox*, published in 1907 (before the name was changed to schizophrenia) is to my mind one of the most profound books ever written on this topic. I consult it from time to time still and am amazed to continue finding gems of psychological wisdom.

Discovering Jung eventually led me to John Weir Perry, a psychiatrist who applied Jungian psychological concepts at Diabasis, an experimental therapeutic community for acutely psychotic individuals he set up in San Francisco in the late 1970s. Dr Perry was the first contemporary psychiatrist I came across who alluded to the possibility some psychotic episodes may involve visionary aspects, a phenomenon I had encountered and been intrigued by many times on the wards: the young men and women whose "illness" seemed to transform them temporarily into saints or mystics with uncannily radiant auras. His words brought back memories of experiences I and my hippy confreres were familiar with and had, in fact, actively pursued in our naïve spiritual questing:

> What do we make of the fact that, when out of their senses, some people have experiences perhaps of beauty, perhaps of terror, but always with implications of awesome depth, and that when they re-emerge out of their craze and into their so-called normal ego, they may shut the trapdoor after them and close out their vision once more and become prosaic in the extreme, straitened in a bland and shallow usualness? What goes wrong when someone becomes a visionary, looking into the heart of his cosmos and of his fellow beings around him, only when he is "sick", only to become blind, constricted, and timid, understanding nothing, when he is "well" again, dependent for the rest of his days perhaps on a drug to keep this soul and its vision dampened down and safely out of reach?[4]

Dr Perry's questions resonated deeply within me. They still do.

The Road Goes Ever On

With Jung as a starting point I continued my search, confident I was at last on the right path. Unexpectedly, this evolved into a decades-long expedition – with many twists and turns and not a few blind alleys – and has involved delving into areas I could hardly have anticipated when I set out. The vast range of subjects I have investigated includes (in no particular order): spirituality, comparative religion, dreams, symbology, mythology, near death experiences, parapsychology, traditional healing, alchemy, yoga, shamanism, ritual, altered states of consciousness, philosophy, psychopharmacolgy, meditation, UFOlogy, art, music, creativity, folklore, mysticism, anthropology, astrology, ethnopharmacology, perinatal phenomena, reincarnation, transpersonal psychology, somatic psychotherapy and many more (the list goes ever on).

I count myself extremely fortunate to have encountered some of the most brilliant minds ever to have dared venture off psychiatry's well-worn track. As well as furnishing priceless insights into the nature of psychosis and mental health, my life has been greatly enriched –

personally and professionally – as a result of studying the work of luminaries such as Anton Boisen, Ronald Laing, John Perry, Loren Mosher, Stanislav Grof, Edward Podvoll, Manfred Bleuler and others. Their guidance and support has been invaluable. Not only do they provide keys to unlocking the mysteries of psychosis, to my mind the views of Jung and these other visionaries are indispensable to anyone with a serious interest in human psychology.

Along my journey's way I have at times been excited, overwhelmed, awestruck, fearful, enthusiastic, depressed, burnt-out, frustrated, angry, sad, ecstatic, lost, confused, resigned, and alone. And, while I believe I have sometimes been adventurous, courageous and bold, I know I've also been fearful, cowardly, avoidant, in denial, and stuck.

Many years of observation and experience have convinced me of the correctness of Jung's assertion that *self-knowledge* is a prerequisite for understanding the mysteries of the psyche in general, and of psychosis in particular. It became clear to me very early that if we don't understand ourselves – what makes *us* "tick" psychologically – we are hardly in a position to understand others. Furthermore, if we are not able to deal constructively with our *own* problems, how can we possibly assist others to cope with their often more difficult ones? Jung warned that close involvement with persons in extreme mental states such as psychosis may induce "psychic infections" in individuals of unstable emotional disposition.[5] All the more reason to attend to our own woundedness before attempting to deal with anyone else's. There is much wisdom in Dr Larry Dossey's observations:

> There was a time in the West, prior to the extreme objectification of nature that occurred with the advent of modern science, when the cultivation of one's inner life was generally considered to be valuable. Looking inward was not only advised for the common man, it was deemed crucial for the specialist in any area of learning. Ignoring the importance of cultivating one's inner life has resulted in disastrous consequences … Something has been lost as a result, something vital, something that is crucial to the mission of the healer … The overwhelming external focus on illness, the view that it can be treated as a totally objective, outer event, simply has not worked … it is no secret that something is wrong. It is not only the patient who is sick, but the healers … Unless the healer is healed, there can be no healing of anyone else.[6]

An unexplored psyche is a potential disease. Over the years I have experimented with a wide variety of methods and techniques designed to promote self-understanding and facilitate personal growth. While these endeavours were motivated in part by the hope of gaining knowledge, beneath this was a raw fact: I simply could not bear the prospect of going through life a prisoner of my moods, forever bound by the constricting strait-jacket of my fears and insecurities. Facing one's "inner demons" is not something to be undertaken lightly. There were times I was certain I would go totally and permanently insane – a state I feared would be so severe in my case that nothing, not even the strongest medication, would save me. I look back on that period with humble gratitude. Although there were some extremely harrowing times, I will be forever thankful I managed to free myself from many personal bonds. This road, no doubt, goes ever on, as Tolkien suggested.

Psychophobia

Is it really true that most people would rather not think about the matters this book deals with, as stated at the beginning of the chapter? More than three decades after I took my first tentative steps on the road to exploring the inner world it is sad to acknowledge that few people have heard of the pioneers mentioned above, let alone had an opportunity to benefit from their accumulated wisdom. Unfortunately this is also true of many whose lives have been directly affected by psychosis. It is doubly unfortunate most mental health professionals remain blithely ignorant in this regard. Jung's numerous brilliant insights are still glossed over, if not summarily dismissed, in most academic psychology courses. (I've noticed those responsible generally possess an extremely limited understanding of Jungian concepts and have rarely even heard of his psychological heirs.)

No matter how valid or truthful it might be, a body of knowledge which does not fit the dominant paradigm may be treated as though it simply didn't exist. Years after his revolutionary book *The Exploration of the Inner World* was published, Anton Boisen lamented the fact that it had "in large measure fallen by the wayside".[7] Half a century after his first book on schizophrenia was published Jung acknowledged it "had practically no influence at all". Regarding *Symbols of Transformation*, a subsequent, more in-depth work on the same subject, Jung opined:

"One could not say it had any noticeable influence on psychiatry."[8] I can only imagine the loneliness and frustration with which these pioneers had to contend – and admire their resolve in the face of the obstinate resistance of their professional colleagues.*

Many factors are responsible for this state of affairs, prominent among them being the well-known human desire for simple solutions to complex problems. One of the most important influences, a phenomenon I refer to as *psychophobia*, was long ago recognised by Jung: "Wherever there is a reaching down into innermost experience, into the nucleus of personality, most people are overcome by fright, and many run away."[9] Jung believed fear of the unconscious psyche not only impedes self-knowledge but is a major obstacle to psychological understanding generally. Although psychophobia is rarely acknowledged – "Often the fear is so great that one dares not admit it even to oneself", said Jung[10] – it has profound consequences. On an individual level it can result in people choosing to live on the surface of their being, scrupulously avoiding anything which might expose them to the anxiety-provoking mysteries of their inner selves. John Perry alludes to this situation:

> The fact of the matter is that in all of us, only a hairsbreadth below the level of conscious rational functioning, there is quite another state of being with an altogether different view of the world and an altogether different way of growing to meet it. And that state of being, or that world, since it is experienced in terms of images and symbols, metaphors and myths, is considered mad and worthy only of banishment from the sane world of common sense. We find ourselves being very fussy about allowing it to appear only on certain terms.[11]

Psychophobia has critical implications for the clinical arena. If those who work in psychiatry, psychology, and allied mental health professions are ignorant of the deeper workings of their own minds – and fearful of them – they are unlikely to be at ease when encountering

---

* In light of the tremendous resistance his new theories encountered, pioneer quantum physicist Max Planck commented: "A new scientific truth does not triumph by convincing its opponents and making them see the light, but rather because its opponents eventually die, and a new generation grows up that is familiar with it." Planck, M. (1949) *Scientific Autobiography and Other Papers*. Westport, Conn: Greenwood Press.

individuals in mental states such as psychosis where these aspects are often laid bare in graphic fashion. As psychologist Janet Dallett explains, instead of empathising with such persons, clinicians driven by fear of their own unconscious propensities might experience a powerful urge – conveniently rationalised as therapeutically appropriate – to use all available means to suppress them:

> Crazy people strip us of defences and confront us with truths we would prefer to avoid. We hospitalise and drug them beyond recognition because we are afraid of what they activate in us, not because it will help them. Everyone goes a little crazy in the presence of insanity. If we were willing to acknowledge and suffer the madness in ourselves, we could participate in its healing, but it is infinitely easier to make scapegoats of those who have been overwhelmed by it.[12]

Clinicians by no means have a monopoly on psychophobia. Individuals who have experienced psychosis, and others involved such as relatives and friends, are just as prone to these fears. The sealing-over coping style discussed in *Chapter Eleven* is one possible manifestation of psychophobia, as are concealment reactions (described by Anton Boisen) and defensive use of the mechanism of projection. Another is the determined search for some "magic pill" that will abolish all troublesome inner experiences.

Psychiatrist Edward Podvoll believes fear of madness and the loss of control that accompanies it is one of the factors that drives psychiatric materialism and the associated tendency toward therapeutic aggression:

> The realisation that psychosis may be an ever-present possibility in the human condition seems to trigger an instinctive fear and dread in many. John Perceval urgently tried to call attention to this singular fear because he witnessed it in all of his caretakers and he felt that it was having profound consequences on the way insane people were being treated and would always be treated. This fear of "losing control" of one's mind causes a great resistance to any kind of exchange or identification with, or genuine empathy for, a person in psychosis. From that has stemmed the neglect, therapeutic aggression, and the many impersonal theories of treatment that are now so prevalent.[13]

Epilogue

So obsessed has psychiatry become with trying to explain every-thing in biological terms – the familiar litany of genetics, chemical imbalances, cerebral dysfunction, and the beguiling hi-tech phrenology of computerised brain imaging – that the psyche, the soul or spirit, appears to have gone missing in action. Jung provides a sorely needed antidote to this insane hyper-materialism. Unlike most mainstream psychiatrists, he never lost sight of the fact that the psyche is central to our concerns:

> Psychiatry, the art of healing the soul, still stands at the door, seeking in vain to weigh and measure as in other departments of science. We have long known that we have to do with a definite organ, the brain; but only beyond the brain, beyond the anatomical substrate, do we reach what is important for us – the psyche, as indefinable as ever, still eluding all explanation, no matter how ingenious ... Psychiatry has been charged with gross materialism. And quite rightly, for it is on the road to putting the organ, the instrument, above the function ... In modern psychiatry the psyche has come off very badly. While immense progress has been made in cerebral anatomy, we know practically nothing about the psyche, or even less than we did before. Modern psychiatry behaves like someone who thinks he can decipher the meaning and purpose of a building by a mineralogical analysis of its stones.[14]

I have had a personal taste of the consequences of collective psychophobia. How else to explain the fact that I have been totally ignored for two decades by my erstwhile profession (psychiatric nursing) despite having spent a good part of this time researching matters of great relevance to that discipline? How else to account for the fact I am rarely invited to teach (and *never* in conventional academic courses) or to speak at mental health conferences – which, in the main, tend to focus on worthy though psychologically shallow matters? And, in an ironic historical reprise, my own books can now be found languishing on the shelves of the mental health library.*

---

* The last time I addressed a group of hospital nurses I was approached by a recent graduate deeply moved by what I spoke about. "That was awesome!" she said. She went on to explain that she had chosen a career in mental health expecting that the kind of holistic approach I described would be standard procedure. Sadly this had proven not to be the case: "All we do here is dish out pills", she explained forlornly. I struggled through my sense of déjà vu to offer her some encouragement. Though initially asked to present a series of lectures to this audience, I wasn't invited back. Whatever became of that idealistic young woman?

303

There can be no doubt that psychophobia is partly responsible for the ascendancy of biomedical psychiatry and the therapeutic aggression which desperately endeavours to banish rather than understand psychosis. Doubtless it also contributed to the collective fear of psychedelic drugs and subsequent banning of scientific research on these enigmatic substances since the 1960s. What might occur if we – people in general and mental health professionals in particular – were able to free ourselves from our limiting fears?

Simple Human Presence

While working as a nurse I often had to dispense medications. To perform this task safely and effectively I learned the names of the bewildering assortment of drugs in routine use, their indications (which kind of patient got what kind of drug), common side effects, and typical dosages. I was also taught that a psychiatric nurses' principal responsibilities could be encapsulated in the simple formula, "Watch, wait and medicate". I spent a great deal of time watching, waiting and medicating in those days.

When a floridly psychotic individual had finally been compre-hensively subdued with massive doses of tranquilisers, staff would watch for the appearance of some sign, however slight at first, indicating that change – "improvement" – was taking place. I often felt like a child beginning the hopeful wait for a magical butterfly to emerge from its dark cocoon. Nurses and others watched closely, all the while attending to the physical needs of persons temporarily incapacitated and ensuring they continued to receive visitors (even if these poor folk were only met with vacant, senseless eyes). Although it often took many weeks of patient watching, some people eventually emerged from their zombie-like state more grounded, and in a more balanced frame of mind, than they had previously been. While no doubt worthy of mute celebration, this outcome was invariably attributed solely to the therapeutic power of whatever medication the person concerned happened to have been receiving – as if some mysterious alchemical process had miraculously transformed leaden madness into the gold of normality!

I witnessed such events often enough over the years for the medications to earn my grudging respect, but still I wondered what was going on. Was it really just a matter of rectifying an unfortunate chemical imbalance in the brain, as my colleagues seemed happy to believe? ("That psychosis needs more medication" was a phrase I recall being used in regard to patients who weren't improving as expected.) Although the evidence was scant, they insisted this was the *scientific* explanation for these miraculous transformations. But I wasn't convinced. Then one day a story spoke so profoundly it challenged me to unlearn much of what I had been taught and long taken for granted.

This anecdote concerns an incident that occurred in the 1950s when the effects of chlorpromazine, the first neuroleptic (anti-psychotic) drug to be employed in psychiatry, were being assessed. George, a long-term patient diagnosed with "chronic schizophrenia", was given an experimental dose of chlorpromazine (Thorazine) every day as a part of this research:

> No one had paid George any attention for years. Now doctors, attendants and nurses all talked to him and watched eagerly to see what effect the drug would have. His condition improved rapidly. After only two weeks of the drug treatment, he was moved to a ward for less disturbed patients where he took part in a number of activities. Soon he was doing so well that he was promoted again. By this time he had lively relationships with the other patients and many members of the hospital staff. He began to spend several hours a day with paints and clay, using them to express the rich fantasy life that had previously interested no one. His doctors marvelled. Attendants praised his skill. George was released from the hospital thirty-eight days after his first dose of Thorazine. While he was signing out he remembered that he had left something behind, went back to his room, and returned with an old sock. The puzzled attendant who asked to see it found thirty-eight Thorazine pills carefully stashed inside the sock. Why, then, had George suddenly come to life?[15]

Why indeed. Though my colleagues thought me naïve, I suspected the interest and kindly attention of others played an important role in George's unexpected recovery, as it did in many instances I had been personally involved with. I already knew Ronald Laing believed in the healing power of *simple human presence*. In his view, a feeling connection with another human being serves as a bridge to those adrift in isolating mental states such as psychosis:

A component in the distress in people who are in a mental state is the feeling of being cut off from ordinary human relationships – a two way chasm or abyss. That in itself is a nightmarish feeling. As time goes on it's rather like blood being cut off. You feel like a hungry ghost. The main factor is presence – making contact – feeling the presence of another human being in itself. If that doesn't happen, nothing does. If that does happen, there's a ground, a basis. But there is no one way for everybody. Other people withdraw from people with extreme or unusual states of mind. To make contact is the most powerful drug there is. That can transform a person's state of mind.[16]

Is it possible, I wondered, that the most powerful therapeutic tool at our disposal is not the potent medications we often use reflexively (and which sometimes help), but our human presence? Subsequent experience has convinced me of the truth of this deceptively simple-sounding proposition. But as I continued working on the wards it became clear not everyone was motivated or equipped to provide this. Perhaps an inner sense of insecurity (possibly unconscious) impels some people to wear their personality, or their professional persona, or their intellectual knowledge (all of these in some cases) like a suit of armour. The frenetic pace of contemporary psychiatric services often rules out any possibility of therapeutic intimacy – besides, maintaining a discreet distance is easily justified as being professionally "appropriate" and conducive to "clinical objectivity". But there are costs associated with an alienating stance – on *both* sides – for, as Jung stressed, therapists can only be effective with their clients when they are open to being affected by them.

A Story That Is Not Told

Psychiatric diagnoses are a two-edged sword. While they may suggest a starting point and general orientation, they can easily get in the way by filling the mind with pre-conceived ideas and limiting expectations. Experience has taught me that people differ greatly from one another, even if they happen to have the same diagnosis. I have come to feel that the notion of distinct "mental illnesses", as enshrined in concepts such as "schizophrenia" and "bipolar disorder", is outmoded, not scientifically valid, and generally unhelpful. In the end what really matters is the kind of relationship two people are able to form together and what each may learn as a result of walking side-by-side for a time.

Entering a therapeutic relationship is akin to embarking on a journey. Neither I nor the person with who I am involved can know beforehand where it might lead or what kind of experiences might occur along the way. It is truly a journey into the unknown for both parties, at once shadowed with a sense of excitement and foreboding. For this undertaking to become a truly creative venture would-be helpers require an open-minded attitude and freedom from prejudice, as Oliver Sacks understood:

> One must drop all presuppositions and dogmas and rules – for these only lead to stalemate or disaster; one must cease to regard all patients as replicas, and honour each with individual attention, attention to how *he* is doing, to *his* individual reactions and propensities; and, in this way, with the patient as one's equal, one's co-explorer, not one's puppet, one may find therapeutic ways which are better than other ways, tactics which can be modified as occasion requires … an intuitive "feel" is the only safe guide: and in this the patient may well surpass his physician.[17]

Rather than applying any sort of standardised treatment or technique I have found it more useful to adapt my approach to the specific needs and circumstances of the person I am hoping to under-stand and assist. In such endeavours every "case" is new and unique. In some instances it may be helpful to explore a person's early life experiences, especially if emotional wounds linked to these have contributed to their psychological vulnerability and ensuing proneness to psychosis. On the other hand, it is sometimes more appropriate to commence at the opposite end, as it were. I have no hesitation delving into a person's spiritual beliefs or metaphysical speculations, no matter how "way out" or "bizarre" they might seem, for I have learnt that something of great personal significance is very often concealed within them.

If both parties are able to remain sufficiently open, sooner or later a unique story begins to emerge. I agree with Jung's assertion that it is crucial for this story to be heard and understood, for it alone provides the human background and context for all that has subsequently taken place:

In many cases in psychiatry, the patient who comes to us has a story that is not told, and which as a rule no one knows of. To my mind, therapy only really begins after the investigation of that wholly personal story. It is the patient's secret, the rock against which he is shattered. If I know his secret story, I have a key to the treatment.[18]

In the course of my inquiries I never forget that I, like every other helper – lay or professional – also have a "wholly personal story", its unique pattern of hurts and wounds intertwined with an abiding history of goodness and sanity.

What If?

This book encapsulates the findings of a lifetime of intensive research, exploration, and reflection. Interestingly, many of the principles I have come to believe are most relevant to a correct understanding of psychosis, and that have most to contribute to the provision of helpful forms of assistance to those in need, are not actually new: some are decades old, others go back much further. However, much of this precious knowledge has either been lost or is systematically overlooked or dismissed as it is considered passé, irrelevant, or unscientific by the reigning arbiters of psychiatric truth. I have found enough evidence to convince me of its validity, and find myself wondering what might occur if these ideas were adopted and implemented.

Many acute psychotic crises are actually problem-solving experiences

Some contemporary investigators have begun to recognise that psychotic phenomena can encompass constructive as well as destructive potential.[19] What if the prevailing "broken brain" ideology misses the mark and that, in fact, "Many of the more serious psychoses are essentially problem-solving experiences closely related to certain kinds of religious experience", as Anton Boisen long ago suggested?[20] What implications does this have for how best to respond to those in the throes of such crises? What does it suggest about the kinds of treatment likely to be of true and lasting benefit?

The psyche is a self-regulating system with an innate self-healing capacity

What if the healing power of the mind has been seriously underestimated and the psyche is indeed a self-regulating system with innate self-healing tendencies, as Jung maintained? Instead of imposing harsh physical treatment, what if our most important task is simply to support natural healing processes and/or remove any obstacles that get in their way?

An environment of sanity can facilitate natural healing of psychosis

What if many acutely psychotic individuals can recover within a short time if they receive adequate emotional support in the context of an "environment of sanity", as the empirical research of psychiatrists Loren Mosher (Soteria), John Perry (Diabasis), and Luc Ciompi (Soteria-Berne) demonstrated? What implications do their findings have for conventional medication-centred treatment?

Spirituality is one of the keys to understanding and treating psychosis

Spirituality is belatedly being recognised as an integral component of mental health and an important facet of many psychotic episodes.[21] What if spirituality plays a critical role in many psychotic crises, and in ensuing healing processes, as ancient wisdom suggests? What if it is true that "Healing never starts at the place of the symptom ... First you have to be healed in your soul."?[22] Jung considered psychiatry "the place where the collision of nature and spirit became a reality."[23] What if psychiatry's rightful mission is indeed the healing of the soul, as it was originally understood to be?

Psychedelic drugs are powerful tools for exploring the human mind/psyche

What if early perceptions were correct and, rather than being primarily "psychotogenic" (psychosis-inducing), psychedelic drugs are indeed mind-expanding or even entheogenic (revealing the divine within), as contemporary research has demonstrated?[24] What if these drugs are powerful amplifiers of unconscious mental processes which could serve as the psychological equivalent of the microscope for observing and studying the deepest levels of the human mind, as Stanislav Grof suggests? What if Dr Grof's "extended cartography of the psyche" – an integration of traditional spiritual wisdom with the findings of modern consciousness research – is a true and accurate representation of the facts?

What are the consequences of failing to give serious consideration to these challenging propositions? What opportunities could be lost, possibly irretrievably? How many people who might have experienced genuine healing and lasting recovery will fail to do so, not because of the inherently destructive nature of their "psychotic illness", but as a result of our personal and collective failure to follow the courageous lead of true pioneers of the art of healing the soul?

Wisdom Of The Heart

Like so many idealistic souls early in their careers I once entertained grandiose fantasies about the difference my personal contributions would one day make. However, I am under no illusion that this book will bring about any of the changes so badly needed in the way psychosis is viewed and treated. What I now know but could not see then is that truth is not, in itself, enough – there are simply too many with vested interests in preserving the status quo, too much unconscious psychological resistance, too many deeply-ingrained habits of thought and behaviour. And the multi-billion dollar pharmaceutical industry will go on aggressively promoting the biomedical paradigm that underpins the industrialisation of mental health and proliferation of McDonald's-style psychiatry.

But I will end on a hopeful note. Picture this: a storm has abated and the shoreline is littered with millions of brightly coloured starfish tossed up by the crashing waves and now helplessly stranded upon the sand. A small boy and his father walk along the beach hand-in-hand. Deeply troubled by this melancholic sight, the boy carefully threads his way through the scattered starfish, gently picking up one after another and returning it to the water. His world-weary father looks on. "I'm afraid you're wasting your time, son", he says knowingly. "There are just too many of them. What you're doing isn't going to make any difference." Gently placing another starfish in the softly rolling tide the boy turns to his father and says, "It makes a difference to *this* one".

Appendix

Archetypal Imagery in Acute Schizophrenia

*Schizophrenia presents us with a problem that
leads down to the very roots of the psyche.*

HG Baynes[1]

Carl Jung received his preliminary training at Burghölzli Mental Hospital in Zürich under the tutelage of Professor Eugen Bleuler, the renowned Swiss psychiatrist who coined the term schizophrenia. From the very beginning of his psychiatric career Jung was fascinated by the richness and inscrutability of his patients' psychotic experiences and struck by the resemblance of hallucinations and delusions to the normal phenomenon of dreaming. He was especially intrigued by the frequent occurrence of religious and mythical themes and imagery in the symptomatology of patients diagnosed with schizophrenia, but at a loss to explain its origins since individuals having these experiences often had no prior exposure to such arcane matters nor any particular interest in them.

Jung eventually came to feel that, just as the structure of the human body reflects the accretions of its long evolutionary history, so too does that of the mind: "The psyche, like the body, is an extremely historical structure".[2] In his view this immensely old psyche forms the basis of the modern-day human mind and continues to affect it. Jung's research led him to conclude that, in addition to a *personal unconscious* containing forgotten or repressed memories and fantasies related to an individual's biographical history, the mind has a deeper, ancient, impersonal level he called the *collective unconscious*:

> Its contents are not personal but collective; that is, they do not belong to one individual alone but to a whole group of individuals, and generally to a whole nation, or even to the whole of mankind. These contents are not acquired during the individual's lifetime

311

but are products of innate forms and instincts ... In the brain the instincts are preformed, and so are the primordial images which have always been the basis of man's thinking – the whole treasure-house of mythological motifs. It is, of course, not easy to prove the existence of the collective unconscious in a normal person, but occasionally mythological ideas are represented in his dreams. These contents can be seen most clearly in cases of mental derangement, especially in schizophrenia, where mythological images often pour out in astonishing variety. Insane people frequently produce combinations of ideas and symbols that could never be accounted for by experiences in their individual lives, but only by the history of the human mind.[3]

Jung believed the collective unconscious to be the repository of primordial mental patterns he called archetypes: "These motifs are not invented so much as discovered", he said. "They are typical forms that appear spontaneously all over the world, independently of tradition, in myths, fairy-tales, fantasies, dreams, visions, and the delusional systems of the insane."[4] Archetypes belong not to the domain of personal memory but to the secrets of the mental history of humankind:

There are present in every individual, besides his personal memories, the great "primordial" images ... inherited possibilities of human imagination as it was from time immemorial. The fact of this inheritance explains the truly amazing phenomenon that certain motifs from myths and legends repeat themselves the world over in identical forms. It also explains why it is that our mental patients can reproduce exactly the same images and associations that are known to us from the old texts ... I do not by any means assert the inheritance of ideas, but only of the possibility of such ideas, which is something very different ... when fantasies are produced which no longer rest on personal memories, we have to do with manifestations of a deeper layer of the unconscious where the primordial images common to humanity lie sleeping. I have called these images or motifs "archetypes" ... primordial images are the most ancient and the most universal "thought-forms" of humanity. They are as much feelings as thoughts; indeed, they lead their own independent life in the manner of part-souls.[5]

Archetypes manifest in unconscious symbolism in the form of recurring themes and images possessing a mythological or religious character.* Familiar archetypal themes include Death and Rebirth, Cosmic Dualism (Light versus Dark, Good versus Evil), and advent of a Prophet or Religious Saviour. These and other archetypes manifest in a variety of ways and are invariably personified, i.e. have the character of personalities (human or otherwise). Personified archetypal images give rise to the basic forms assumed by various gods and goddesses of religion, the heroes and heroines of mythology, innocent or evil characters in fairytales, and beguiling figures encountered in dreams. The Self, Wise Old Man, Great Mother, Maiden, Divine Child, Hero/Saviour, and Trickster are but a few of the many archetypes of the collective unconscious.[6] Jung especially emphasised the role played by the archetypes he called anima (the feminine image within a man's psyche) and animus (the masculine image in a woman's psyche).

When they enter consciousness archetypal images have a powerful effect. A sure sign of their influence is the occurrence of dreams or fantasies with vivid religious and/or mythological motifs and other "cosmic" characteristics, e.g. temporal and spatial infinity, enormous speed and extension of movement, lunar, telluric, and solar aspects, astrological associations, dramatic changes in bodily proportions. Dreams carrying archetypal imagery are invariably profoundly moving. Sometimes referred to as "big dreams", they are readily distinguished from dreams originating in the personal unconscious:

> Whenever collective material prevails under normal conditions it produces important dreams. Primitives call them "big dreams" and consider them of tribal significance. You find the same thing in the Greek and Roman civilisations, where such dreams were reported to the Areopagus or to the Senate. One meets these dreams frequently in the decisive moments or periods of life: in childhood from the third to the sixth year; at puberty, from fourteen to sixteen; in the period of maturity from twenty to twenty-five; in middle life from thirty-five to forty; and before death. They also occur in particularly important psychological situations ... We may safely

---

* Joseph Campbell, widely regarded as the world's foremost authority on mythology, has said: "All my life, as a student of mythologies, I have been working with these archetypes, and I can tell you, they *do* exist and are the same all over the world." Campbell, J. (1985) *Myths To Live By*. London: Paladin. p.168.

assume that important personal matters and worries account for personal dreams. We are not so sure of our ground when we come to collective dreams, with their often weird and archaic imagery, which cannot be traced back to personal sources. The history of symbols, however, yields the most surprising and enlightening parallels, without which we could never follow up the remarkable meaning of such dreams.[7]

Jung explained that people always know when they have had a "big dream" due to its powerful emotional impact:

[The dreamer] knows it by an instinctive feeling of significance. He feels so overwhelmed by the impression it makes that he would never think of keeping the dream to himself. He *has* to tell it ... the collective dream has a feeling of importance about it that impels communication.[8]

Characteristics shared by dreams and psychosis were described in *Chapter Four*. Most dreams are derived from material such as memories, wishes, and fears that was once conscious. By contrast, dreams originating in the collective unconscious involve material that has never been conscious – hence it is described as "archaic" or "primordial". Dreams of the former kind have an exclusively personal meaning and significance. Insofar as they involve mythological imagery, those of the second kind have a collective character. Jung's investigations led him to believe that a distinguishing characteristic of schizophrenia was the preponderance of collective and archetypal material in this type of psychosis:

Both types of dream are reflected in the symptomatology of schizophrenia. There is a mixture of personal and collective material just as there is in dreams. But in contradistinction to normal dreams, the collective material seems to predominate ... *Schizophrenia in particular yields an immense harvest of collective symbols* ... The fact that schizophrenia disrupts the foundations of the psyche accounts for the abundance of collective symbols, because it is the latter material that constitutes the basic structure of the personality. From this point of view we might conclude that the schizophrenic state of mind, so far as it yields archaic material, has all the characteristics of a "big dream" – in other words, that it is an important event, exhibiting the same "numinous" quality which in primitive cultures is attributed to a magic ritual.[9]

Some of the archetypal themes which may appear during certain varieties of acute psychosis were described in *Chapter Six*. They include embarking on a heroic journey or being involved in a titanic "cosmic" battle between universal forces of Good and Evil. If acute psychosis resembles a dream which occurs while a person is awake (*Chapter Four*), psychoses involving archetypal imagery could be likened to experiencing a "big dream" while awake. And, whereas the contents of the personal unconscious are felt to belong to one's own psyche, images originating in the collective unconscious are experienced as alien, as if they came from outside of oneself. The mind may fall under their influence as if under a magical spell:

> The archetypes have, when they appear, a distinctly numinous character which can only be described as "spiritual", if "magical" is too strong a word ... In its effects it is anything but unambiguous. It can be healing or destructive, but never indifferent ... This aspect deserves the epithet "spiritual" above all else. It not infrequently happens that the archetype appears in the form of a *spirit* in dreams or fantasy-products, or even comports itself like a ghost. There is a mystical aura about its numinosity, and it has a corresponding effect upon the emotions. It mobilises philosophical and religious convictions in the very people who deemed themselves to be miles above any such fits of weakness. Often it drives with unexampled passion and remorseless logic towards its goal and draws the subject under its spell, from which despite the most desperate resistance he is unable, and finally no longer even willing, to break free, because the experience brings with it a depth and fullness of meaning that was unthinkable before ... The essential content of all mythologies and all religions and all "isms" is archetypal.[10]

The way a person responds to the presence of archetypal images can have decisive consequences. Identifying with a favoured image may result in a person feeling he or she has actually *become* it, e.g. rather than experiencing a vision or sensing a divine presence one feels one *is* Christ, Virgin Mary, omniscient Prophet, or some such exalted personage. In contrast to such inflationary effects, projecting unfavoured images onto the surrounding environment may result in development of a paranoid outlook, e.g. person feels threatened by malevolent external forces or agencies. The result, in either case, is an erroneous and distorted perception of reality: "Here we see the characteristic effect of the archetype: it seizes hold of the psyche with a kind of primeval force and compels it to transgress the bounds of humanity. It causes exaggeration, a puffed-up attitude (inflation), loss of free will, delusion."[11] Jung regarded succumbing to the fascination of archetypal imagery to be particularly dangerous:

> The forces that burst out of the collective psyche have a confusing and blinding effect. One result … is a release of involuntary fantasy, which is apparently nothing else than the specific activity of the collective psyche. This activity throws up contents whose existence one had never suspected before. But as the influence of the collective unconscious increases, so the conscious mind loses its power of leadership. Imperceptibly it becomes the led, while the unconscious and impersonal process gradually takes control. Thus, without noticing it, the conscious personality is pushed about like a figure on a chess-board by an invisible player.[12]

Jung believed that providing an explanation of the universal, impersonal meaning of archetypal images can help free people from their spell: "I vividly recall the case of a professor who had a sudden vision and thought he was insane. He came to see me in a state of complete panic. I simply took a 400-year-old book from the shelf and showed him an old woodcut depicting his very vision. 'There's no reason for you to believe that you're insane,' I said to him. 'They knew about your vision 400 years ago.' Whereupon he sat down entirely deflated, but once more normal."[13]

Jung's concepts of the collective unconscious and archetypes furnish precious keys with which to unlock the mysteries of psychosis. Without them quintessential aspects of psychotic experience remain totally incomprehensible. Ignorance of these concepts often results in phenomena of great psychological significance being treated as meaningless, or causes well-meaning therapists to subject such experiences to incorrect interpretation as a result of attempts to fit them to wholly inadequate interpretive frameworks (e.g. cognitive behaviour therapy, Freudian psychoanalysis).

Carl Jung's pioneering approach to psychosis has been adopted and extended by a number of contemporary researcher/clinicians, most notably psychiatrists John Weir Perry and Stanislav Grof. Dr Perry in particular has been at the forefront of efforts to implement an approach to schizophrenia and other psychoses based on Jungian concepts. His books *The Far Side of Madness* and *Trials of the Visionary Mind* provide a detailed account of the practical application of these ideas.[14] Dr Perry played an instrumental role in setting up Diabasis, an experimental therapeutic community for acutely psychotic individuals that operated successfully in San Francisco during the late 1970s.

References

Chapter One. Psychosis Defined

1   Menninger, K. (1967) *The Vital Balance: The Life Process in Mental Health and Illness*. New York: Viking Press. p.9.
2   American Psychiatric Association (1994) *Diagnostic and Statistical Manual of Mental Disorders - Fourth Edition (DSM-IV)*. Washington, DC: American Psychiatric Association.
3   Ibid. p.311.
4   Ibid. p.291.

Chapter Two. Myths of Mental Illness

1   Healy, D. (1990) *The Suspended Revolution: Psychiatry and Psychotherapy Re-Examined*. London: Faber and Faber. p.xiv.
2   Cosgrove, L. et al. (2006) Financial Ties between *DSM-IV* Panel Members and the Pharmaceutical Industry. *Psychotherapy and Psychosomatics*, Vol.75, No.3: 154-160.
3   Moyniham, R. et al. (2002) Selling Sickness: The Pharmaceutical Industry and Disease Mongering. *British Medical Journal*, Vol.324: 886-890.
4   Bentall, R. (1990) The Syndromes and Symptoms of Psychosis. In Bentall, R. (ed) *Reconstructing Schizophrenia*. London: Routledge. p.32.
5   Bentall, R. (2003) *Madness Explained*. London: Allen Lane.
6   Boyle, M. (1993) *Schizophrenia: A Scientific Delusion?* London: Routledge; Read, J. et al. (eds) (2004) *Models Of Madness*. New York: Brunner-Routledge.
7   Kubie, L. (1971) Multiple Fallacies in the Concept of Schizophrenia. *Journal of Nervous and Mental Disease*, Vol.15, No.5: 331-342. p.331 (emphasis added).
8   Ciompi, L. (1980) The Natural History of Schizophrenia in the Long Term. *British Journal of Psychiatry*, Vol.136: 413-420. p.420.
9   Strauss, J. (1969) Hallucinations and Delusions as Points on Continua Function. *Archives of General Psychiatry*, Vol.21: 581-586. p.585 (emphasis added).
10 Bleuler, M. (1979) My Sixty Years With Schizophrenics. In Bellak, L. (ed) *Disorders of the Schizophrenic Syndrome*. New York: Basic Books. p.viii.
11 Bleuler, M. (1978) *The Schizophrenic Disorders: Long-Term Patient and Family Studies*. Newhaven: Yale University Press. p.484 (emphasis added).

12   Van Os, J. et al. (2000) Strauss (1969) Revisited: A Psychosis
      Continuum in the General Population? *Schizophrenia Research*,
      Vol.45: 11-20; Johns, L. and van Os, J. (2001) The Continuity of
      Psychotic Experiences in the General Population. *Clinical Psychology
      Review*, Vol.21: 1125-1141.
13   Watkins, J. (2008) *Hearing Voices: A Common Human Experience*.
      Melbourne: Michelle Anderson.
14   Bentall, R. (2003) *Madness Explained*. London: Allen Lane. p.132.
15   Warner, R. (1985) *Recovery from Schizophrenia*. London: Routledge
      and Kegan Paul.
16   Jablensky, A. et al. (1992) Schizophrenia: Manifestations, Incidence
      and Course in Different Cultures: A WHO Ten-Country Study,
      Psychological Medicine, Suppl.20: 1-97.
17   Nemiah, J. (1989) The Varieties of Human Experience. *British Journal
      of Psychiatry*, Vol.154: 459-466. p.460 (emphasis in original).
18   Jung, C.G. (1982) *The Psychogenesis of Mental Disease*. Princeton:
      Princeton University Press. p.165.
19   Harrison, P. (1999) The Neuropathology of Schizophrenia: A Critical
      Review of the Data and Their Interpretation. *Brain*, Vol.122:
      593-624. p.593.
20   Bentall, R. (ed) (1990) *Reconstructing Schizophrenia*. London:
      Routledge; Boyle, M. (1993) *Schizophrenia: A Scientific Delusion?*
      London: Routledge.
21   Valenstein, E. (1998) *Blaming the Brain: The Truth About Drugs and
      Mental Health*. New York: The Free Press. p.125.
22   Torrey, E. (1988) *Surviving Schizophrenia: A Family Manual (Revised
      Edition)*. New York: Harper and Row.
23   Weinberger, D. et al. (1982) Computer Tomography in
      Schizophreniform Disorder and Other Acute Psychiatric Disorders.
      Archives of General Psychiatry, Vol.39: 778-783.
24   Seidman, L. (1983) Schizophrenia and Brain Dysfunction: An
      Integration of Recent Neurodiagnostic Findings. *Psychological Bulletin*,
      Vol.94: 195-238.
25   Frith, C. and Johnstone, E. (2003) *Schizophrenia: A Very Short
      Introduction*. Oxford: Oxford University Press. p.102.
26   Claridge, G. (1985) *The Origins of Mental Illness*. Oxford: Blackwell.
27   Iversen, S. (1995) Interactions Between Excitatory Amino Acids and
      Dopamine Systems in the Forebrain: Implications for Schizophrenia
      and Parkinson's Disease. *Behavioural Pharmacology*, Vol.6: 478-491.
28   Doidge, N. (2008) *The Brain That Changes Itself*. Melbourne: Scribe.
29   Nelson, J. (1990) *Healing the Split*. Los Angeles, CA: Jeremy Tarcher.
      p.129 (emphasis in original).

30   Ross, C. (1989) *Multiple Personality Disorder: Diagnosis, Clinical Features, and Treatment.* New York: John Wiley and Sons. p. 161 (emphasis in original).
31   Boisen, A. (1971) *The Exploration of the Inner World: A Study of Mental Disorder and Religious Experience.* Philadelphia: University of Philadelphia Press. p.314.
32   Ciompi, L (1984) Is There Really a Schizophrenia? The Long-Term Course of Psychotic Phenomena. *British Journal of Psychiatry*, Vol.145: 636-640. p.636.
33   Bentall, R. (2003) *Madness Explained.* London: Allen Lane. p.141 (emphasis in original).

Chapter Three. The Roots of Psychosis
1   Jung, C.G. (1982) *The Psychogenesis of Mental Disease.* Princeton: Princeton University Press. p.162.
2   Ibid. p.162.
3   Podvoll, E. (2003) *Recovering Sanity: A Compassionate Approach to Understanding and Treating Psychosis.* Boston: Shambhala. p.2.
4   Sharfstein, S. (2005) Big Pharma and American Psychiatry: The Good, the Bad, and the Ugly. *Psychiatric News*, Vol.40, No.16, p.3.
5   Frith, C. and Johnstone, E. (2003) *Schizophrenia: A Very Short Introduction.* Oxford: Oxford University Press. p.96 (emphasis added).
6   Zubin, J. and Steinhauer, S. (1981) How to Break the Logjam in Schizophrenia: A Look Beyond Genetics. *Journal of Nervous and Mental Disease*, Vol.169, No.8: 477-492. p.479.
7   Kaplan, H. and Sadock, B. (eds) (1981) *Modern Synopsis of Comprehensive Textbook of Psychiatry/III (Third Edition).* Baltimore: Williams and Wilkins. p.310.
8   Leete, E. (1993) The Interpersonal Environment: A Consumer's Personal Recollection. In Hatfield, A. and Lefley, H. *Surviving Mental Illness: Stress, Coping and Adaptation.* New York: The Guildford Press. p.119.
9   Claridge, G. (1985) *Origins of Mental Illness.* Oxford: Blackwell.
10   Heston, L. (1966) Psychiatric Disorders in Foster Home Reared Children of Schizophrenic Mothers. *British Journal of Psychiatry*, Vol.112: 819-826.
11   A Recovering Patient (1986) "Can We Talk?" The Schizophrenic Patient in Psychotherapy. *American Journal of Psychiatry*, Vol.143: 68-70. p.68.
12   Arieti, S. (1981) *Understanding and Helping the Schizophrenic: A Guide for Family and Friends.* Harmondsworth: Penguin Books. p.89.
13   Lovejoy, M. (1982) Expectations and the Recovery Process. *Schizophrenia Bulletin*, Vol.8, No.4: 605-609. p.605.

References

14 Goodman, L. et al. (1997) Physical and Sexual Assault History in
Women with Serious Mental Illness. *Schizophrenia Bulletin*, Vol.23:
685-696; Hyun, M. et al. (2000) Relationship of Childhood Physical
and Sexual Abuse to Adult Bipolar Disorder. *Bipolar Disorder*, Vol.2:
121-135.

15 Morrison, A. et al. (2003) Relationships Between Trauma and
Psychosis: A Review and Integration. *British Journal of Clinical
Psychology*, Vol.42: 331-353; Read, J. et al. (2005) Childhood Trauma,
Psychosis and Schizophrenia: A Literature Review with Theoretical
and Clinical Implications. *Acta Psychiatrica Scandinavica*, Vol.112:
330-350.

16 Morrison, A. et al. (2005) Trauma and Psychosis: Theoretical and
Clinical Implications. *Acta Psychiatrica Scandinavica*, Vol.112: 327-
329. p.328.

17 Meares, A. (1977) *The Introvert*. Melbourne: Hill of Content. p.18.

18 Grinker, R. and Holzman, P. (1973) Schizophrenic Pathology in Young
Adults: A Clinical Study. *Archives of General Psychiatry*, Vol.28: 168-175.

19 Arieti, S. (1981) *Understanding and Helping the Schizophrenic*.
Harmondsworth: Penguin Books. p.92.

20 Nelson, J. (1990) *Healing the Split*. Los Angeles, CA: Jeremy Tarcher.
p.41.

21 McGrath, M. (1984) First Person Account: Where Did I Go?
Schizophrenia Bulletin, Vol.10: 638-640. p.638.

22 Luhrmann, T. (2000) *Of Two Minds: The Growing Disorder in
American Psychiatry*. New York: Alfred Knopf. p.120.

23 Podvoll, E. (2003) *Recovering Sanity*. Boston: Shambhala. p.99
(emphasis in original).

24 Bowers, M. (1974) *Retreat From Sanity: The Structure of Emerging
Psychosis*. New York: Human Services Press.

25 Arieti, S. (1981) *Understanding and Helping the Schizophrenic*.
Harmondsworth: Penguin Books. p.95.

26 Jung, C.G. (1982) *The Psychogenesis of Mental Disease*. Princeton:
Princeton University Press. p.218 (emphases added).

27 Jung, C.G. (1987) Foreword to Perry, J. *The Self in Psychotic Process*.
Dallas, Texas: Spring Publications.

28 Podvoll, E. (2003) *Recovering Sanity*. Boston: Shambhala. p.99.

29 Nelson, J. (1990) *Healing the Split*. Los Angeles, CA: Jeremy Tarcher.
pp.42-44 (emphasis in original).

Chapter Four. Dreaming While Awake

1 Cited in Fischman, L. (1983) Dreams, Hallucinogenic Drug States,
and Schizophrenia: A Psychological and Biological Comparison.

Schizophrenia Bulletin, Vol.9, No.1: 73-89. p.73.

2   Freud, S. (1940) An Outline of Psychoanalysis. In Strachey, J. (ed.) *Standard Edition of the Complete Psychological Works of Sigmund Freud (Vol.23)*. London: Hogarth Press. p.172.

3   Freud, S. (1996) *The Interpretation of Dreams*. New York: Gramercy Books. p.66.

4   Jung, C.G. (1974) *The Psychology of Dementia Praecox*. Princeton: Princeton University Press. p.163.

5   Freud, S. (1996) *The Interpretation of Dreams*. New York: Gramercy Books. p.390fn.

6   Rycroft, C. (1991) *The Innocence of Dreams*. London: Hogarth Press. p.3.

7   Chapman, J. (1966) The Early Symptoms of Schizophrenia. *British Journal of Psychiatry*, Vol.112: 225-251. p.240.

8   MacDonald, N. (1960) Living with Schizophrenia. *Canadian Medical Association Journal*, Vol.82. Cited in Kaplan, B. (ed.) (1964) *The Inner World of Mental Illness*. New York: Harper and Row. p.175.

9   Bowers, M. and Freedman, D. (1966) "Psychedelic" Experiences in Acute Psychoses. *Archives of General Psychiatry*, Vol.15: 240-248.

10   Leete, E. (1993) The Interpersonal Environment. In Hatfield, A. and Lefley, H. *Surviving Mental Illness*. New York: The Guildford Press. p.117.

11   Conrad, K. (1958) *Die Beginnende Schizophrenie*. Thieme: Stuttgart. p.53. Cited in Ciompi, L. (1988) *The Psyche and Schizophrenia*. Cambridge, Massachusetts: Harvard University Press. p.210.

12   Bleuler, E. (1950) *Dementia Praecox or The Group of Schizophrenias*. New York: International Universities Press. p.351.

13   Ibid. p.350.

14   Bleuler, M. (1978) *The Schizophrenic Disorders*. Newhaven: Yale University Press. p.482 (emphasis added).

15   Fischman, L. (1983) Dreams, Hallucinogenic Drug States, and Schizophrenia: A Psychological and Biological Comparison. *Schizophrenia Bulletin*, Vol.9, No.1: 73-89.

16   Zubin, J. and Steinhauer, S. (1981) How to Break the Logjam in Schizophrenia: A Look Beyond Genetics. *Journal of Nervous and Mental Disease*, Vol.169, No.8: 477-492.

17   Jung, C.G. (1974) *The Psychology of Dementia Praecox*. Princeton: Princeton University Press. p.163

18   Kaplan, H. and Sadock, B. (1981) *Modern Synopsis of Comprehensive Textbook of Psychiatry/III (Third Edition)*. Baltimore: Williams and Wilkins. p.311.

19   Podvoll, E. (2003) *Recovering Sanity*. Boston: Shambhala. p.158.

20 Farr, E. (1982) A Personal Account of Schizophrenia. In Tsuang, M. *Schizophrenia: The Facts*. Oxford: Oxford University Press. pp.1-5.

21 Corday, R. (1989) The Experience of Psychosis. *Journal of Contemplative Psychotherapy*. Vol.6: 63-78. p.68.

22 Rollin, H. (ed) (1980) *Coping With Schizophrenia*. London: National Schizophrenia Fellowship of Britain. p.149.

23 Jung, C.G. (1994) *Man and His Symbols*. New York: Anchor Press. p.53.

24 Jung, C.G. (1974) *The Psychology of Dementia Praecox*. Princeton: Princeton University Press. p.124.

25 Bleuler, E. (1950) *Dementia Praecox or The Group of Schizophrenias*. New York: International Universities Press. p. 405.

26 Freud, S. (1991) *The Interpretation of Dreams*. Harmondsworth: Penguin. p.163 (emphasis in original).

27 Jung, C.G. (1982) *The Psychogenesis of Mental Disease*. Princeton: Princeton University Press. p.144.

28 Arieti, S. (1981) *Understanding and Helping the Schizophrenic*. Harmondsworth: Penguin Books. p.55.

29 Bleuler, M. (1974) The Long-Term Course of the Schizophrenic Psychoses. *Psychological Medicine*, Vol.4: 244-254.

30 Sohl, R. and Carr, A. (eds) (1970) *The Gospel According to Zen*. New York: New American Library. p.117.

31 McGorry, P. et al. (1991) Posttraumatic Stress Disorder Following Recent-Onset Psychosis. *Journal of Nervous and Mental Disease*, Vol.179, No.5: 253-258.

32 McGlashan, T. and Carpenter, W. (1976) Postpsychotic Depression in Schizophrenia. *Archives of General Psychiatry*, Vol.33: 231-239; Mackinnon, B. (1977) Postpsychotic Depression and the Need for Personal Significance. *American Journal of Psychiatry*, Vol.134, No.4: 427-429.

33 Jung, C.G. (1982) *The Psychogenesis of Mental Disease*. Princeton: Princeton University Press. p.178.

Chapter Five. The Varieties of Psychotic Experience I: Psychological Crises

1 Boisen, A. (1971) *The Exploration of the Inner World*. Philadelphia: University of Philadelphia Press. p.53.

2 Podvoll, E. (1979) Psychosis and the Mystic Path. *The Psychoanalytic Review*, Vol.66, No.4: 575-594. p.576.

3 Ciompi, L (1988) *The Psyche and Schizophrenia*. Cambridge, Massachusetts: Harvard University Press. p.201.

4 Jung, C.G. (1974) *The Psychology of Dementia Praecox*. Princeton: Princeton University Press. p.162.

5   Bleuler, E. (1950) *Dementia Praecox or The Group of Schizophrenias.* New York: International Universities Press. p.460.
6   Jefferson, L. (1964) I Am Crazy Wild This Minute. How Can I Learn To Think Straight? In Kaplan, B. (ed) *The Inner World of Mental Illness.* New York: Harper and Row. p.31.
7   Arieti, S. (1974) *Interpretation of Schizophrenia (Second Edition).* New York: Basic Books. p.698.
8   Arieti, S. (1981) *Understanding and Helping the Schizophrenic.* Harmondsworth: Penguin Books. p.95.
9   Ibid. p.51.
10   Ibid. p.97 (emphasis added).
11   Zigler, E. and Glick, M. (1988) Is Paranoid Schizophrenia Really Camouflaged Depression? *American Psychologist*, Vol.43, No.4: 284-290.
12   Jackson, M. and Williams, P. (1996) *Unimaginable Storms: A Search for Meaning in Psychosis.* London: Karnac Books. p.43.
13   Arieti, S. (1981) *Understanding and Helping the Schizophrenic.* Harmondsworth: Penguin Books. p.51 (emphasis added).
14   Jung, C.G. (1982) *The Psychogenesis of Mental Disease.* Princeton: Princeton University Press. p.224.
15   Sanford, J. (1977) *Healing and Wholeness.* New York: Paulist Press. p.95.
16   Jung, C.G. (1982) *The Psychogenesis of Mental Disease.* Princeton: Princeton University Press. p.239.
17   Ibid. p.207.
18   Jung, C.G. (1974) *The Psychology of Dementia Praecox.* Princeton: Princeton University Press. p.166.
19   Laing, R.D. (1965) *The Divided Self.* Harmondsworth: Penguin. p.99 (emphasis added).
20   Boisen, A. (1971) *The Exploration of the Inner World.* Philadelphia: University of Philadelphia Press. p.158.

Chapter Six. The Varieties of Psychotic Experience II: Psychospiritual Crises

1   Podvoll, E. (2003) *Recovering Sanity.* Boston: Shambhala. p.64.
2   Assagioli, R. (1975) *Psychosynthesis: A Manual of Principles and Techniques.* Wellingborough: Turnstone Press. p.39 (emphasis added).
3   Podvoll, E. (1979) Psychosis and the Mystic Path. *The Psychoanalytic Review*, Vol.66, No.4: 575-594. p.593.
4   Bowers, M. (1974) *Retreat From Sanity.* New York: Human Services Press; Nelson, J. (1990) *Healing the Split.* Los Angeles, CA: Jeremy Tarcher.

5   Perry, J. (1999) *Trials of the Visionary Mind: Spiritual Emergency and the Renewal Process.* New York: State University of New York Press. p.4.

6   Bleuler, E. (1950) *Dementia Praecox or The Group of Schizophrenias.* New York: International Universities Press. p.257.

7   In Silverman, J. (1970) When Schizophrenia Helps. *Psychology Today,* Vol.4: 63-65. p.63.

8   Boisen, A. (1971) *The Exploration of the Inner World.* Philadelphia: University of Philadelphia Press. pp.59-60.

9   Boisen, A. (1947) Onset in Acute Schizophrenia. *Psychiatry,* Vol.10: 159-166. p.161 (emphasis added).

10   Perry, J. (2005) *The Far Side of Madness.* (Second Edition) Putnam, CT: Spring Publications Inc. p.27 (emphasis added).

11   Podvoll, E. (2003) *Recovering Sanity.* Boston: Shambhala. p.174.

12   Dallett, J. (1988) *When The Spirits Come Back.* Toronto: Inner City Books. p.17.

13   Boisen, A. (1971) *The Exploration of the Inner World.* Philadelphia: University of Philadelphia Press. p.54.

14   Bleuler, E. (1950) *Dementia Praecox or The Group of Schizophrenias.* New York: International Universities Press. p.464.

15   Perry, J. (1987) *The Self in Psychotic Process.* Dallas, Texas: Spring Publications; Perry, J. (1999) *Trials of the Visionary Mind.* New York: State University of New York Press; Perry, J. (2005) *The Far Side of Madness.* (Second Edition) Putnam, CT: Spring Publications Inc.

16   Sanford, J. (1977) *Healing and Wholeness.* New York: Paulist Press. p.96.

17   Boisen, A. (1971) *The Exploration of the Inner World.* Philadelphia: University of Philadelphia Press. p.170.

18   Ibid. p.169.

19   Anonymous (1955) An Autobiography of a Schizophrenic Experience. *Journal of Abnormal and Social Psychology,* Vol.51: 677-689. p.679.

20   Boisen, A. (1971) *The Exploration of the Inner World.* Philadelphia: University of Philadelphia Press. p.115.

21   Perry, J. (1956) A Jungian Formulation of Schizophrenia. *American Journal of Psychotherapy,* Vol.10, No.1, 54-65. p.59.

22   Ibid. p.59.

23   Edinger, E. (1955) Archetypal Patterns in Schizophrenia. *American Journal of Psychiatry,* Vol.121: 354-357. p.356.

24   Boisen, A. (1971) *The Exploration of the Inner World.* Philadelphia: University of Philadelphia Press. p.48.

25   Anonymous (1955) An Autobiography of a Schizophrenic Experience. *Journal of Abnormal and Social Psychology,* Vol.51: 677-689. p.679.

26   Ibid. p.684.

27 Boisen, A. (1971) *The Exploration of the Inner World*. Philadelphia: University of Philadelphia Press. p.315.
28 Assagioli, R. (1975) *Psychosynthesis*. Wellingborough: Turnstone Press. pp.43-45.
29 Grof, C. and Grof, S. (1990) *The Stormy Search for the Self. A Guide to Personal Growth through Transformational Crisis*. Los Angeles, CA: Tarcher. p.31 (emphasis in original).
30 Ibid. p.35 (emphasis added).
31 Fenwick, P. and Fenwick, E. (2008) *The Art of Dying: A Journey to Elsewhere*. London: Continuum.
32 Lukoff, D. (1991) Divine Madness: Shamanistic Initiatory Crisis and Psychosis. *Shaman's Drum*, Vol.22: 24-29.
33 Jung, C.G (1972) *Synchronicity: An Acausal Connecting Principle*. London: Routledge and Kegan Paul.
34 Mack, J. (1994) *Abduction: Human Encounters with Aliens*. New York: Charles Scribner's Sons.
35 Thompson, K. (1989) The UFO Encounter as a Crisis of Transformation. In Grof, C. and Grof, S. (eds) *Spiritual Emergency: When Personal Transformation Becomes A Crisis*. Los Angeles: Jeremy Tarcher.
36 Grof, C. and Grof, S. (eds) (1989) *Spiritual Emergency: When Personal Transformation Becomes A Crisis*. Los Angeles: Jeremy Tarcher. p.25.
37 Miller, J. (1990) Mental Illness and Spiritual Crisis: Implications for Psychiatric Rehabilitation. *Psychosocial Rehabilitation Journal*, Vol.14, No.2: 29-47; Watson, K. (1994) Spiritual Emergency: Concepts and Implications for Psychotherapy. *Journal of Humanistic Psychology*, Vol.34, No.2: 22-45; Ankrah, L. (2002) Spiritual Emergency and Counselling: An Exploratory Study. *Counselling and Psychotherapy Research*, Vol.2, No.1: 55-60; Collins, M. (2008) Spiritual Emergency: Transpersonal, Personal, and Political Dimensions. *Psychotherapy and Politics International*, Vol.6, No.1: 3-16.
38 Sullivan, H.S. (1974) *Schizophrenia As A Human Process*. New York: W.W. Norton.
39 Handel, M. (1987) *A Personal Account of Schizophrenia* (Unpublished).

Chapter Seven. The Varieties of Psychotic Experience III: Drug-Induced Experiences

1 Hayes, C. (2000) *Tripping: An Anthology of True Life Psychedelic Adventures*. New York: Penguin Compass. p.4.
2 Spinella, M. (2001) *The Psychopharmacology of Herbal Medicine: Plant Drugs that Alter Mind, Brain, and Behaviour*. Cambridge, Massachusetts: The MIT Press.

References

3   Julien, R. (2001) *A Primer of Drug Action: A Concise, Non-Technical Guide to the Actions, Uses, and Side Effects of Psychoactive Drugs (9th edition)*. New York: Worth Publishers.

4   Glaser, F. (1966) Inhalation Psychosis and Related States. *Archives of General Psychiatry*, Vol.17: 315-322.

5   Thompson, P. et al. (2004) Structural Abnormalities in the Brains of Human Subjects Who Use Methamphetamine. *Journal of Neuroscience*, Vol.24: 6028-6034.

6   de Win, M. et al. (2008) Neurotoxic Effects of Ecstasy on the Thalamus. *British Journal of Psychiatry*, Vol.193: 289-296.

7   Topp, L. et al. (1999) Ecstasy Use in Australia: Patterns of Use and Associated Harm. *Drug and Alcohol Dependence*, Vol.55: 105-115.

8   Morgan, M. (2000) Ecstasy (MDMA): A Review of its Possible Persistent Psychological Effects. *Psychopharmacology*, Vol.152: 230-248.

9   Rounsaville, B. et al. (1991) Psychiatric Diagnoses of Treatment-Seeking Cocaine Abusers. *Archives of General Psychiatry*, Vol.48: 43-51.

10 Little, K. et al. (2003) Loss of Striatal Vesicular Monoamine Transporter Protein (VMAT2) in Human Cocaine Users. *American Journal of Psychiatry*, Vol.160, No.1: 47-65.

11 Schultes, R. and Hofmann, A. (1992) *Plants of the Gods: Their Sacred, Healing and Hallucinogenic Powers*. Rochester, Vermont: Healing Arts Press.

12 Castle, D. and Murray, R. (eds) (2004) *Marijuana and Madness. Psychiatry and Neurobiology*. Cambridge: Cambridge University Press.

13 Linszen, D. et al. (2004) Cannabis Abuse and the Course of Schizophrenia. In Castle, D. and Murray, R. (eds) *Marijuana and Madness*. Cambridge: Cambridge University Press.

14 Phillips, L. et al. (2002) Cannabis Use is Not Associated with the Development of Psychosis in an "Ultra" High-Risk Group. *Australian and New Zealand Journal of Psychiatry*, Vol.36: 800-806.

15 Moore, T. et al. (2007) Cannabis Use and Risk of Psychotic and Affective Mental Health Outcomes. *Lancet*, Vol.370: 319-328.

16 Arseneault, L. et al. (2004) Causal Association Between Cannabis and Psychosis: Examination of the Evidence. *British Journal of Psychiatry*, Vol.184: 110-117. p.115.

17 Ellison, G. et al. (1996) The Neurotoxic Effects of Continuous Cocaine and Amphetamine in Habenula: Implications for the Substrate of Psychosis. *National Institute on Drug Abuse Research Monograph Series*, Vol 163: 117-145.

18 Topp, L. et al. (1999) Ecstasy Use in Australia: Patterns of Use and Associated Harm. *Drug and Alcohol Dependence*, Vol.55: 105-115.

19   American Psychiatric Association (1994) *Diagnostic and Statistical Manual of Mental Disorders - Fourth Edition (DSM-IV)*. Washington, DC: American Psychiatric Association. p.310.

20   Podvoll, E. (2003) *Recovering Sanity*. Boston: Shambhala. pp.174-176 (emphasis added).

21   Baudelaire, C. (1860) *Les Paradis Artificiels*. Paris: Poulet-Malassis.

22   Hofmann, A. (1983) *LSD: My Problem Child: Reflections on Sacred Drugs, Mysticism, and Science*. Los Angeles: Jeremy Tarcher. p.69.

23   Hayes, C. (2000) *Tripping*. New York: Penguin Compass. p.24.

24   Wang, G-J., et al. (2004) Partial Recovery of Brain Metabolism in Methamphetamine Abusers After Protracted Abstinence. *American Journal of Psychiatry*, Vol.161, No.2: 242-248.

Chapter Eight. Psychedelic Experience – Mysticism and Madness

1   Hayes, C. (2000) *Tripping*. New York: Penguin Compass. p.42.

2   Lewin, L. (1998) *Phantastica: A Classic Survey on the Use and Abuse of Mind-Altering Plants*. Vermont: Park Street Press. p.80.

3   Ludlow, F.H. (1857) *The Hasheesh Eater*. New York: Harper and Brothers.

4   James, W. (1929) *The Varieties of Religious Experience*. New York: The Modern Library. p.378.

5   Ibid. p.378.

6   Huxley, A. (1959) *The Doors of Perception*. Harmondsworth: Penguin. pp.16-19.

7   Wasson, R. (1957) Seeking the Magic Mushroom. *Life*, 13th May, 49:100.

8   Hofmann, A. (1983) *LSD: My Problem Child*. Los Angeles: Jeremy Tarcher. p.109.

9   Wasson, R. (1963) The Hallucinogenic Fungi of Mexico. *The Psychedelic Review*, Vol.1 No.1. p.30.

10   Hofmann, A. (1983) *LSD: My Problem Child*. Los Angeles: Jeremy Tarcher. p.17.

11   Ibid.

12   Ibid. p.47.

13   Sandison, R. (1954) Psychological Aspects of the LSD Treatment of the Neuroses. *Journal of Mental Science*, 100:508.

14   Busch, A. and Johnson, W. (1950) Lysergic Acid Diethylamide (LSD-25) as an Aid in Psychotherapy. *Diseases of the Nervous System*, Vol.11:204.

15   Pahnke, W. (1969) LSD and Religious Experience. In DeBold, R. and Leaf, R. (eds) *LSD, Man & Society*. London: Faber and Faber. p.71.

16   Kurland, A. et al. (1969) The Therapeutic Potential of LSD in Medicine. In DeBold, R. and Leaf, R. (eds) *LSD, Man & Society*. London: Faber and Faber.

17   Masters, R. and Houston, J. (1966) *The Varieties of Psychedelic Experience*. New York: Dell Publishing Co., Inc. p.132.

18   Pahnke, W. (1969) LSD and Religious Experience. In DeBold, R. and Leaf, R. (eds) *LSD, Man & Society*. London: Faber and Faber. p. 70-71.

19   Greenfield, R. (2006) *Timothy Leary: A Biography*. Orlando, Florida: Harcourt. p.113.

20   Leary, T. (1970) *The Politics of Ecstasy*. London: Paladin

21   Cohen, S. and Ditman, K. (1963) Prolonged Adverse Reactions to Lysergic Acid Diethylamide. *Archives of General Psychiatry*, Vol.8:475.

22   Louria, D. (1969) The Abuse of LSD. In DeBold, R. and Leaf, R. (eds) *LSD, Man & Society*. London: Faber and Faber. p.38.

23   Masters, R. and Houston, J. (1966) *The Varieties of Psychedelic Experience*. New York: Dell Publishing Co., Inc. p.3.

24   Strassman, R. (1991) Human Hallucinogenic Drug Research in the United States: A Present-Day Case History and Review of the Process. *Journal of Psychoactive Drugs*, 23:29-38.

25   Strassman, R. (1984) Adverse Reactions to Psychedelic Drugs: A Review of the Literature. *Journal of Nervous and Mental Disease*, Vol.172: 577-595.

26   Stevens, J. (1987) *Storming Heaven: LSD and the American Dream*. New York: Grove Press, p.57.

27   Grof, S. (1994) *LSD Psychotherapy*. Alameda, CA: Hunter House. p.309 (emphasis added).

28   Grof, S. (1985) *Beyond the Brain*. New York: State University of New York Press.

29   Hofmann, A. (1983) *LSD: My Problem Child*. Los Angeles: Jeremy Tarcher. pp.66-67 (emphasis added).

30   Nelson, J. (1990) *Healing the Split*. Los Angeles, CA: Jeremy Tarcher. p.148.

31   Grof, S (1979) *Realms of the Human Unconscious: Observations from LSD Research*. London: Souvenir Press.

32   Klüver, H. (1928) *Mescal: The "Divine" Plant and Its Psychological Effects*. London: Kegan Paul, Trench, Trubner and Company. Cited in De Ropp, R. (1957) *Drugs and the Mind*. London: The Scientific Book Club. p.57.

33   Hayes, C. (2000) *Tripping*. New York: Penguin Compass. p.253.

34   Ibid. p.21.

35   Weil, A. (1975) *The Natural Mind*. Harmondsworth: Penguin. p.150.

36   Hayes, C. (2000) *Tripping*. New York: Penguin Compass. p.150.

37   Ibid. p.348

38   Ibid. p.366.

39   Huxley, A. (1959) *The Doors of Perception*. Harmondsworth: Penguin. p.47.

40   Masters, R. and Houston, J. (1966) *The Varieties of Psychedelic Experience*. New York: Dell Publishing Co., Inc. p.51 (emphasis added).

41   Grof, S. (1994) *LSD Psychotherapy*. Alameda, CA: Hunter House. p.156.

42   Ibid. p.309.

43   Ibid. p.157.

44   Ibid. p.45.

45   Ibid. p.156.

46   Halpern, J. and Pope, H. (1999) Do Hallucinogens Cause Residual Neurotoxicity? *Drug and Alcohol Dependence*, Vol.53: 247-256.

47   Strassman, R. (2001) *DMT: The Spirit Molecule*. Vermont: Park Street Press. p.222.

48   Masters, R. and Houston, J. (1966) *The Varieties of Psychedelic Experience*. New York: Dell Publishing Co., Inc. p.320 (note 28).

49   Hayes, C. (2000) *Tripping*. New York: Penguin Compass. p.378.

50   Schultes, R. and Hofmann, A. (eds) (1992) *Plants of the Gods*. Vermont: Healing Arts Press.

51   De Ropp, R. (1957) *Drugs and the Mind*. London: The Scientific Book Club. p.29.

52   Hofmann, A. (1983) *LSD: My Problem Child*. Los Angeles: Jeremy Tarcher. p.108.

53   Wasson, R. (1957) Seeking the Magic Mushroom. *Life*, 13th May, 49:100.

54   Eliade, M. (1989) *Shamanism: Archaic Techniques of Ecstasy*. Harmondsworth: Penguin.

55   Elkin, A. (1977) *Aboriginal Men of High Degree (Second Edition)*. St Lucia: University of Queensland Press.

56   Harner, M. (ed) (1973) *Hallucinogens and Shamanism*. London: Oxford University Press.

57   Letcher, A. (2006) *Shroom: A Cultural History of the Magic Mushroom*. London: Faber and Faber. p.100.

58   Hofmann, A. (1983) *LSD: My Problem Child*. Los Angeles: Jeremy Tarcher. p.xii.

59   Pahnke, W. (1969) LSD and Religious Experience. In DeBold, R. and Leaf, R. (eds) *LSD, Man & Society*. London: Faber and Faber.

60   Griffiths, R. et al. (2006) Psilocybin Can Occasion Mystical-Type Experiences Having Substantial Personal Meaning and Spiritual Significance. *Psychopharmacology*, Vol.187, No.3: 268-283. p.282.

61   Strassman, R. (2001) *DMT: The Spirit Molecule*. Vermont: Park Street Press. p.27.

References

62   Grof, S. (1979) *Realms of the Human Unconscious: Observations from LSD Research*. London: Souvenir Press. p.32.
63   Grof, S. (1985) *Beyond the Brain*. New York: State University of New York Press.
64   Fischman, L. (1983) Dreams, Hallucinogenic Drug States, and Schizophrenia: A Psychological and Biological Comparison. *Schizophrenia Bulletin*, Vol.9, No.1: 73-89.

Chapter Nine. Psychosis – Breakdown or Breakthrough?

1   Lukoff, D. (1985) The Diagnosis of Mystical Experiences with Psychotic Features. *Journal of Transpersonal Psychology*, Vol.17, No.2: 155-181. p.158
2   Vollenweider, F. et al. (1998) Psilocybin Induces Schizophrenia-Like Psychosis in Humans Via a Serotonin-2 Agonist Action. *Neuroreport*, Vol.9: 3897-3902.
3   Boisen, A. (1971) *The Exploration of the Inner World*. Philadelphia: University of Philadelphia Press. p.28.
4   Kaplan, H. and Sadock, B. (eds) (1981) *Modern Synopsis of Comprehensive Textbook of Psychiatry/III* (*Third Edition*). Baltimore: Williams and Wilkins. p.321.
5   American Psychiatric Association (1994) *Diagnostic and Statistical Manual of Mental Disorders - Fourth Edition (DSM-IV)*. Washington, DC: American Psychiatric Association. p.280.
6   Jung, C.G. (1982) *The Psychogenesis of Mental Disease*. Princeton: Princeton University Press. p.177.
7   Boisen, A. (1971) *The Exploration of the Inner World*. Philadelphia: University of Philadelphia Press. p.29.
8   Ibid. p.157.
9   Ibid. p.30.
10   Ibid. p.31.
11   Ibid. p.39.
12   Boisen, A. (1964) *A Little Known Country*. In Kaplan, B. (ed) *The Inner World of Mental Illness*. New York: Harper and Row. p.122.
13   Ibid. p.122.
14   Ibid. p.123.
15   Boisen, A. (1971) *The Exploration of the Inner World*. Philadelphia: University of Philadelphia Press. p.1.
16   Ibid. p.115.
17   Farr, E. (1982) A Personal Account of Schizophrenia. In Tsuang, M. *Schizophrenia: The Facts*. Oxford: Oxford University Press. p.2.
18   Ibid. p.3.
19   Ibid. p.7.

20   Ibid. p.4.
21   Ibid. p.9.
22   Keil.J. (1986) Journey Within. In Garson, S. *Out Of Our Minds.* Buffalo, New York: Prometheus Books. p.98.
23   Ibid. p.97.
24   Ibid. p.98.
25   Ibid. p.99.
26   Ibid. p.98.
27   Ibid. p.99 (emphasis in original).
28   Ibid. p.100.
29   Frese, F. (1993) Cruising the Cosmos, Part Three: Psychosis and Hospitalisation. A Consumer's Personal Recollection. In Hatfield, A. and Lefley, H. *Surviving Mental Illness.* New York: The Guildford Press. p.68.
30   Ibid. p.70.
31   Ibid. p.71.
32   Ibid. p.71.
33   Ibid. p.71.
34   Ibid. p.72.
35   Ibid. p.72.
36   Ibid. p.76.
37   Lukoff, D. (1990) Divine Madness: Shamanistic Initiatory Crisis and Psychosis. *Shaman's Drum*, Winter, 1990-1991: 24-29. p.24.
38   Ibid. p.26.
39   Kulkarni, J. et al. (1991) Biological Investigations. In Kosky, R. et al. (eds) *Mental Health and Illness.* Sydney: Butterworth-Heinemann.
40   American Psychiatric Association (1994) *Diagnostic and Statistical Manual of Mental Disorders - Fourth Edition (DSM-IV).* Washington, DC: American Psychiatric Association. p.310.
41   Boisen, A. (1971) *The Exploration of the Inner World.* Philadelphia: University of Philadelphia Press. p.56.
42   Sass, L. (1992) *Madness and Modernism.* New York: BasicBooks. p.303.
43   Perry, J. (1999) *Trials of the Visionary Mind.* Albany: State University of New York Press. p.25.
44   Ibid. p.14.
45   Boisen, A. (1971) *The Exploration of the Inner World.* Philadelphia: University of Philadelphia Press. p.57.
46   Ibid. p.39 (emphasis added).
47   Ibid. p.159.
48   Ibid. p.159.
49   Boisen, A. (1947) Onset in Acute Schizophrenia. *Psychiatry*, Vol.10: 159-166. p.165.

50   Boisen, A. (1971) *The Exploration of the Inner World*. Philadelphia: University of Philadelphia Press. p.81.

51   Pinches, A. (1998) Sane In A Crazy, Crazy World: At Least It's A Learning Experience! *New Paradigm* (April), 10-15. pp.10, 11, 15.

52   Rakfeldt, J. and Strauss, J. (1989) The Low Turning Point. A Control Mechanism in the Course of Mental Disorder. *Journal of Nervous and Mental Disease*, Vol.177, No.1: 32-37.

53   Chadwick, P. (1997) *Schizophrenia: The Positive Perspective*. London: Routledge. p.50 (emphases in original).

Chapter Ten. Psychosis and Spirituality

1   Podvoll, E. (2003) *Recovering Sanity*. Boston: Shambhala. p.28.

2   Bolen, J. (1996) *Close To The Bone: Life-Threatening Illness and the Search for Meaning*. New York: Scribner. pp.14-16.

3   Clifford, T. (1989) *The Diamond Healing: Tibetan Buddhist Medicine and Psychiatry*. Wellingsborough, England: The Aquarian Press. p.137.

4   Larson, D. and Larson, S. (2003) Spirituality's Potential Relevance to Physical and Emotional Health: A Brief Review of Quantitative Research. *Journal of Psychology and Theology*. Vol.31, No.1: 37-51.

5   Larson, D. et al. (1992) Associations Between Dimensions of Religious Commitment and Mental Health Reported in the American Journal of Psychiatry and Archives of General Psychiatry: 1978-1989. *American Journal of Psychiatry*, Vol.149: 557-559.

6   Sullivan, P. (1993) "It Helps Me to be a Whole Person": The Role of Spirituality Among the Mentally Challenged. *Psychosocial Rehabilitation Journal*. Vol.16, No.3: 125-134.

7   Tepper, L. et al. (2001) The Prevalence of Religious Coping Among Persons with Persistent Mental Illness. *Psychiatric Services*, Vol.52, No.5: 660-665.

8   D'Souza, R. (2002) Do Patients Expect Psychiatrists to be Interested in Spiritual Issues? *Australasian Psychiatry*, Vol.10, No.1: 44-47. p.46.

9   Kirov, G. et al. (1998) Religious Faith After Psychotic Illness. *Psychopathology*. Vol.31: 234-245.

10   Dodds, E. (1951) *The Greeks and the Irrational*. Berkeley: University of California Press. p.61.

11   Boisen, A. (1971) *The Exploration of the Inner World*. Philadelphia: University of Philadelphia Press. p.7.

12   Ibid. p.139.

13   Jaspers, K. (1963) *General Psychopathology*. Chicago: University of Chicago Press. p.108.

14   Lukoff, D. (1985) The Diagnosis of Mystical Experiences with Psychotic Features. *The Journal of Transpersonal Psychology*, Vol.17, No.2: 155-181.

15   Scotton, B. et al. (eds) (1996) *Textbook of Transpersonal Psychiatry and Psychology.* New York: BasicBooks.

16   Podvoll, E. (2003) *Recovering Sanity.* Boston: Shambhala. p.6.

17   Stifler, K. et al. (1993) An Empirical Investigation of the Discriminability of Reported Mystical Experiences Among Religious Contemplatives, Psychotic Inpatients, and Normal Adults. *Journal for the Scientific Study of Religion*, Vol.32, No.4: 366-372. p.371.

18   Vonnegut, M. (1976) *The Eden Express.* New York: Bantam. p.98.

19   Coate, M. (1964) *Beyond All Reason.* London: Constable.

20   Podvoll, E. (2003) *Recovering Sanity.* Boston: Shambhala. p.17.

21   Clay, S. (1987) Stigma and Spirituality. *Journal of Contemplative Psychotherapy*, Vol.4: 87-94.

22   Coate, M. (1964) *Beyond All Reason.* London: Constable.

23   Hegel, G.W.F. (1971) *Philosophy of Mind.* Oxford: Clarendon Press. p.143.

24   Boisen, A. (1971) *The Exploration of the Inner World.* Philadelphia: University of Philadelphia Press. p.29.

25   Ibid. p.122.

26   Sheehan, W. and Kroll, J. (1990) Psychiatric Patients' Belief in General Health Factors and Sin as Causes of Illness. *American Journal of Psychiatry*, Vol.147: 112-113.

27   Jaspers, K. (1963) *General Psychopathology.* Chicago: University of Chicago Press. p.425.

28   Fierz, H. (1991) *Jungian Psychiatry.* Einsiedeln, Switzerland: Daimon Verlag. p.178.

29   Farr, E. (1982) A Personal Account of Schizophrenia. In Tsuang, M. *Schizophrenia: The Facts.* Oxford: Oxford University Press. p.4.

30   Kroll, J. and Bachrach, B. (1982) Medieval Visions and Contemporary Hallucinations. *Psychological Medicine*, Vol.12: 709-721.

31   Singer, J. (1973) *Boundaries of the Soul.* New York: Anchor Books. p.223.

32   Bucke, R. (1961) *Cosmic Consciousness. A Study in the Evolution of the Human Mind.* Secaucus, NJ: Citadel Press.

33   Vonnegut, M. (1976) *The Eden Express.* New York: Bantam. p.99.

34   Assagioli, R. (1975) *Psychosynthesis.* Wellingborough, Northamptonshire: Turnstone Press.

35   Keil, J. (1986) Journey Within. In Garson, S. *Out Of Our Minds.* Buffalo, New York: Prometheus Books. p.99 (emphasis in original).

36   Saint John of the Cross (1959) *Dark Night of the Soul.* New York: Image Books.

37   James, W. (1929) *The Varieties of Religious Experience.* New York: The Modern Library. p.417.

References

38 Boisen, A. (1971) *The Exploration of the Inner World*. Philadelphia: University of Philadelphia Press. p.11.

39 I Thessalonians, 5:21 (RSV).

40 I John 4:1 (RSV).

41 Boisen, A. (1971) *The Exploration of the Inner World*. Philadelphia: University of Philadelphia Press. p.119.

42 Galations 5:22-23 (RSV).

43 Clifford, T. (1989) *The Diamond Healing: Tibetan Buddhist Medicine and Psychiatry*. Wellingsborough, England: The Aquarian Press. p.151.

44 Grof, S. (2006) *When The Impossible Happens*. Boulder, CO: Sounds True, Inc. p.26.

45 Morgan, B. (2007) *I Celebrate Myself: The Somewhat Private Life of Allen Ginsberg*. New York: Penguin. p.324.

46 Stifler, K. et al. (1993) An Empirical Investigation of the Discriminability of Reported Mystical Experiences Among Religious Contemplatives, Psychotic Inpatients, and Normal Adults. *Journal for the Scientific Study of Religion*, Vol.32, No.4: 366-372. p.371.

47 Clay, S. (1994) Reins of Wild Horses. *Psychiatry*, Vol.57: 376-384. p.381.

48 Podvoll, E. (2003) *Recovering Sanity*. Boston: Shambhala. p.86.

49 Boisen, A. (1971) *The Exploration of the Inner World*. Philadelphia: University of Philadelphia Press. p.116.

50 Podvoll, E. (2003) *Recovering Sanity*. Boston: Shambhala. p.309 (emphasis in original).

Chapter Eleven. An Environment of Sanity

1 Podvoll, E. (2003) *Recovering Sanity*. Boston: Shambhala. p.253.

2 Ciompi, L. (1983) How to Improve the Treatment of Schizophrenics: A Multicausal Illness Concept and Its Therapeutic Consequences. In Stierlin, H. et al. (eds) *Psychosocial Intervention in Schizophrenia: An International View*. Berlin: Springer Verlag. p.62.

3 Havens, L. (1989) *A Safe Place*. New York: Ballantine Books. p.168.

4 Ciompi, L. (1988) *The Psyche and Schizophrenia*. Cambridge, MA: Harvard University Press. p.255.

5 Podvoll, E. (2003) *Recovering Sanity*. Boston: Shambhala. p.152.

6 Mosher, L. (1991) Soteria: A Therapeutic Community for Psychotic Persons. *International Journal of Therapeutic Communities*, Vol. 12, No. 1: 53-67.

7 Mosher, L. and Menn, A. (1978) The Surrogate "Family", An Alternative to Hospitalisation. In: Shershow, J. (ed) *Schizophrenia: Science and Practice*. Cambridge, MA: Harvard University Press.

8 Ibid. p. 237.

9   Bola, J. and Mosher, L. (2003) Treatment of Acute Psychosis Without Neuroleptics: Two-Year Outcomes From The Soteria Project. *Journal of Nervous and Mental Disease*, Vol. 191: 219-229. p.226.

10   Mosher, L. (1999) Soteria and Other Alternatives to Acute Psychiatric Hospitalisation: A Personal and Professional Review. *Journal of Nervous and Mental Disease*, Vol.187: 142-149.

11   Ciompi, L. et al. (1992) The Pilot Project 'Soteria Berne': Clinical Experiences and Results. *British Journal of Psychiatry*, Vol. 161, (suppl.18): 145-153. p.147.

12   Ciompi, L. (1994) Affect Logic: An Integrative Model of the Psyche and Its Relations to Schizophrenia. *British Journal of Psychiatry*, Vol.164 (suppl. 23): 51-55. p.54

13   Calton, T. et al. (2008) A Systematic Review of the Soteria Paradigm for the Treatment of People Diagnosed with Schizophrenia. *Schizophrenia Bulletin*, Vol.34, No.1: 181-192.

14   Podvoll, E. (2003) *Recovering Sanity*. Boston: Shambhala. p.128.

15   Perry, J. (2005) *The Far Side of Madness*. (Second Edition) Putnam, CT: Spring Publications Inc. pp.173-174.

16   Jung, C.G. (1987) Foreword to Perry, J. *The Self in Psychotic Process*. Dallas, Texas: Spring Publications. p.v.

17   Mosher, L. et al. (1973) Characteristics of Non-Professionals Serving as Primary Therapists for Acute Schizophrenics. *Hospital and Community Psychiatry*, Vol.24, No.6: 391-396.

18   Mosher, L. and Menn, A. (1978) The Surrogate "Family", An Alternative to Hospitalisation. In: Shershow, J. (ed) *Schizophrenia: Science and Practice*. Cambridge, MA: Harvard University Press. p.231.

19   Ciompi, L. (1988) *The Psyche and Schizophrenia*. Cambridge, MA: Harvard University Press. p.268.

20   Bleuler, M. (1978) *The Schizophrenic Disorders*. Newhaven: Yale University Press.

21   Boisen, A. (1971) *The Exploration of the Inner World*. Philadelphia: University of Philadelphia Press. p.314.

22   Zubin, J. and Spring, B. (1977) Vulnerability: A New View of Schizophrenia. *Journal of Abnormal Psychology*, Vol.86: 103-126.

23   Nuechterlein, K. and Dawson, M. (1984) A Heuristic Vulnerability/Stress Model of Schizophrenic Episodes. *Schizophrenia Bulletin*, Vol.10, No.2: 300-312.

24   Brown, G. and Birley, J. (1968) Crises and Life Changes and the Onset of Schizophrenia. *Journal of Health and Social Behaviour*, Vol.9: 203-214.

25   Kavanagh, D. (1992) Recent Developments in EE and Schizophrenia. *British Journal of Psychiatry*, Vol.160: 601-620.

26   Vaughan, C. and Leff, J. (1976) The Influence of Family Life and
      Social Factors on the Course of Psychiatric Illness. *British Journal of
      Psychiatry*, Vol.129: 125-137.

27   Docherty, J. et al. (1978) Stages of Onset of Schizophrenic Psychosis.
      American Journal of Psychiatry, Vol.135, No.4: 420-426.

28   Ciompi, L. (1988) *The Psyche and Schizophrenia*. Cambridge, MA:
      Harvard University Press. p.256.

29   McGlashan, T. et al. (1975) Integration and Sealing Over: Clinically
      Distinct Recovery Styles From Schizophrenia. *Archives of General
      Psychiatry*, Vol. 32: 1269-1272.

30   McGlashan, T. et al. (1977) Art and Recovery Style From
      Psychosis. *Journal of Nervous and Mental Disease*, Vol.164, No.3:
      182-190.

31   McGlashan, T. et al. (1975) Integration and Sealing Over: Clinically
      Distinct Recovery Styles From Schizophrenia. *Archives of General
      Psychiatry*, Vol. 32: 1269-1272. p.1271.

32   Keil, J. (1986) Journey Within. In Garson, S. *Out Of Our Minds*.
      Buffalo, New York: Prometheus Books. p.100.

33   McGlashan, T. and Carpenter, W. (1981) Does Attitude Toward
      Psychosis Relate to Outcome? *American Journal of Psychiatry*, Vol.138,
      No.6: 797-801.

34   Bleuler, M. (1979) On Schizophrenic Psychoses. *American Journal of
      Psychiatry*, Vol.136, No.11: 1403-1409. p.1404.

35   Bleuler, M. (1978) *The Schizophrenic Disorders*. Newhaven: Yale
      University Press. p.480.

36   Bleuler, M. (1979) My Sixty Years With Schizophrenics. In Bellak, L.
      (ed) *Disorders of the Schizophrenic Syndrome*. New York: Basic Books.
      p.vii.

37   Bleuler, M. (1978) The Long-Term Course of Schizophrenic
      Psychoses. In Wynne, L. et al. (eds) *The Nature of Schizophrenia: New
      Approaches to Research and Treatment*. New York: John Wiley and
      Sons. p.633.

38   Podvoll, E. (2003) *Recovering Sanity*. Boston: Shambhala.

39   Ibid. pp.209-211.

40   Cited in Whitaker, R. (2002) *Mad In America: Bad Science,
      Bad Medicine and the Enduring Mistreatment of the Mentally Ill*.
      Cambridge, MA: Perseus Books. p.221.

41   Perry, J. (2005) *The Far Side of Madness*. (Second Edition) Putnam,
      CT: Spring Publications Inc. p.2.

42   Ibid. p.16.

43   Boisen, A. (1971) *The Exploration of the Inner World*. Philadelphia:
      University of Philadelphia Press. p.30.

44   Mosher, L. and Menn, A. (1978) The Surrogate "Family", An Alternative to Hospitalisation. In: Shershow, J. (ed) *Schizophrenia: Science and Practice*. Cambridge, MA: Harvard University Press. p. 237.

45   Grof, C. and Grof, S. (1990) *The Stormy Search for the Self*. Los Angeles, CA: Tarcher. p.43 (emphasis in original).

46   Jung, C.G. (1982) *The Psychogenesis of Mental Disease*. Princeton: Princeton University Press. p.260.

47   Handel, M. (1987) *A Personal Account of Schizophrenia* (Unpublished).

48   Ciompi, L. (1989) The Dynamics of Complex Biological-Psychosocial Systems. *British Journal of Psychiatry*, Vol.155 (suppl.5): 15-21.

49   Boisen, A. (1971) *The Exploration of the Inner World*. Philadelphia: University of Philadelphia Press. p.54 (emphasis added).

50   McGlashan, T. and Carpenter, W. (1981) Does Attitude Toward Psychosis Relate to Outcome? *American Journal of Psychiatry*, Vol.138, No.6: 797-801. p.800 (emphasis in original).

51   Jung, C.G. (1967) *Memories, Dreams, Reflections*. London: Fontana. p.214.

52   Pierce, E. (1987) *Ordinary Insanity*. Dulwich Hill, NSW: P.E.Pierce. pp.91-93.

53   Hayward, M. and Taylor, E. (1956) A Schizophrenic Patient Describes the Action of Intensive Psychotherapy. *Psychiatric Quarterly*, Vol.30: 211-248. p.221.

54   A Recovering Patient (1986) "Can We Talk?" The Schizophrenic Patient in Psychotherapy. *American Journal of Psychiatry*, Vol.143: 68-70. p.70.

55   Rogers, C. (1980) *A Way of Being*. Boston: Houghton Mifflin. p.152.

Chapter Twelve. Healing and Recovery
1   Podvoll, E. (2003) *Recovering Sanity*. Boston: Shambhala. p.40.
2   Boisen, A. (1947) Onset in Acute Schizophrenia. *Psychiatry*, Vol.10: 159-166.
3   Scott, R. (1973) The Treatment Barrier: Part Two. The Patient as an Unrecognised Agent. *British Journal of Medical Psychology*, Vol.46: 57-67; Strauss, J. et al. (1987) The Role of the Patient in Recovery from Psychosis. In Strauss, J. et al. (eds) *Psychosocial Treatment of Schizophrenia*. Toronto: Hans Huber.
4   Brier, A. and Strauss, J. (1983) Self-Control in Psychotic Disorders. *Archives of General Psychiatry*, Vol.40: 1141-1145; Carr, V. (1988) Patients' Techniques for Coping with Schizophrenia: An Exploratory Study. *British Journal of Medical Psychology*, Vol.61: 339-352.

References

5   Tooth, B. et al. (2003) Factors Consumers Identify As Important
      To Recovery From Schizophrenia. *Australasian Psychiatry*, Vol. 11
      (supplement): 70-77.

6   Leete, E. (1993) The Interpersonal Environment. In Hatfield, A. and
      Lefley, H. *Surviving Mental Illness.* New York: The Guildford Press.
      p.125.

7   Weingarten, R. (1994) The Ongoing Processes of Recovery. *Psychiatry*,
      Vol. 57: 369-375. pp. 369, 372.

8   Podvoll, E. (2003) *Recovering Sanity.* Boston: Shambhala. p.243.

9   Carr, V. (1983) Recovery From Schizophrenia: A Review of Patterns
      of Psychosis. *Schizophrenia Bulletin*, Vol.9, No.1: 95-121.

10   Podvoll, E. (2003) *Recovering Sanity.* Boston: Shambhala. p.209.

11   Jaspers, K. (1963) *General Psychopathology.* Chicago: University of
      Chicago Press. p.422.

12   McGlashan, T. and Keats, C. (1989) *Schizophrenia: Treatment Process
      and Outcome.* Washington, DC: American Psychiatric Press. p.67.

13   Podvoll, E. (2003) *Recovering Sanity.* Boston: Shambhala. p.209.

14   Bowers, M. (1974) *Retreat From Sanity.* New York: Human Services
      Press. p.187.

15   Podvoll, E. (2003) *Recovering Sanity.* Boston: Shambhala. p.152.

16   Ibid. pp.240-243 (emphasis in original).

17   Sharfstein, S. (2005) Big Pharma and American Psychiatry: The
      Good, the Bad, and the Ugly. *Psychiatric News*, Vol.40, No.16, p.3.

18   Jones, P. et al. (2006) Randomised Controlled Trial of the Effect on
      Quality of Life of Second- vs First-Generation Antipsychotic Drugs
      in Schizophrenia: Cost Utility of the Latest Antipsychotic Drugs in
      Schizophrenia Study (CUtLASS 1). *Archives of General Psychiatry*,
      Vol.63: 1079-1087.

19   Lewis, S. and Lieberman, J. (2008) CATIE and CUtLASS: Can We
      Handle the Truth? *British Journal of Psychiatry*, Vol.192: 161-163;
      Leucht, S. et al. (2009) Second-Generation Versus First-Generation
      Antipsychotic Drugs for Schizophrenia: A Meta-Analysis. *The Lancet*,
      Vol.373: 31-41.

20   Tyrer, P. and Kendall, T. (2009) The Spurious Advance of
      Antipsychotic Drug Therapy. *The Lancet*, Vol.373: 4-5. p.4.

21   Bleuler, M. (1986) Introduction and Overview. In: Burrows, G. et al.
      (eds) *Handbook of Studies on Schizophrenia.* Amsterdam: Elsevier. p. 8
      (emphasis added).

22   Healy, D. (1993) *Psychiatric Drugs Explained.* London: Mosby. p.15.

23   Podvoll, E. (2003) *Recovering Sanity.* Boston: Shambhala. p.228.

24   Rappaport, M. et al. (1978) Are There Schizophrenics for Whom
      Drugs May be Unnecessary or Contraindicated? *International*

Pharmacopsychiatry, Vol.13: 100-111; Buckley, P. (1982) Identifying Schizophrenic Patients Who Should Not Receive Medication. *Schizophrenia Bulletin*, Vol.8, No.3: 429-432; Fenton, W. and McGlashan, T. (1987) Sustained Remission in Drug-Free Schizophrenic Patients. *American Journal of Psychiatry*, Vol.144, No.10: 1306-1309.

25   Van Putten, T. et al. (1984) Response to Antipsychotic Medication: The Doctor's and the Consumer's View. *American Journal of Psychiatry*, Vol. 141, No. 1: 16-19.

26   Van Putten, T. and May, P. (1978) Subjective Response as a Predictor of Outcome in Pharmacotherapy: The Consumer Has a Point. *Archives of General Psychiatry*, Vol. 35: 477-480.

27   Awad, A. and Hogan, T. (1994) Subjective Response to Neuroleptics and the Quality of Life: Implications for Treatment Outcome. *Acta Psychiatrica Scandinavica*, Vol. 89 (suppl. 380): 27-32.

28   Bentall, R. (2003) *Madness Explained*. London: Allen Lane. p.499 (emphasis in original).

29   Haddock, G. and Slade, P. (1996) *Cognitive-Behavioural Interventions with Psychotic Disorders*. London: Routledge.

30   Hoffman, R. et al. (2000) Transcranial Magnetic Stimulation and Auditory Hallucinations in Schizophrenia. *Lancet*, 355: 1073-1075; Hoffman, R. et al. (2003) Transcranial Magnetic Stimulation of Left Temporoparietal Cortex and Medication-Resistant Auditory Hallucinations. *Archives of General Psychiatry*, Vol.60: 49-56.

31   Carr, V. (1988) Patients' Techniques for Coping with Schizophrenia: An Exploratory Study. *British Journal of Medical Psychology*, Vol.61: 339-352.

32   Watkins, J. (2008) *Hearing Voices: A Common Human Experience*. Melbourne: Michelle Anderson.

33   Watkins, J. (1996) *Living With Schizophrenia. An Holistic Approach to Understanding, Preventing and Recovering from Negative Symptoms*. Melbourne: Hill of Content.

34   McEvoy, J. et al. (1991) Optimal Dose of Neuroleptic in Acute Schizophrenia: A Controlled Study of the Neuroleptic Threshold and Higher Haloperidol Dose. *Archives of General Psychiatry*, Vol. 38: 776-784.

35   Schooler, N. (1991) Maintenance Medication for Schizophrenia: Strategies for Dose Reduction. *Schizophrenia Bulletin*, Vol. 17, No. 2: 311-324.

36   Torrey, E. (1988) *Surviving Schizophrenia: A Family Manual (Revised Edition)*. New York: Harper and Row, p.192.

References

37   Baldessarini, R. and Viguera, A. (1995) Neuroleptic Withdrawal in Schizophrenic Patients. *Archives of General Psychiatry*, Vol. 52: 189-191; Viguera, A. et al. (1997) Clinical Risk Following Abrupt and Gradual Withdrawal of Maintenance Neuroleptic Treatment. *Archives of General Psychiatry*, Vol.54: 49-55.

38   Podvoll, E. (2003) *Recovering Sanity*. Boston: Shambhala.

39   Grof, C. and Grof, S. (1990) *The Stormy Search for the Self*. Los Angeles, CA: Tarcher. p.44.

40   Carpenter, W. and Heinrichs, D. (1983) Early Intervention, Time-Limited, Targeted Pharmacotherapy of Schizophrenia. *Schizophrenia Bulletin*, Vol. 9, No. 4: 533-542.

41   Harding, C. and Zahniser, J. (1994) Empirical Correction of Seven Myths about Schizophrenia with Implications for Treatment. *Acta Psychiatrica Scandinavica*, Vol.90 (suppl 384): 140-146; Harrow, M. and Jobe, T. (2007) Factors Involved in Outcome and Recovery in Schizophrenia Patients Not on Antipsychotic Medications: A 15-Year Multifollow-Up Study. *Journal of Nervous and Mental Disease*, Vol.195: 406-414.

42   Gardos, G. and Cole, J. (1978) Maintenance Antipsychotic Therapy: Is the Cure Worse than the Disease? *American Journal of Psychiatry*, Vol. 133, No. 1: 32-36. pp. 34, 35, 36 (emphasis in original).

43   Carpenter, W. (1999) Diazepam Treatment for Early Signs of Exacerbation in Schizophrenia. *American Journal of Psychiatry*, Vol. 156: 299-303.

44   Lingjaerde, O. (1985) Antipsychotic Effect of Benzodiazepines. In: Burrows, G. et al. (eds) *Antipsychotics*. Amsterdam: Elsevier.

45   Nestoros, J. (1980) Benzodiazepines in Schizophrenia: Need for a Reassessment. *International Pharmacopsychiatry*, Vol. 15: 171-179.

46   Csernansky, J. et al. (1988) Double-Blind Comparison of Alprazolam, Diazepam, and Placebo for the Treatment of Negative Schizophrenic Symptoms. *Archives of General Psychiatry*, Vol. 45: 655-659.

47   Menza, M. and Harris, D. (1989) Benzodiazepines and Catatonia: An Overview. *Biological Psychiatry*, Vol. 26: 842-846.

48   Warner, R. (1985) *Recovery from Schizophrenia*. London: Routledge and Kegan Paul. p. 264.

49   Packer, L. and Colman, C. (1999) *The Antioxidant Miracle*. New York: John Wiley and Sons.

50   Shiriqui, C. and Jones, B. (1990) Free Radicals and Tardive Dyskinesia. *Canadian Journal of Psychiatry*, Vol. 35; Tsai, G. et al. (1998) Markers of Glutamatergic Neurotransmission and Oxidative Stress Associated with Tardive Dyskinesia. *American Journal of Psychiatry*, Vol. 155, No. 9: 1207-1213.

51   Mahadik, S. et al. (2006) Prevention of Oxidative Stress-Mediated Neuropathology and Improved Clinical Outcome by Adjunctive Use of a Combination of Antioxidants and Omega-3 Fatty Acids in Schizophrenia. *International Review of Psychiatry*, Vol.18, No.2: 119-131.

52   Brighthope, I. (1994) The Therapeutic Potential of Antioxidants in the Prevention and Treatment of Degenerative Diseases. *Journal of the Australasian College of Nutritional and Environmental Medicine*, Vol. 13, No. 1: 15-25.

53   Stoll, A. (2002) *The Omega-3 Connection*. London: Simon and Schuster. p.209.

54   Arvindakshan, M. et al. (2003) Supplementation with a Combination of Omega-3 Fatty Acids and Antioxidants (Vitamins E and C) Improves the Outcome of Schizophrenia. *Schizophrenia Research*, Vol.62: 195-204.

55   Amminger, G. et al. (2007) Randomised Controlled Trial of Omega-3 Fatty Acids in Adolescents at Ultra-High-Risk for Psychosis [Abstract]. *Australian and New Zealand Journal of Psychiatry*, Vol.41 (suppl 2). p.A257. Presented at World Psychiatric Association International Congress, Melbourne, Australia, 28th November-2nd December, 2007.

56   Ciompi, L. (1988) *The Psyche and Schizophrenia*. Cambridge, MA: Harvard University Press. p.292.

57   Boisen, A. (1947) Onset in Acute Schizophrenia. *Psychiatry*, Vol.10: 159-166. p.166.

58   Jaspers, K. (1963) *General Psychopathology*. Chicago: University of Chicago Press. p.425.

59   Podvoll, E. (2003) *Recovering Sanity*. Boston: Shambhala. p.207.

60   Ibid. p.128.

61   Pierce, E. (1988) *Passion for the Possible*. Gladesville, NSW: P.E.Pierce. p.109.

Epilogue. Unshrinking Psychosis

1   Jung, C.G. (1987) Foreword to Perry, J. *The Self In Psychotic Process*. Dallas, Texas: Spring Publications. p.iv.

2   Jung, C.G. (1973) *Memories, Dreams, Reflections*. London: Random House. p.135.

3   Jung, C.G. (1987) Foreword to Perry, J. *The Self In Psychotic Process*. Dallas, Texas: Spring Publications. pp.iii-v (emphasis in original).

4   Perry, J. (2005) *The Far Side of Madness*. (Second Edition) Putnam, CT: Spring Publications Inc. p.8.

5   Jung, C.G. (1982) *The Psychogenesis of Mental Disease*. Princeton: Princeton University Press. p.265.

References

6 Dossey, L. (1988) The Inner Life Of the Healer: The Importance of Shamanism for Modern Medicine. In Doore, G. (ed) *Shaman's Path: Healing, Personal Growth, and Empowerment.* Boston: Shambhala. p.90.

7 Boisen, A. (1971) *The Exploration of the Inner World.* Philadelphia: University of Philadelphia Press. p.x.

8 Jung, C.G. (1987) Foreword to Perry, J. *The Self In Psychotic Process.* Dallas, Texas: Spring Publications. p.iv.

9 Jung, C.G. (1973) *Memories, Dreams, Reflections.* London: Random House. p.164.

10 Jung, C.G. (1975) *The Undiscovered Self.* London: Routledge and Kegan Paul. p.48.

11 Perry, J. (2005) *The Far Side of Madness.* (Second Edition) Putnam, CT: Spring Publications Inc. p.9.

12 Dallett, J. (1988) *When The Spirits Come Back.* Toronto: Inner City Books. p.14.

13 Podvoll, E. (2003) *Recovering Sanity.* Boston: Shambhala. p.132.

14 Jung, C.G. (1982) *The Psychogenesis of Mental Disease.* Princeton: Princeton University Press. pp.158-160.

15 Dallett, J. (1988) *When The Spirits Come Back.* Toronto: Inner City Books. p.15.

16 Fields, R. (1986) R.D. Laing and The Psychology of Simple Presence. *The Vajradhatu Sun,* Vol.8, No.5. p.3.

17 Sacks, O. (1991) *Awakenings.* London: Pan Books. p.259 (emphases in original).

18 Jung, C.G. (1973) *Memories, Dreams, Reflections.* London: Random House. p.138.

19 Jackson, M. and Fulford, K. (2002) Psychosis Good and Bad: Values-Based Practice and the Distinction Between Pathological and Non-pathological Forms of Psychotic Experience. *Philosophy, Psychiatry and Psychology,* Vol.9, No.4: 387-394.

20 Boisen, A. (1971) *The Exploration of the Inner World.* Philadelphia: University of Philadelphia Press. p.53.

21 Clarke, I. (ed) (2001) *Psychosis and Spirituality: Exploring The New Frontier.* London: Whurr Publishers.

22 Kreinheder, A. (1980) The Healing Power of Illness. *Psychological Perspectives.* Vol.11, No.1: 9-18. p.13.

23 Jung, C.G. (1973) *Memories, Dreams, Reflections.* London: Random House. p.130.

24 Griffiths, R. et al. (2006) Psilocybin Can Occasion Mystical-Type Experiences Having Substantial Personal Meaning and Spiritual Significance. *Psychopharmacology,* Vol.187, No.3: 268-283.

Appendix. Archetypal Imagery in Acute Schizophrenia

1   Baynes, H. (1969) *Mythology of the Soul*. London: Rider and
     Company. p.xvii.
2   Jung, C.G. (1987) Foreword to Perry, J. *The Self In Psychotic Process*.
     Dallas, Texas: Spring Publications. p.vi.
3   Jung, C.G. (1977) *Psychology and the Occult*. Princeton: Princeton
     University Press. p.117.
4   Jung, C.G. (1982) *The Psychogenesis of Mental Disease*. Princeton:
     Princeton University Press. p.261.
5   Jung, C.G. (1966) *Two Essays on Analytical Psychology*. Princeton:
     Princeton University Press. p.65.
6   Jung, C.G. (1968) *The Archetypes and the Collective Unconscious*.
     Princeton: Princeton University Press.
7   Jung, C.G. (1982) *The Psychogenesis of Mental Disease*. Princeton:
     Princeton University Press. p.242.
8   Jung, C.G. (1966) *Two Essays on Analytical Psychology*. Princeton:
     Princeton University Press. p.178.
9   Jung, C.G. (1982) *The Psychogenesis of Mental Disease*. Princeton:
     Princeton University Press. p.242 (emphasis added).
10   Jung, C.G. (1969) *On the Nature of the Psyche*. Princeton: Princeton
     University Press. p.115 (emphasis in original).
11   Jung, C.G. (1966) *Two Essays on Analytical Psychology*. Princeton:
     Princeton University Press. p.70.
12   Ibid. p.160.
13   Jung, C.G. (ed) (1988) *Man And His Symbols*. New York: Anchor
     Press. p.69.
14   Perry, J. (2005) *The Far Side of Madness*. (Second Edition) Putnam,
     CT: Spring Publications Inc.; Perry, J. (1999) *Trials of the Visionary
     Mind*. New York: State University of New York Press.

Index

doubts (islands of clarity) 270
dreams, and psychosis 48ff;
psychosis as waking 56; lucid
51fn; and schizophrenia 54-56;
themes and images in waking
61-64; "big" dreams 313-315
drifting reaction (Boisen) 167-169
drug-induced psychosis 5, 107ff,
135ff; *see also* substance-induced
psychotic disorder
drugs, illicit: and psychosis 5, 80,
107ff; set and setting 120, 122;
tolerance to 111, 113, 119, 121,
147; neurological effects of
125-127; psychological and
social effects of 127-130;
spiritual and existential effects of
131-133; pro-psychotic effects
of 126, 134; *see also* psychedelic
drugs
drugs, social 109
drugs, therapeutic 109
DSM-IV, psychotic disorders listed
in 5-12; value of 12; influence of
pharmaceutical industry on 13;
artificial nature of disorders in 16
dyskinesia 285
dystonia 286

"early" psychosis 224, 282
echolalia 11
echopraxia 11
Ecstasy (MDMA): as empathogen
112, 147fn; neurological toxicity
of 113fn; lack of hallucinogenic
effect 147fn
ego: weakness of as vulnerability
factor 71; dissolution of 87,
98; death of 140, 150; loss of
boundaries of 252
elation 6
emergence of "past life" memories
100

emergence/emergency, spiritual –
see spiritual emergency
emotional shut-down 38, 71, 285
entheogens – *see* psychedelic drugs
environment: of sanity 223ff;
healing 246-260
episodes of unitive consciousness 98
erotomania 7
euphoria 7
experiences of close encounters with
UFOs 103
The Exploration of the Inner World
(Boisen) 173
expressed emotion (EE) 238
extended cartography of psyche
(Grof) 164, 309
extrapyramidal symptoms 286
extrasensory perception (ESP) 101

façade of normality 40, 72, 128
false self 40, 41, 80, 128
The Far Side of Madness (Perry) 317
flashbacks 156
flight of ideas 8, 191, 192
formal thought disorder 9
free radicals 287, 288
functional mental disorders 4

genes: and predisposition to
psychosis 30, 31; disharmonious
combinations of as factor
in schizophrenia 31fn;
hypersensitivity and 32
ghosts 219
Good Friday Experiment 162
Grof, Stanislav 80, 97, 98, 102,
104, 148, 152, 155, 156, 164,
219, 252, 282, 299, 309

hallucinations: definition 2, 9;
auditory 2, 10; visual 2; tactile
7; olfactory 7; non-auditory 4,
124, 189, 236; commanding